Anticoagulants

Editor

JERROLD H. LEVY

CLINICS IN LABORATORY MEDICINE

www.labmed.theclinics.com

September 2014 • Volume 34 • Number 3

ELSEVIER

1600 John F. Kennedy Boulevard ● Suite 1800 ● Philadelphia, Pennsylvania, 19103-2899

http://www.theclinics.com

CLINICS IN LABORATORY MEDICINE Volume 34, Number 3
September 2014 ISSN 0272-2712, ISBN-13: 978-0-323-32329-1

Editor: Joanne Husovski
Developmental Editor: Yonah Korngold

Reprints. For copies of 100 or more, of articles in this publication, please contact the Commercial Reprints Department, Elsevier Inc., 360 Park Avenue South, New York, New York 10010-1710. Tel. 212-633-3874, Fax: 212-633-3820, E-mail: reprints@elsevier.com.

Clinics in Laboratory Medicine (ISSN 0272-2712) is published quarterly by Elsevier Inc., 360 Park Avenue South, New York, NY 10010-1710. Months of issue are March, June, September, and December. Business and Editorial offices: 1600 John F. Kennedy Blvd., Suite 1800, Philadelphia, PA 19103-2899. Periodicals postage paid at NewYork, NY and additional mailing offices. Subscription prices are $250.00 per year (US individuals), $419.00 per year (US institutions), $135.00 per year (US students), $305.00 per year (Canadian individuals), $510.00 per year (Canadian institutions), $185.00 per year (Canadian students), $390.00 per year (foreign individuals), $510.00 per year (foreign institutions), $185.00 (foreign students). Foreign air speed delivery is included in all Clinics subscription prices. All prices are subject to change without notice. POSTMASTER: Send address changes to *Clinics in Laboratory Medicine*, Elsevier Health Sciences Division, Subscription Customer Service, 3251 Riverport Lane, Maryland Heights, MO 63043. **Customer Service: 1-800-654-2452 (US). From outside of the US and Canada, call 1-314-447-8871. Fax: 1-314-447-8029. E-mail: journalscustomerservice-usa@elsevier.com (for print support) or journalsonlinesupport-usa@elsevier.com (for online support).**

Clinics in Laboratory Medicine is covered in *EMBASE/Exerpta Medica, MEDLINE/PubMed (Index Medicus), Cinahl, Current Contents/Clinical Medicine, BIOSIS* and *ISI/BIOMED.*

Contributors

EDITOR

JERROLD H. LEVY, MD, FAHA, FCCM
Professor of Anesthesiology; Associate Professor of Surgery; CoDirector, Cardiothoracic
ICU, Department of Anesthesiology, Duke University School of Medicine, Durham, North
Carolina

AUTHORS

AHMED AL-BADRI, MD
Department of Medicine, Lenox Hill Hospital, North Shore-LIJ Health System, New York,
New York

ERIC ANDERSON, MD
Department of Surgery, University of North Dakota School of Medicine and Health
Sciences, Grand Forks, North Dakota

GERHARD DICKNEITE, PhD
CSL Behring, Preclinical R&D, Marburg, Germany

WULF DIETRICH, MD, PhD
Institute for Research in Cardiac Anesthesia, Munich, Germany

CORNELIUS DYKE, MD
Assistant Professor of Surgery, Department of Surgery, University of North Dakota School
of Medicine and Health Sciences, Grand Forks, North Dakota; Attending Surgeon,
Department of Cardiothroacic Surgery, Sanford Health Fargo, Fargo, North Dakota

DAVID FARAONI, MD, FCCP
Department of Anesthesiology, Queen Fabiola Children's University Hospital, Brussels,
Belgium

OLIVER GROTTKE, MD, PhD
Department of Anesthesiology, RWTH Aachen University Hospital, Aachen, Germany

SOLVEIG HORSTMANN, MD
Neurologist, Department of Neurology, University of Heidelberg, Heidelberg, Germany

JAMES M. HUNTER Jr, MD
Assistant Professor, Department of Anesthesiology, University of Alabama at Birmingham,
Birmingham, Alabama

JEFFREY H. LAWSON, MD, PhD
Professor of Surgery, Division of Vascular Surgery, Department of Surgery, Duke
University Medical Center, Duke University, Durham, North Carolina

MARCEL LEVI, MD, PhD, FRCP
Professor of Medicine; Dean, Faculty of Medicine, Academic Medical Center, University of
Amsterdam, Amsterdam, The Netherlands

JERROLD H. LEVY, MD, FAHA, FCCM
Professor of Anesthesiology; Associate Professor of Surgery; CoDirector, Cardiothoracic ICU, Department of Anesthesiology, Duke University School of Medicine, Durham, North Carolina

MARISA B. MARQUES, MD
Professor, Department of Pathology, University of Alabama at Birmingham, Birmingham, Alabama

C. CAMERON MCCOY, MD
Resident, Department of Surgery, Duke University Medical Center, Duke University, Durham, North Carolina

SADIA MEDDAHI, PharmD
Department of Biological Hematology, Cochin Hôtel-Dieu University Hospitals, Paris, France; BIOMNIS Laboratories, Ivry-sur-Seine, France

MARCO RANUCCI, MD, FESC
Director of Clinical Research, Vascular Anesthesia and Intensive Care, IRCCS Policlinico San Donato, San Donato Milanese, Milan, Italy

ARUN SAINI, MD, FAAP
Clinical Fellow, Division of Critical Care Medicine, Department of Pediatrics, Washington School of Medicine in St Louis, St Louis, Missouri

CHARLES MARC SAMAMA, MD, PhD, FCCP
Professor, Department of Anesthesia and Intensive Care Medicine, Cochin Hôtel-Dieu University Hospitals, Paris, France

MEYER MICHEL SAMAMA, MD, PharmD
Department of Biological Hematology, Cochin Hôtel-Dieu University Hospitals, Paris, France; BIOMNIS Laboratories, Ivry-sur-Seine, France

RAVI SARODE, MD
Professor of Pathology and Director of Transfusion Medicine and Hemostasis, Department of Pathology, University of Texas Southwestern Medical Center, Dallas, Texas

MARK L. SHAPIRO, MD
Associate Professor of Surgery, Division of Trauma & Critical Care, Department of Surgery, Duke University Medical Center, Duke University, Durham, North Carolina

PHILIP C. SPINELLA, MD, FCCM
Associate Professor and Director, Critical Care Translational Research Program, Division of Critical Care Medicine, Department of Pediatrics, Washington School of Medicine in St Louis, St Louis, Missouri

JENNA L. SPRING, MD
Department of Medicine, University of Toronto, Ontario, Canada

HENRI SPRONK, PhD
Assistant Professor, Department of Internal Medicine, Cardiovascular Research Institute Maastricht, Maastricht University Medical Center, Maastricht, The Netherlands

ALEX C. SPYROPOULOS, MD, FACP, FCCP, FRCPC
Department of Medicine, Lenox Hill Hospital, North Shore-LIJ Health System, New York, New York

FANIA SZLAM, MMSc
Emory University Hospital, Emory University School of Medicine, Atlanta, Georgia

JOANNE VAN RYN, PhD
Department of Cardiometabolic Disease Research, Boehringer Ingelheim Pharma GmbH & Co KG, Biberach, Germany

ROLAND VELTKAMP, MD, FESO
Neurologist, Department of Stroke Medicine, Charing Cross Hospital, Imperial College London, London, United Kingdom; Neurologist, Department of Neurology, University of Heidelberg, Heidelberg, Germany

THOMAS R. VETTER, MD, MPH
Professor, Department of Anesthesiology, University of Alabama at Birmingham, Birmingham, Alabama

LANCE A. WILLIAMS III, MD
Assistant Professor, Department of Pathology, University of Alabama at Birmingham, Birmingham, Alabama

ANNE WINKLER, MD, MSc
Assistant Professor, Department of Pathology & Laboratory Medicine, Emory University Hospital, Atlanta, Georgia

ALISA S. WOLBERG, PhD, FAHA
Department of Pathology and Laboratory Medicine, University of North Carolina at Chapel Hill, Chapel Hill, North Carolina

Contents

New oral anticoagulants (NOACs) are increasingly replacing vitamin K antagonists and older parenteral agents in clinical practice. NOACs offer several advantages compared with standard agents, including rapid onset of action, fixed dosing, and no requirement for routine coagulation monitoring. However, like all anticoagulants, NOACs carry a risk of bleeding. Here, we discuss the pharmacology and safety of NOACs, with particular emphasis on the risks of bleeding associated with NOACs versus standard anticoagulants, and we provide an overview of current bleeding management strategies.

Although the activated partial thromboplastin time, prothrombin time, and international normalized ratio are widely used in routine preoperative testing, these hemostatic tests are not reliable predictors of perioperative bleeding in patients without known bleeding risk factors. In contrast, a preoperative bleeding history and physical examination are usually obtained in an attempt to identify important bleeding risk factors. However, these coagulation tests are used extensively for monitoring anticoagulation with different pharmacologic agents.

Dabigatran, a direct thrombin inhibitor, is increasingly used clinically as one of the new oral anticoagulants. This review summarizes the assays available to measure its activity and includes the relative sensitivity of the different assays for this agent. In addition to plasma-based clotting tests, assays commonly used in surgical/emergency settings, such as activated clotting time and thromboelastometry/thromboelastography, are reviewed. In addition, the thrombin generation assay is discussed as an important method to determine the potential risk of thrombosis or bleeding and its relevance to the measurement of direct thrombin inhibitors.

New oral factor Xa inhibitors are intended to progressively substitute the oral vitamin K antagonists and parenteral indirect inhibitors of factor Xa in the prevention and treatment of venous and arterial thromboembolic episodes. This article focuses on the main clinical studies and on biological measurements of new oral factor Xa inhibitors, and addresses several safety issues. These newer agents do not require any routine laboratory monitoring of blood coagulation; however, biological tests have been developed in order to assess the plasma concentration of these drugs in several clinical settings. This article reviews these 4 oral direct factor Xa inhibitors.

Venous thromboembolism covers a range of conditions from deep vein thrombosis to pulmonary embolism. Treatment aims to alleviate symptoms, minimize acute morbidity and mortality by preventing the extension or potentially fatal embolization of the initial thrombus, and avoid post-thrombotic syndrome. Anticoagulant therapy is the mainstay of treatment, but treatment decisions and the choice of an appropriate anticoagulation agent are modified according to the predisposition for venous thromboembolism, the site and extent of thrombus, the presence or absence of symptomatic embolism, and patient's bleeding risk. Newer oral anticoagulants have been developed to overcome the drawbacks of other agents, improve patient care, and simplify and improve management.

Patients undergoing thoracic and cardiac procedures are at the highest risk for postoperative atrial fibrillation (POAF). POAF is associated with poor short-term and long-term outcomes, including high rates of early and late stroke, and late mortality. Patients with POAF that persists for longer than 48 hours should be anticoagulated on warfarin. Three new oral anticoagulants are available for the treatment of nonvalvular atrial fibrillation and have been found to be as efficacious or superior to warfarin in the prevention of stroke in high-risk patients, with similar to lower rates of major bleeding, and lower rates of intracranial hemorrhage.

A lack of consensus on anticoagulant reversal during acute trauma is compounded by an aging population and the expanding spectrum of new anticoagulation agents. Developments in laboratory assays and transfusion medicine, including thromboelastography, recombinant factors, and factor concentrates, have revolutionized care for anticoagulated trauma patients. Accordingly, clinicians must be fully aware of drug mechanisms, assays to determine drug activity, and appropriate reversal strategies for patients on anticoagulants. Drugs include vitamin K antagonists, direct thrombin inhibitors, direct factor Xa inhibitors, low molecular weight heparin, and antiplatelet agents. This article discusses the appropriate assessment and management of trauma patients receiving these agents.

> Bleeding is a significant complication of anticoagulant therapy. With the emergence of new oral anticoagulants (NOACs; ie, direct factor IIa or Xa inhibitors), this risk is further compounded by the lack of validated reversal strategies for these agents. Emerging postmarketing evidence suggests that the bleeding risks are in line with results observed in head-to-head clinical trials of NOACs versus traditional anticoagulants. Several guidelines have recommended the use of hemostatic agents for NOAC reversal in patients with life-threatening bleeding. Ultimately, adequately powered studies will be crucial for full assessment of the effectiveness and safety of any proposed reversal strategies.

> Intracerebral hemorrhage (ICH) associated with the use of oral anticoagulants (OAC-ICH) results in particularly severe strokes. A key target for the treatment of OAC-ICH is rapid restoration of effective coagulation. In patients receiving vitamin K antagonists, hemostatic factors such as prothrombin complex concentrate (PCC), fresh frozen plasma, and recombinant activated factor VII, in addition to vitamin K, can be used for anticoagulation reversal. However, emergency management of ICH during treatment with the new direct OACs (NOACs) is a major challenge. In the absence of specific antidotes, PCCs are recommended for NOAC reversal, mainly based on preclinical data.

> Every year, new studies are undertaken to address the complex issue of periprocedural management of patients on anticoagulants and antiplatelet medications. In addition, newer drugs add to the confusion among clinicians about how to best manage patients taking these agents. Using the most recent data, guidelines, and personal experience, this article discusses recommendations and presents simplified algorithms to assist clinicians in the periprocedural management of patients on anticoagulants.

> Vitamin K antagonist (VKA) therapy is a mainstay of treatment for patients at risk of thromboembolic events. Despite widespread use, a major limitation of VKA therapy is the substantial risk of serious bleeding complications, which often require rapid reversal of anticoagulation. A recent randomized multicenter comparison between a 4-factor prothrombin complex concentrate (4F-PCC) and plasma in patients with acute major bleeding has provided important new evidence of the benefit of 4F-PCC over plasma for urgent VKA reversal.

Although new oral anticoagulants (NOACs) represent an advance in anticoagulant therapy over vitamin K antagonists (VKAs), they nevertheless
have a low, but significant risk for bleeding complications. Reversal agents
for VKAs, such as prothrombin complex concentrates (PCCs), are currently being evaluated in preclinical studies for NOAC reversal. This article
reviews the preclinical data for the most extensively studied PCC for
NOAC reversal, Beriplex, a 4-factor PCC. The results from the Beriplex
studies are also compared with those obtained with other reversal agents,
including different nonactivated PCCs, activated PCCs, and recombinant
activated factor VII.

New oral anticoagulants (NOACs) are increasingly replacing standard
anticoagulants. These new drugs have been recently introduced in clinical
practice, and specific knowledge regarding preoperative interruption, anticoagulation assessment, and reversal therapies is needed. In this article, 3
main areas related to perioperative NOACs management are discussed:
(1) physicians' knowledge, (2) current practices, and (3) perspectives to
improve management of patients treated with NOACs.

Compared to in situ vascular physiology where pro and anti-hemostatic
processes are in balance to maintain hemostasis, the use of ECMO in a
critically ill child increases the risk of hemorrhagic or thromboembolic
events due to a perturbation in the balance inherent of this complex system. The ECMO circuit has pro-hemostatic effects due to contact activation of hemostasis and inflammatory pathways. In addition, the critical
illness of the child can cause dysregulation of hemostasis that may shift
between hyper and hypocoagulable states over time.

This study examines the relationship between D-dimer concentration and
patient age, gender, race, and renal function, and the role of D-dimer concentration as a predictor of in-hospital mortality, in a critically ill patient
population. The results demonstrate there is a correlation between
increased D-dimer concentration and renal impairment in critically ill
patients, with patients in renal failure having the highest D-dimer concentrations. Peak D-dimer levels were higher among female patients than in

male patients, but there was no association between peak D-dimer levels and other patient characteristics. D-dimer concentration was also not predictive of in-hospital mortality.

CLINICS IN LABORATORY MEDICINE

RELATED INTEREST

Critical Care Clinics July 2012 (Vol. 28, No. 3)
Newer Anticoagulants in Critically Ill Patients
Anita Rajasekhar, Rebecca Beyth, and Mark A. Crowther, *Editors*

**DOWNLOAD
Free App!**

Review Articles
THE CLINICS

NOW AVAILABLE FOR YOUR iPhone and iPad

Preface

Anticoagulants

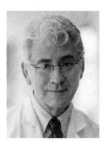

Jerrold H. Levy, MD, FAHA, FCCM
Editor

Anticoagulants have increasingly become a therapeutic mainstay in the management of patients for multiple prophylactic and therapeutic reasons. Warfarin and other vitamin K antagonists (VKAs) are still extensively used for multiple indications and will likely continue to be the agents of choice for patients with valvular heart disease, mechanical heart valves, and ventricular assist devices. However, with the advent of new oral anticoagulation agents (NOACs), newer paradigms for patient management have also emerged. The NOACs provide additional therapeutic approaches to anticoagulation for patients in multiple settings, including inpatient and outpatient, surgical, and medically managed patient populations, as extensively reviewed in this issue.

New pharmacologic agents provide novel approaches for patient management but, as with all therapies, they have associated risk and benefit profiles that must be considered to optimize patient management. For all anticoagulation agents, the major risk is of course bleeding. However, while bleeding can occur with any anticoagulation therapy, there has been increasing attention on NOAC-associated bleeding, as therapeutic approaches for managing bleeding in NOAC-treated patients are different than those validated for use in warfarin-treated patients. Despite widespread criticism that "antidotes" for the NOACs don't exist, until 2013 there were no four-factor prothrombin complex concentrates available for warfarin/VKA reversal in the United States. Plasma/ fresh frozen plasma (FFP) is still widely used despite the fact that the lowest international normalized ratio obtainable with FFP is 1.6,[1] and recent studies have shown that the use of FFP is a leading cause of volume overload.[2–4] In addition, while the use of male-only plasma has reduced the number of antibody-mediated cases of transfusion-related acute lung injury (TRALI), and associated mortality, TRALI still remains a concern.[5] Furthermore, despite the ongoing extensive use of low-molecular-weight heparin (LMWH) in surgical patients and in a hospital setting, there is no reversal agent available to treat a life-threatening bleed in LMWH-treated patients.

Clin Lab Med 34 (2014) xiii–xv
http://dx.doi.org/10.1016/j.cll.2014.06.016
0272-2712/14/$ – see front matter © 2014 Elsevier Inc. All rights reserved.

In this issue of *Clinics in Laboratory Medicine*, the focus is on anticoagulation. For this publication, I have assembled many of the world experts to review and discuss critical aspects of both older and newer anticoagulants and their management, including patient monitoring, evaluating laboratory testing, and evaluating what coagulation test results mean. In addition to discussion on monitoring and managing patients receiving factor Xa and direct thrombin inhibitors, there are extensive discussions on bleeding management in these patients. As part of this important topic, I have included anticoagulation and bleeding management in a spectrum of important settings, including postoperative atrial fibrillation, intracranial hemorrhage, extracorporeal membrane oxygenation, trauma, and perioperative management. The idea for the content of this supplement came in part from a 2013 satellite symposium sponsored by CSL Behring at the International Society of Thrombosis and Haemostasis (ISTH), entitled "Bleeding Emergencies: Strategies for the Reversal of Old- and New-Generation Oral Anticoagulants"; five of the articles were developed from the presentations given at this meeting. I also invited other experts on anticoagulation management, who will share their understanding of management and urgent reversal of anticoagulation in a complex set of in-hospital settings, from adult to pediatrics (extracorporeal membrane oxygenation), in the perioperative setting, and from other therapeutic settings. I have also included an article on understanding the extensive use (and abuse) of prothrombin and partial thromboplastin times in patients as monitoring tools for both anticoagulation and potential bleeding.

The evolution of cardiovascular medicine and therapeutic approaches has been greatly facilitated with the development of multiple pharmacologic strategies for anticoagulation, including both parenteral and oral agents. However, as previously mentioned, all of these agents are associated with a risk of bleeding, and multiple factors can influence bleeding in anticoagulated patients. This supplement on anticoagulation provides an updated and important review of management approaches in this patient population. Of importance is also the development of purified and recombinant factors and factor concentrates to manage complex bleeding paradigms, which will be discussed in several articles, and other agents currently under investigation.

In summary, my view is that *new drugs create new paradigms*. In addition to the new anticoagulation agents, new strategies for monitoring and managing patients are important and are extensively addressed in the 15 articles included in this issue. I would like to thank the authors, who are busy physicians, clinicians, and scientists, for taking the time to write these articles. Dr Steven Shafer once told me that friends don't ask friends to write articles. However, these articles together represent a collective insight from experts who manage anticoagulation and its side effects on a daily basis, who have contributed to our understanding and to the availability of therapeutic agents for both anticoagulation and urgent bleeding management, and who took the time to make their important contributions. I am most appreciative of their efforts. I would also like to thank Dr Michael Thimme, from CSL Behring, whose ongoing vision and support of important educational programs, including our previous symposium at the ISTH meeting, is most appreciated.

Jerrold H. Levy, MD, FAHA, FCCM
Duke University Medical Center
2301 Erwin Road, 5691H HAFS
Box 3094, Durham, NC 27710, USA

E-mail address:
jerrold.levy@duke.edu

REFERENCES

1. Holland LL, Brooks JP. Toward rational fresh frozen plasma transfusion: the effect of plasma transfusion on coagulation test results. Am J Clin Pathol 2006;126: 133–9.
2. Ageno W, Gallus AS, Wittkowsky A, et al. Oral anticoagulant therapy: antithrombotic therapy and prevention of thrombosis, 9th edition: American College of Chest Physicians evidence-based clinical practice guidelines. Chest 2012; 141(Suppl 2):e44S–88S.
3. Magee G, Peters C, Zbrozek A. Analysis of inpatient use of fresh frozen plasma and other therapies and associated outcomes in patients with major bleeds from vitamin K antagonism. Clin Ther 2013;35(9):1432–43.
4. Magee G, Zbrozek A. Fluid overload is associated with increases in length of stay and hospital costs: pooled analysis of data from more than 600 US hospitals. Clinicoecon Outcomes Res 2013;5:289–96.
5. Silliman CC, Fung YL, Ball JB, et al. Transfusion-related acute lung injury (TRALI): current concepts and misconceptions. Blood Rev 2009;23(6):245–55.

Pharmacology and Safety of New Oral Anticoagulants

The Challenge of Bleeding Persists

Jerrold H. Levy, MD, FAHA, FCCM

KEYWORDS

- Bleeding • Safety • Dabigatran • Rivaroxaban • Apixaban
- Prothrombin complex concentrates

KEY POINTS

- Owing to benefits in ease of administration, safety, and efficacy demonstrated in clinical trials, the use of new oral anticoagulants (NOACs) in clinical practice is increasing.
- Compared with standard anticoagulants, these new agents offer a number of advantages, including rapid onset of action, fixed dosing, and no requirement for routine coagulation monitoring.
- There are currently no validated NOAC-specific reversal agents and there is a lack of clinical data assessing the efficacy and safety of existing protocols for bleeding management in NOAC-treated patients. However, an increasing number of studies are being undertaken and new therapeutic approaches developed, as discussed elsewhere in this supplement.
- With all anticoagulation agents, the management of life-threatening bleeding presents a significant challenge, and will continue to evolve as new therapeutic approaches and data emerge.

INTRODUCTION AND BACKGROUND

The prevalence of cardiovascular diseases, such as atrial fibrillation (AF) and venous thromboembolism (VTE), sustains a demand for safe and effective anticoagulation therapies. In the United States alone, AF is estimated to affect approximately 2.3 million people,[1] whereas projections suggest that the number of adults with VTE

Conflict of Interest Statements: Prof. J.H. Levy serves on steering committees for Boehringer Ingelheim, CSL Behring AG, Grifols, Janssen Pharmaceuticals, and The Medicines Company. Editorial assistance was provided by Fishawack Communications Ltd, with a grant from CSL Behring, Marburg, Germany.
Duke University School of Medicine, Divisions of Cardiothoracic Anesthesiology and Critical Care, Duke University Hospital, 2301 Erwin Road, Durham, NC 27710, USA
E-mail address: jerrold.levy@duke.edu

in the United States may exceed 1.5 million by 2050.[2] Warfarin has long been a standard of antithrombotic therapy; however, there is a growing trend toward replacing it and the older parenteral agents, such as unfractionated and low molecular weight heparin (UFH and LMWH, respectively), with new oral anticoagulants (NOACs) that are perceived to offer better efficacy, safety, and ease of administration with oral use.[3]

Four NOACs are currently approved worldwide. The thrombin (factor IIa [FIIa]) inhibitor dabigatran (Pradaxa) is used primarily for stroke prevention in patients with nonvalvular AF and is approved for this indication in the United States and Canada,[4,5] European Union (EU),[6] Australia,[7] and Japan.[8] In Europe, Canada, and Australia, dabigatran also is approved for the prevention of VTE in patients undergoing hip or knee surgery.[5–7] Three different factor Xa (FXa) inhibitors also are approved. Apixaban (Eliquis) is approved in the EU, United States, and Canada for the prevention of stroke and systemic embolism in patients with nonvalvular AF[9–11] and in the EU and Canada for the prevention of VTE after hip or knee replacement surgery.[9,11] Rivaroxaban (Xarelto) is approved in the United States and Canada for stroke prevention in patients with nonvalvular AF and for the treatment and prevention of VTE,[12,13] but has EU approval only for coadministration (with acetylsalicylic acid and/or other agents) for the prevention of atherothrombotic events in acute coronary syndrome.[14] Edoxaban (Lixiana) is currently approved only in Japan, where it is indicated for the prevention of VTE after hip or knee replacement.[15] Other oral anticoagulants are in development, including the FXa inhibitor betrixaban, which is currently under investigation in a phase III clinical trial (NCT01583218).[16]

Compared with standard anticoagulants, such as UFH, LMWH, and vitamin K antagonists (VKAs), NOACs offer several advantages. These include rapid onset of action, predictable pharmacokinetics, a predictable anticoagulant effect (which obviates the need for routine laboratory monitoring), and few food or drug interactions.[3] Furthermore, the risk of bleeding is generally lower compared with VKAs.[17,18] However, bleeding associated with all anticoagulants remains a significant challenge. For the NOACs, major bleeding rates of 2.1% to 3.6% per year have been reported in clinical trials.[19–22] In another trial, in which short-term treatment with apixaban was evaluated for thromboprophylaxis after hip replacement, 0.8% of patients in the apixaban arm experienced major bleeding during a treatment and evaluation period of approximately 5 weeks.[23] In these trials, the definition of major bleeding was based on that proposed by the International Society on Thrombosis and Haemostasis (ISTH) (fatal outcome, involvement of a critical anatomic site, fall in hemoglobin concentration of ≥ 2 g/L, or transfusion of ≥ 2 units of blood or red cells),[24] with minor variations from the ISTH definition in some of the studies.[19,22,23] Clearly, when bleeding occurs or patients require surgery, therapeutic approaches are important to consider.[3] A lack of NOAC-specific reversal agents compounds the challenge, whereas some standard anticoagulants (eg, UFH and warfarin) have accepted, validated, acute reversal agents (protamine sulfate and 4-component prothrombin complex concentrates [PCCs], respectively). However, it was not until late 2013 that a 4-component PCC became available in the United States.[25]

This article reviews the available safety data, including bleeding profile, and major strategies for NOAC-induced bleeding management associated with the 3 NOACs approved in North America: dabigatran, rivaroxaban, and apixaban.

SUMMARY OF PHARMACOLOGY

Dabigatran is a reversible direct thrombin (FIIa) inhibitor that binds clot-bound and free thrombin without the need for antithrombin.[3,4] It is administered as the prodrug, dabigatran etexilate, which is rapidly converted via esterase-mediated hydrolysis to the active form, dabigatran.[4] Both rivaroxaban and apixaban are oral, direct FXa inhibitors that selectively block the active site of FXa (**Fig. 1**).[10,12] Drugs in both categories offer significant advantages over warfarin and LMWHs. Although warfarin dosing must be individualized based on each patient's international normalized ratio, NOACs allow fixed oral dosing with a predictable anticoagulant effect, eliminating the need for routine testing and dosage adjustment. In addition, they have predictable pharmacokinetics, including a rapid onset of anticoagulation within 4 hours and a half-life ranging from 5 to 17 hours. Warfarin typically takes at least 3 to 5 days to establish a therapeutic anticoagulant effect, often requires intermittent bridging with other agents, and has a substantially longer half-life than the NOACs (**Table 1**).[26] The pharmacokinetic properties of warfarin and the LMWH enoxaparin are compared with NOACs in **Table 1**.[27,28] LMWHs require parenteral, rather than oral, administration, which limits their long-term use.[29] In addition, studies suggest that administration of protamine only partially reverses LMWH-induced anticoagulation,[30] highlighting the lack of an effective antidote for LMWHs.[29]

BLEEDING CHALLENGE

The risk of bleeding is associated with all anticoagulation therapy. In a systematic review of 43 randomized controlled trials, Holster and colleagues[31] compared the use of NOACs with standard care (defined as either LMWH, VKA, antiplatelet therapy, or no therapy/placebo) in multiple indications, observing that the risk of gastrointestinal (GI) bleeding with NOACs was only slightly greater (odds ratio [OR] 1.45; 95% confidence interval [CI] 1.07–1.97); however, there was considerable heterogeneity among the trials ($I^2 = 61\%$).[31] This was also reflected in clinically relevant bleeding, which was observed to be at only a slightly higher risk with NOAC treatment than

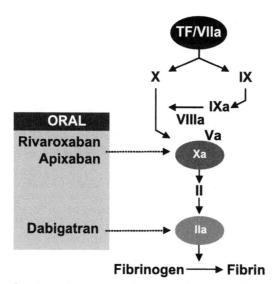

Fig. 1. Effect sites of anticoagulant agents. The new oral anticoagulation agents inhibit one of two major targets in the coagulation cascade. Rivaroxaban and apixaban directly inhibit factor Xa, and dabigatran directly inhibits thrombin. (*From* Levy JH, Faraoni D, Spring JL, et al. Managing new oral anticoagulants in the perioperative and intensive care unit setting. Anesthesiology 2013;118(6):1467; with permission.)

Table 1
Key pharmacodynamic/pharmacokinetic attributes of NOACs currently approved in North America compared with warfarin

Parameter	Dabigatran	Rivaroxaban	Apixaban	Warfarin	Enoxaparin
Target	FIIa	FXa	FXa	Vitamin K-dependent clotting factors (factors II, VII, IX, and X and anticoagulant proteins C and S)	FXa and FIIa
Time to maximum inhibition	1–3 h	2–4 h	3–4 h	Generally within 24 h; may be delayed to 72–96 h after administration	3–5 h after injection
Half-life[a]	12–17 h	5–13 h	~12 h	20–60 h (mean ~40 h)	4.5–7 h
Plasma protein binding	35%	92%–95%	87%	99%	Antithrombin binding required for activity

[a] In healthy subjects. In clinical practice, NOAC recipients (especially the frail elderly) would be expected to have multiple comorbidities, altering the pharmacokinetic profile of the agent. For example, in patients with age-related or other renal impairment, dabigatran and rivaroxaban have been shown to have significantly longer half-lives. The half-life of dabigatran is 18–27 hours in patients with moderate-to-severe renal impairment[4] and that of rivaroxaban is 11–13 hours in elderly patients.[12]

Data from Refs.[3,4,10,12,26–28,58]

with standard care (OR 1.16; 95% CI 1.00–1.34), with some degree of heterogeneity ($I^2 = 83\%$).[31] However, defining standard care in these cases is complex, with the variability of anticoagulation that may occur with VKA agents. In another analysis of trials of NOACs in patients with nonvalvular AF, Mitchell and colleagues[32] also found that rivaroxaban and dabigatran 150 mg were associated with a higher risk of GI bleeding than warfarin; however, most GI bleeds are not life-threatening, and can be resolved by stopping anticoagulation treatment and implementing the appropriate corrective measures (**Fig. 2**).[3] This finding also may reflect the more consistent anticoagulation produced by the NOACs due to their minimal interactions with food or other drug interactions.

Anticoagulation Therapy and Elderly Patients

Anticoagulation therapy and the associated bleeding risk is of particular concern in frail elderly patients and individuals with mechanical valves.[33,34] RE-ALIGN, a trial comparing the use of dabigatran and warfarin in patients with mechanical heart valves, noted that dabigatran is not an appropriate alternative to warfarin in these patients, as mechanical heart valves may require more intense anticoagulation with warfarin, which inhibits factors II, VII, IX, and X.[34] However, in 2012, the US Food and Drug Administration (FDA) evaluated postmarketing reports of dabigatran-related bleeding,[35,36] using insurance claims and administrative data, and indicated that the incidence of bleeding was not higher with dabigatran compared with warfarin.[36]

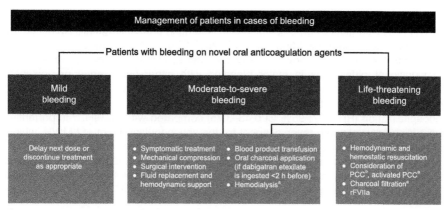

Fig. 2. Management strategies for NOAC-treated patients in cases of bleeding. [a]For dabigatran. [b]For rivaroxaban and apixaban. (*From* Levy JH, Faraoni D, Spring JL, et al. Managing new oral anticoagulants in the perioperative and intensive care unit setting. Anesthesiology 2013;118(6):1472; with permission.)

Evidence of Increased Bleeding Risk with NOACs Versus Standard Anticoagulants

The evidence of increased bleeding risk with NOACs versus standard anticoagulants must be weighed against a substantial body of evidence that shows the newer agents have lower rates of major and potentially fatal bleeding than standard agents such as warfarin.[19–23,37–41] A systematic review and meta-analysis by Dentali and colleagues[18] showed reduced rates of both major bleeding and intracranial bleeding with NOACs versus VKAs, which has been further highlighted in a number of other similar reviews and meta-analyses. It also has been suggested by Dogliotti and colleagues[42] that the incidence of intracerebral bleeding may be lower with NOACs than with warfarin, as evidenced by a reduction of almost half in the risk of hemorrhagic stroke (relative risk [RR] 0.51; 95% CI 0.41–0.64; $P<.0001$) in NOAC-treated patients with AF. This conclusion is reinforced by a systematic review by Baker and Phung,[17] which reported a significantly lower risk of hemorrhagic stroke with NOACs in general (RR 0.46; 95% CI 0.27–0.77) and, among NOACs, with dabigatran compared with rivaroxaban (RR 0.45; 95% CI 0.21–0.98).[17] Analysis suggests that the risk of major bleeding with NOACs varies among the different agents. There are no large, head-to-head studies of NOACs[17,43]; however, using warfarin as a common comparator, adjusted indirect comparisons provide insight into bleeding risk among them.[17,18,42–44]

In a retrospective analysis of 5 phase III trials involving almost 30,000 patients, Majeed and colleagues[45] compared the management and prognosis of major bleeding in patients treated with dabigatran or warfarin. Importantly, they found that patients on dabigatran who experienced major bleeds (627 [3.7%] of 16,755) generally had a higher propensity to bleed than those who experienced major bleeds on warfarin (407 [4.1%] of 10,002), because they were older, had lower creatinine clearance, and more frequently used acetylsalicylic acid or nonsteroidal anti-inflammatory agents. This suggests that dabigatran may have a higher bleeding threshold compared with warfarin.[45] Although more patients who experienced major bleeding on dabigatran required red blood cell transfusions, fewer of these patients received plasma transfusions, their stay in intensive care was shorter (mean 1.6 vs 2.7 nights; $P = .01$) and there was a trend toward lower 30-day mortality (9.1% vs 13.0%; $P = .057$) compared with those who had major bleeding on warfarin.

Comparing oral direct FXa inhibitors, including rivaroxaban and apixaban, with LMWH in postsurgical thromboprophylaxis, Neumann and colleagues[46] identified an increased risk of major bleeding (OR 1.27; 95% CI 0.98–1.65; equivalent to 2 more events per 1000 patients); however, several other systematic reviews have reported no significant differences in major bleeding with either rivaroxaban or apixaban compared with LMWH.[47] With dabigatran, no significant difference was found either in major bleeding events (RR 0.94; 95% CI 0.58–1.52)[46] or in bleeding leading to rehospitalization (RR 1.27; 95% CI 0.43–3.75) compared with LMWH.[48] Importantly, there is no fully validated reversal agent for the anticoagulant effect of LMWH, which can lead to problems in clinical situations. Although protamine sulfate has been suggested as an antidote for LMWH, it is not an effective reversal agent.[30,49,50] Thus, for all anticoagulation agents, major bleeding remains a significant challenge in clinical practice for which effective management strategies are crucial.

BLEEDING TREATMENT STRATEGIES

There is a lack of clinical data assessing the efficacy and safety of anticoagulant reversal protocols in either bleeding patients or those undergoing emergency surgery. However, guidelines on NOAC-related bleeding management have been published; these are based on clinical studies of volunteers who were anticoagulated with NOACs, experts' opinions, and laboratory end points.[51–53] Potential therapeutic approaches are shown in **Fig. 2**. For elective surgery, the first step to control bleeding is to delay or discontinue NOAC treatment, as appropriate.[3,51,52] The recommended interval between administration of the last NOAC dose and an invasive procedure varies with the level of bleeding risk associated with the procedure and, in the case of dabigatran, with the patient's renal function, but in general is not less than 24 hours (**Table 2**). Although cessation of NOAC treatment can be effective before a planned procedure, given the required length of discontinuation intervals, specific therapeutic approaches are needed when patients require urgent surgery or experience an acute bleeding event.

While coagulation testing is not routinely required in NOAC-treated patients, in patients who need emergency treatment, such as those who develop an acute bleed, have a suspected overdose, or require emergency surgery, testing is necessary to determine whether to proceed with urgent procedures.[3] Following evaluation of anticoagulation status, initial treatment measures for significant bleeding should include hemodynamic and hemostatic resuscitation and, if possible, local hemostatic control.[3,52–54] To prevent further NOAC absorption, activated charcoal may be considered if the drug was taken within 2 hours of admission; however, options to remove NOACs are limited. Dabigatran can be dialyzed because of its low protein binding, but this is not an option with rivaroxaban or apixaban, both of which are highly protein-bound

Table 2
Summary of recommended presurgical discontinuation intervals for NOACs

Agent	Timing of Last Dose Before Surgical Procedure
Dabigatran	1–2 d (CrCl ≥50 mL/min); 3–5 d (CrCl <50 mL/min)
Rivaroxaban	≥24 h
Apixaban	≥48 h (moderate-to-high bleeding risk); ≥24 h (low bleeding risk)

Bleeding risks are those associated with the surgical procedure under consideration.
Abbreviation: CrCl, creatinine clearance.
Data from Refs.[4,10,12]

(see **Table 1**). Dialysis also is not possible with a patient in shock. In cases of severe bleeding, off-label treatment with prohemostatic agents may be considered.[3,52,53] These include nonactivated PCC, activated PCC (FEIBA [Factor VIII Inhibitor Bypassing Activity; Baxter Healthcare Corp, Westlake Village, CA]) or recombinant FVIIa. More detail on the use of PCCs in the reversal of NOAC-related bleeding can be found elsewhere in this issue by Dickneite and colleagues.

Although there is a lack of evidence about when to restart patients on anticoagulation therapy after a bleeding event or surgical procedure, it is generally agreed that the time without anticoagulation should be minimized and anticoagulant therapy restarted when clinically appropriate after adequate hemostasis has been achieved.[4,12] It is widely agreed that warfarin therapy can be resumed as early as the evening of, or day after, most types of surgery[55] and LMWH after 24 hours following most procedures (but potentially longer after major surgery).[55] The FDA also recently recommended that clinicians carefully consider the timing of enoxaparin therapy resumption in patients undergoing spinal catheter placement, to avoid the risk of spinal column bleeding and subsequent paralysis.[56] NOAC therapy can, in general, resume 6 to 8 hours after the intervention (and after complete hemostasis has been achieved),[53] whereas dabigatran can generally be restarted with a single capsule (110 mg or 150 mg depending on the dose prescribed) 1 to 4 hours after surgery, with the usual regimen started the next day.[57] In all cases, the bleeding risk associated with resumption of anticoagulation therapy after a bleeding event or surgical procedure must be carefully weighed against the risk of thromboembolic events.[52]

SUMMARY

Owing to benefits in ease of administration, safety, and efficacy demonstrated in clinical trials, the use of NOACs in clinical practice is increasing. Compared with standard anticoagulants, these new agents offer a number of advantages, including rapid onset of action, fixed dosing, and no requirement for routine coagulation monitoring. There are currently no validated NOAC-specific reversal agents and there is a lack of clinical data assessing the efficacy and safety of existing protocols for bleeding management in NOAC-treated patients. However, an increasing number of studies are being undertaken and new therapeutic approaches developed, as discussed by Levy and colleagues elsewhere in this issue. With all anticoagulation agents, the management of life-threatening bleeding presents a significant challenge, and will continue to evolve as new therapeutic approaches and data emerge.

REFERENCES

1. Kannel WB, Benjamin EJ. Status of the epidemiology of atrial fibrillation. Med Clin North Am 2008;92(1):17–40, ix.
2. Deitelzweig SB, Johnson BH, Lin J, et al. Prevalence of clinical venous thromboembolism in the USA: current trends and future projections. Am J Hematol 2011; 86(2):217–20.
3. Levy JH, Faraoni D, Spring JL, et al. Managing new oral anticoagulants in the perioperative and intensive care unit setting. Anesthesiology 2013;118(6):1466–74.
4. Dabigatran prescribing information. Ridgefield (CT): Boehringer Ingelheim Pharmaceuticals, Inc; 2013.
5. Dabigatran product monograph. Burlington (Canada): Boehringer Ingelheim Canada Ltd; 2012.
6. Dabigatran summary of product characteristics. Bracknell (United Kingdom): Boehringer Ingelheim Limited; 2012.

7. Dabigatran prescribing information. North Ryde (Australia): Boehringer Ingelheim Pty Limited; 2013.

8. Boehringer Ingelheim pharmaceuticals I. PRAZAXA® (dabigatran etexilate) approved in Japan for stroke prevention in atrial fibrillation 2011. Available at: https://www.boehringer-ingelheim.com/news/news_releases/press_releases/2011/21_january_2011_dabigatranetexilate.html. Accessed July 4, 2014.

9. Apixaban summary of product characteristics. Uxbridge (United Kingdom): Bristol-Myers Squibb/Pfizer EEIG; 2011.

10. Apixaban prescribing information. Princeton (NJ): Bristol-Myers Squibb Company; 2012.

11. Apixaban product monograph. Kirkland (Canada): Pfizer Canada Inc; 2012.

12. Rivaroxaban prescribing information. Titusville (NJ): Janssen Pharmaceuticals, Inc; 2013.

13. Rivaroxaban product monograph. Toronto (Canada): Bayer Inc; 2013.

14. Rivaroxaban summary of product characteristics. Berlin (Germany): Bayer Pharma AG; 2013.

15. Edoxaban package insert. Tokyo (Japan): Daiichi Sankyo Company Ltd; 2011.

16. Available at: http://www.clinicaltrials.gov. Accessed September 30, 2013.

17. Baker WL, Phung OJ. Systematic review and adjusted indirect comparison meta-analysis of oral anticoagulants in atrial fibrillation. Circ Cardiovasc Qual Outcomes 2012;5(5):711–9.

18. Dentali F, Riva N, Crowther M, et al. Efficacy and safety of the novel oral anticoagulants in atrial fibrillation: a systematic review and meta-analysis of the literature. Circulation 2012;126(20):2381–91.

19. Connolly SJ, Ezekowitz MD, Yusuf S, et al. Dabigatran versus warfarin in patients with atrial fibrillation. N Engl J Med 2009;361(12):1139–51.

20. Granger CB, Alexander JH, McMurray JJ, et al. Apixaban versus warfarin in patients with atrial fibrillation. N Engl J Med 2011;365(11):981–92.

21. Lopes RD, Al-Khatib SM, Wallentin L, et al. Efficacy and safety of apixaban compared with warfarin according to patient risk of stroke and of bleeding in atrial fibrillation: a secondary analysis of a randomised controlled trial. Lancet 2012;380(9855):1749–58.

22. Patel MR, Mahaffey KW, Garg J, et al. Rivaroxaban versus warfarin in nonvalvular atrial fibrillation. N Engl J Med 2011;365(10):883–91.

23. Lassen MR, Gallus A, Raskob GE, et al. Apixaban versus enoxaparin for thromboprophylaxis after hip replacement. N Engl J Med 2010;363(26):2487–98.

24. Schulman S, Kearon C. Definition of major bleeding in clinical investigations of antihemostatic medicinal products in non-surgical patients. J Thromb Haemost 2005;3(4):692–4.

25. US Food and Drug Administration approves Kcentra for the urgent reversal of anticoagulation in adults with major bleeding. 2013 Available at: http://www.fda.gov/NewsEvents/Newsroom/Pressannouncements/ucm350026.htm. Accessed November 5, 2013.

26. US Food and Drug Administration. Coumadin official FDA information, side effects and uses. 2011. Available at: http://www.drugs.com/pro/coumadin.html. Accessed September 30, 2013.

27. Fareed J, Hoppensteadt D, Walenga J, et al. Pharmacodynamic and pharmacokinetic properties of enoxaparin: implications for clinical practice. Clin Pharm 2003;42(12):1043–57.

28. sanofi-aventis. Enoxaparin—Highlights of prescribing information. 2008. Available at: http://www.accessdata.fda.gov/drugsatfda_docs/label/2009/020164s083lbl.pdf. Accessed November 5, 2013.

29. Eikelboom JW, Weitz JI. New anticoagulants. Circulation 2010;121(13):1523–32.

30. van Veen JJ, Maclean RM, Hampton KK, et al. Protamine reversal of low molecular weight heparin: clinically effective? Blood Coagul Fibrinolysis 2011;22(7):565–70.

31. Holster IL, Valkhoff VE, Kuipers EJ, et al. New oral anticoagulants increase risk for gastrointestinal bleeding: a systematic review and meta-analysis. Gastroenterology 2013;145(1):105–12. e15.

32. Mitchell SA, Simon TA, Raza S, et al. The efficacy and safety of oral anticoagulants in warfarin-suitable patients with nonvalvular atrial fibrillation: systematic review and meta-analysis. Clin Appl Thromb Hemost 2013;19(6):619–31.

33. Harper P, Young L, Merriman E. Bleeding risk with dabigatran in the frail elderly. N Engl J Med 2012;366(9):864–6.

34. Adam SS, McDuffie JR, Ortel TL, et al. Comparative effectiveness of warfarin and new oral anticoagulants for the management of atrial fibrillation and venous thromboembolism: a systematic review. Ann Intern Med 2012;157(11):796–807.

35. Southworth MR, Reichman ME, Unger EF. Dabigatran and postmarketing reports of bleeding. N Engl J Med 2013;368(14):1272–4.

36. US Food and Drug Administration. Pradaxa (dabigatran etexilate mesylate): drug safety communication—safety review of post-market reports of serious bleeding events. 2012. Available at: http://www.fda.gov/safety/medwatch/safetyinformation/safetyalertsforhumanmedicalproducts/ucm282820.htm. Accessed August 30, 2013.

37. Büller HR, Prins MH, Lensin AW, et al. Oral rivaroxaban for the treatment of symptomatic pulmonary embolism. N Engl J Med 2012;366(14):1287–97.

38. Lassen MR, Raskob GE, Gallus A, et al. Apixaban or enoxaparin for thromboprophylaxis after knee replacement. N Engl J Med 2009;361(6):594–604.

39. Schulman S, Kearon C, Kakkar AK, et al. Dabigatran versus warfarin in the treatment of acute venous thromboembolism. N Engl J Med 2009;361(24):2342–52.

40. Lassen MR, Raskob GE, Gallus A, et al. Apixaban versus enoxaparin for thromboprophylaxis after knee replacement (ADVANCE-2): a randomised double-blind trial. Lancet 2010;375(9717):807–15.

41. Bauersachs R, Berkowitz SD, Brenner B, et al. Oral rivaroxaban for symptomatic venous thromboembolism. N Engl J Med 2010;363(26):2499–510.

42. Dogliotti A, Paolasso E, Giugliano RP. Novel oral anticoagulants in atrial fibrillation: a meta-analysis of large, randomized, controlled trials vs warfarin. Clin Cardiol 2013;36(2):61–7.

43. Biondi-Zoccai G, Malavasi V, D'Ascenzo F, et al. Comparative effectiveness of novel oral anticoagulants for atrial fibrillation: evidence from pair-wise and warfarin-controlled network meta-analyses. HSR Proc Intensive Care Cardiovasc Anesth 2013;5(1):40–54.

44. Ntaios G, Papavasileiou V, Diener HC, et al. Nonvitamin-K-antagonist oral anticoagulants in patients with atrial fibrillation and previous stroke or transient ischemic attack: a systematic review and meta-analysis of randomized controlled trials. Stroke 2012;43(12):3298–304.

45. Majeed A, Hwang HG, Connolly SJ, et al. Management and outcomes of major bleeding during treatment with dabigatran or warfarin. Circulation 2013;128(21):2325–32.

46. Neumann I, Rada G, Claro JC, et al. Oral direct factor Xa inhibitors versus low-molecular-weight heparin to prevent venous thromboembolism in patients

undergoing total hip or knee replacement: a systematic review and meta-analysis. Ann Intern Med 2012;156(10):710–9.

47. Adam SS, McDuffie JR, Lachiewicz PF, et al. Comparative effectiveness of new oral anticoagulants and standard thromboprophylaxis in patients having total hip or knee replacement: a systematic review. Ann Intern Med 2013;159(4): 275–84.

48. Sobieraj DM, Coleman CI, Tongbram V, et al, editors. Venous thromboembolism prophylaxis in orthopedic surgery. Rockville (MD): Agency for Healthcare Research and Quality (US); 2012. Mar. Report No.: 12-EHC020-EF.

49. Garcia DA, Baglin TP, Weitz JI, et al. Parenteral anticoagulants: antithrombotic therapy and prevention of thrombosis, 9th ed: American College of Chest Physicians evidence-based clinical practice guidelines. Chest 2012;141(Suppl 2): e24S–43S.

50. Levi MM, Eerenberg E, Lowenberg E, et al. Bleeding in patients using new anticoagulants or antiplatelet agents: risk factors and management. Neth J Med 2010;68(2):68–76.

51. Pengo V, Crippa L, Falanga A, et al. Questions and answers on the use of dabigatran and perspectives on the use of other new oral anticoagulants in patients with atrial fibrillation. A consensus document of the Italian Federation of Thrombosis Centers (FCSA). Thromb Haemost 2011;106(5):868–76.

52. Turpie AG, Kreutz R, Llau J, et al. Management consensus guidance for the use of rivaroxaban—an oral, direct factor Xa inhibitor. Thromb Haemost 2012;108(5): 876–86.

53. Heidbuchel H, Verhamme P, Alings M, et al. EHRA practical guide on the use of new oral anticoagulants in patients with non-valvular atrial fibrillation: executive summary. Eur Heart J 2013;34(27):2094–106.

54. Lazo-Langner A, Lang ES, Douketis J. Clinical review: clinical management of new oral anticoagulants: a structured review with emphasis on the reversal of bleeding complications. Crit Care 2013;17(3):230.

55. Ortel TL. Perioperative management of patients on chronic antithrombotic therapy. Blood 2012;120(24):4699–705.

56. US Food and Drug Administration. Safety announcement—Updated recommendations to decrease risk of spinal column bleeding and paralysis in patients on low molecular weight heparins. 2013. Available at: http://www.fda.gov/downloads/Drugs/DrugSafety/UCM373735.pdf. Accessed November 5, 2013.

57. Huisman MV, Lip GY, Diener HC, et al. Dabigatran etexilate for stroke prevention in patients with atrial fibrillation: resolving uncertainties in routine practice. Thromb Haemost 2012;107(5):838–47.

58. Young E, Cosmi B, Weitz J, et al. Comparison of the non-specific binding of unfractionated heparin and low molecular weight heparin (Enoxaparin) to plasma proteins. Thromb Haemost 1993;70(4):625–30.

Clinical Use of the Activated Partial Thromboplastin Time and Prothrombin Time for Screening

A Review of the Literature and Current Guidelines for Testing

Jerrold H. Levy, MD, FAHA, FCCM[a],*, Fania Szlam, MMSc[b],
Alisa S. Wolberg, PhD, FAHA[c], Anne Winkler, MD, MSc[d]

KEYWORDS

- Activated clotting time • Anticoagulation • Monitoring
- Activated partial thromboplastin time • Prothrombin time • Surgery

KEY POINTS

- Although the activated partial thromboplastin time (aPTT), prothrombin time (PT), and international normalized ratio (INR) are widely used in routine preoperative testing, these hemostatic tests are not reliable predictors of perioperative bleeding in patients without known bleeding risk factors.
- A preoperative bleeding history and physical examination are usually obtained in an attempt to identify important bleeding risk factors. However, current questionnaires used to assess bleeding history are notoriously poor at characterizing bleeding. In such cases, follow-up hemostatic testing may be appropriate.
- The aPTT is extensively used to monitor therapy with unfractionated heparin and other anticoagulant agents, including direct thrombin inhibitors, whereas the PT and INR are used to monitor the anticoagulant effects of warfarin and other vitamin K antagonists, and to adjust their dosages.

Conflict of Interest Statements: Prof. J.H. Levy serves on steering committees for Boehringer Ingelheim, CSL Behring AG, Grifols, Janssen Pharmaceuticals, and The Medicines Company. F. Szlam, Dr AM Winkler, and Dr A.S. Wolberg have no relevant conflict of interest to disclose.
[a] Duke University School of Medicine, Divisions of Cardiothoracic Anesthesiology and Critical Care, Duke University Hospital, 2301 Erwin Road, Durham, NC 27710, USA; [b] Emory University Hospital, Emory University School of Medicine, 1364 Clifton Road, Atlanta, GA 30322, USA; [c] Department of Pathology and Laboratory Medicine, University of North Carolina at Chapel Hill, 815 Brinkhous-Bullitt Building, CB# 7525, Chapel Hill, NC 27599-7525, USA; [d] Department of Pathology & Laboratory Medicine, Emory University Hospital, 1364 Clifton Road, Atlanta, GA 30322, USA
* Corresponding author.
E-mail address: Jerrold.levy@duke.edu

Clin Lab Med 34 (2014) 453–477
http://dx.doi.org/10.1016/j.cll.2014.06.005
0272-2712/14/$ – see front matter © 2014 Elsevier Inc. All rights reserved.

labmed.theclinics.com

INTRODUCTION

Standard coagulation monitoring is used to manage hemostasis and bleeding in hospitalized patients, including those undergoing surgical procedures and during cardiac surgery with cardiopulmonary bypass (CPB). Multiple factors influence coagulation in hospitalized patients, especially in a perioperative setting. Such factors include type of procedure, previous surgery at the same anatomic site, degree of tissue injury, and the underlying state of the hemostatic system. Surgical procedures that may be associated with increased bleeding potential due to high tissue vascularity include tonsillectomy and vascular and cardiac surgery. In other cases, bleeding risk is associated with the potential for related adverse events, especially if bleeding occurs in the central nervous system or other closed spaces, such as in ophthalmic procedures.

Multiple assessments are routinely undertaken to assess the risk of bleeding in a given patient, including patient history, history of prior procedures with excessive bleeding, and family history. However, laboratory testing is often also extensively used in this evaluation. Tests that are performed most commonly include the activated partial thromboplastin time (aPTT), prothrombin time (PT), international normalized ratio (INR), and activated clotting time (ACT) for patients during cardiac surgery. The ACT is more often used for monitoring anticoagulation for CPB.

Although laboratory testing with the aPTT and PT is appropriate to monitor anticoagulation, and the tests evolved soon after the introduction of warfarin to determine hemostatic abnormalities, the value of these tests to predict bleeding in surgical patients is not well documented despite their widespread use. Their usefulness is further complicated by underlying bleeding disorders, test characteristics, and the potential for false-positive and false-negative results. In the presence of a lupus anticoagulant or factor XII deficiency, for example, the aPTT may be prolonged, but this prolongation is not associated with an increased risk of bleeding.[1]

A systematic review of the literature published in 1997 suggests that preoperative laboratory tests of hemostasis before elective surgery in patients without a positive personal history for abnormal bleeding are not helpful and rarely lead to a change in clinical management of the patient.[2] Furthermore, guidelines on the preoperative assessment of bleeding risk state that hemostatic tests are poor predictors of bleeding and that routine tests in patients without a history indicative of bleeding are not generally recommended.[3,4]

Despite these perspectives, these coagulation tests are frequently used for clinical decision-making in hospitalized patients. The purpose of this review is to examine the clinical applications of the aPTT and PT tests and their role in assessing perioperative bleeding risk for perioperative screening. In addition, the use of the ACT will be considered for anticoagulation monitoring for CPB as it is used extensively in the hospital setting.

aPTT

The aPTT is a global coagulation screening test that is used for assessment of the coagulation status in patients with suspected acquired deficiencies of coagulation factors of the intrinsic and common pathways of the coagulation system. The test is affected by multiple factors, including the levels of factors VIII, IX, XI, XII, X, II, and fibrinogen. The aPTT is widely used for monitoring anticoagulation therapy with low levels of heparin (from 0.1 IU/mL to approximately 1 IU/mL). In a normal population, the aPTT varies, and this interindividual variability is reflected in a wide reference interval. The aPTT reference interval also differs between laboratories that use reagents with different factor sensitivities and different lipid compositions as well as different instrumentation. The aPTT reagent is a mixture of phospholipids and activators (eg, kaolin, silica, or ellagic acid). Studies have shown considerable differences in the responsiveness of various aPTT reagents to mild and moderate deficiencies of coagulation factors, particularly factors VIII and IX.[5] Furthermore, in 1.5% to 3% of the population, aPTT is prolonged because of mild to severe factor XII deficiency; however, this prolongation is not associated with an increased risk of bleeding.[1] In addition, laboratories determine a reference interval to encompass the central 95% of apparently healthy men and women with similar demographics to the hospitalized population.[6] As a result, 5% of normal individuals will fall outside of the reference interval. Last, elevations of biological substances such as C-reactive protein have recently been published to interfere with commonly used aPTT reagents and will cause a false prolongation because of interferences with phospholipids, particularly phosphatidylcholine and phosphatidylethanolamine, which are commonly used in aPTT reagents.[7]

Clinical Uses of the aPTT

The aPTT is extensively used to monitor unfractionated heparin (UFH) therapy and other anticoagulant agents, including direct thrombin inhibitors. The limitations for this test include biological variability, insensitivity to some clinically important bleeding disorders (eg, factor XIII deficiency, α_2-antiplasmin deficiency), variability in instrumentation and reagents, low sensitivity to common pathway deficiencies (fibrinogen, prothrombin), variability due to physiologic changes (eg, in pregnancy, physical stress, or trauma), clinically irrelevant prolongation due to certain factor deficiencies (eg, factor XII [one of the commonest causes of unexpected aPTT prolongation], prekallikrein, and high-molecular-weight kininogen deficiencies), and preanalytical errors such as improper specimen collection.

PT AND INR

The PT measures the time required for clotting to occur after the addition of a source of tissue factor to recalcified citrated plasma in laboratory instruments and on point of care (POC) devices. The PT is measured by adding thromboplastin (a mixture of tissue factor, calcium, and phospholipid) to a patient's citrated plasma sample, and clot formation is determined. It is used also as a screening assay to detect deficiencies of one or more coagulation factors (fibrinogen and factors II, V, VII, and X). The INR was introduced by the World Health Organization to overcome variability in PT results due to differing sensitivities of thromboplastin reagents produced by different manufacturers.[8] The INR is the ratio of the patient's PT value divided by the normal value (geometric mean PT value for non-anticoagulated patients), as determined by the local laboratory, raised to the International Sensitivity Index (ISI) value (usually between 1.0 and 2.0) for the reagent and analytical system used: $INR = (PT_{patient}/PT_{geomean})^{ISI}$.

Clinical Uses of the PT/INR

The PT/INR is used extensively to monitor the anticoagulant effects of warfarin and other vitamin K antagonists and to adjust their dosages. Clinically, it is an in vitro measure of the extrinsic and common coagulation pathways and should therefore detect deficiencies of factors II, V, VII and X, and very low fibrinogen concentrations. As with all coagulation tests, the PT/INR is limited by biological variability, insensitivity to many bleeding disorders (eg, factor XIII deficiency, α_2-antiplasmin deficiency), variability in results due to differences in reagents and coagulation analyzers, and preanalytical errors. In addition, the PT results may be prolonged in young children. A study in healthy subjects categorized into 3 age groups (1–5 years, 6–10 years, and 11–18 years) showed no significant differences between the groups in terms of aPTT; however, children in the youngest age group had significantly higher mean PT compared with adults ($P = .03$).[9] **Table 1** summarizes a range of conditions that may be present based on the results of PT and aPTT testing.

UTILITY OF aPTT AND PT: EVIDENCE FROM THE LITERATURE

Findings of previously published reviews of the literature on coagulation testing are summarized in **Table 2**.[2,10–18] The overwhelming conclusion from these reviews is that routine preoperative hemostatic testing with aPTT and PT is not useful in asymptomatic patients with no known risk factors. Moreover, with aPTT and PT, the high rate of false-positive and false-negative results may lead to inappropriate precautionary measures or false reassurance, respectively.[12]

Individual studies assessing the value of preoperative aPTT and PT (and other tests) for predicting bleeding risk are summarized in **Table 3** (prospective studies[19–35]) and **Table 4** (retrospective studies[36–48]). In most cases, aPTT and PT were not shown to have any significant positive predictive value for postoperative bleeding risk. However, in contrast with the negative findings in most of these studies, there are several case reports in which preoperative testing was considered valuable because it identified individuals with bleeding disorders in whom there was no suggestive history: congenital factor X deficiency,[49] mild hemophilia,[50] and warfarin toxicity.[50]

Table 1
Summary of conditions that may be present based on the results of PT and aPTT testing

PT Result	aPTT Result	Examples of Conditions That May Be Present
Prolonged	Normal	• Liver disease • Vitamin K deficiency • Decreased or defective factor VII • Chronic, low-grade DIC • Vitamin K antagonist (warfarin) therapy
Normal	Prolonged	• Decreased or defective factor VIII, IX XI, XII, prekalikrein, high-molecular-weight kininogen • Type 3 vWD • Presence of lupus anticoagulant
Prolonged	Prolonged	• Decreased or defective fibrinogen, factor II, V, or X • Severe liver disease • Acute DIC
Normal	Normal or slightly prolonged	• May indicate normal hemostasis; however, PT and aPTT can be normal in conditions such as mild deficiencies in other factors and in the mild form of vWD • Further testing may be required to diagnose these conditions

Abbreviations: DIC, disseminated intravascular coagulation; vWD, von Willebrand disease.

Table 2
Published reviews of preoperative coagulation testing

Reference	Age	Conclusions
Any surgery		
Swedish Council on Technology Assessment,[8,10] 1991	Adult	Presurgical hemostatic tests are unnecessary in asymptomatic patients
Munro et al,[2] 1997	Adult/pediatric	Hemostatic tests have no value in predicting perioperative bleeding in the absence of clinical features
Peterson et al,[11] 1998	Adult/pediatric	In the absence of a history of excessive bleeding, the bleeding time fails as a screening test and is not indicated as a routine preoperative test
Chee & Greaves,[12] 2003	Adult/pediatric	Indiscriminate coagulation testing is not useful in a surgical or a medical setting, due to the limited sensitivity and specificity of the tests, and the high rate of false-positive and false-negative results
Eckman et al,[13] 2003	Adult/pediatric	For nonsurgical and surgical patients without synthetic liver dysfunction or a history of oral anticoagulant use, routine testing has no benefit in assessment of bleeding risk
Dzik,[14] 2004	Adult/pediatric	PT/INR had a poor predictive value for bleeding risk. Whether mild or moderate abnormalities of such tests have any clinically relevant predictive value as appropriate triggers for prophylactic transfusions before invasive procedures should be investigated in formal randomized clinical trials
Sié & Steib,[15] 2006	Adult/pediatric	Systematic preoperative screening is poorly efficient. It should be restricted to selected patients based on clinical history and physical examination
Kozek-Langenecker,[16] 2010	Adult/pediatric	Routine perioperative coagulation tests, including aPTT, PT, and INR, are poor predictors of bleeding and mortality. Such testing is still in use due to tradition rather than evidence
Cardiac surgery		
Klopfenstein,[17] 1996	Adult/pediatric	Clinical assessment of hemostatic function before cardiac operations is both effective and efficient. It obviates routine laboratory testing and favors the introduction of blood conservation strategies early on during the process of care
Tonsillectomy		
Krishna & Lee,[18] 2001	Adult/pediatric	There is no difference in the rate of posttonsillectomy bleeding in patients with abnormal compared with normal preoperative coagulation tests

Table 3
Prospective studies assessing preoperative coagulation tests for predicting intraoperative and/or postoperative bleeding risk

Type of Surgery and Reference	Age (n)	Laboratory Tests	PTT/aPTT Predictive	PT Predictive	Other Findings/Conclusions
General/not specified					
Eisenberg et al,[19] 1982	Age not stated (n = 750)	PTT, PT	No	No	PT and PTT detected few unsuspected bleeding disorders preoperatively, and there were a large number of apparently false-positive results
Borzotta & Keeling,[20] 1984	Adult (n = 83)	PTT, PT, PC, BT	Yes, with bleeding history	Yes, with bleeding history	Bleeding history should guide the selection of laboratory tests. Neither history nor laboratory tests alone provide insurance against hemorrhagic mishaps, but together they help the surgeon protect his or her charge from unexpected failure of hemostasis
Rohrer et al,[21] 1988	Adult/pediatric (n = 282)	PTT, PT, PC, BT	No	No	Of 514 screening tests performed, 4.1% were abnormal but none identified a clinically significant coagulopathy. Preoperative screening tests for coagulopathies not suspected on the basis of detailed clinical information are unnecessary and should not be done
Macpherson et al,[22] 1993	Age not stated Study 1, preoperative screening (n = 111, after excluding 45 patients who had taken aspirin in the previous week, and 3 with a history suggesting bleeding risk) Study 2, investigation of disproportionate hemorrhage (n = 1872)	aPTT, PT, BT, PC	No	No	If patients have no relevant history and physical examination is negative, preoperative screening for coagulation defects would seem to be unnecessary

Houry et al,[23] 1995	Adult, age 16–99 y (n = 3242)	PTT, PT, PC, BT	No	No	Preoperative hemostatic screening tests should not be performed routinely but only in patients with abnormal clinical data
Koscielny et al,[24] 2004	Adult, age 17–87 y (n = 5649)	aPTT, PT, PC, including PFA-100 (+vWF and BT in patients with a positive bleeding history)	No	No	The sensitivity of the PFA-100: collagen-epinephrine test was highest (90.8%) in comparison with the other screening tests, with a high positive predictive value (81.8%) and a higher negative predictive value (93.4%)
Spinal					
Murray et al,[25] 1999	Age not stated (n = 156)	aPTT (5 per patient), PT (6 per patient), INR, PT ratio, aPTT ratio	Variable	Variable	Among 16 patients with increased bleeding during surgery, PT and aPTT test results (all performed with the same instrument in the same laboratory) varied markedly. Variability was not reduced by use of the PT or aPTT ratio, or INR, or by incorporation of a measure of PT or aPTT test sensitivity to factor-deficient serum
Cardiac					
Colon-Otero et al,[26] 1987	Adult/pediatric, with congenital heart disease (n = 235)	aPTT, PTT, PT, TT, PC	Yes	Yes	One or more test values were abnormal in 19% of subjects—a significantly higher incidence than that expected in a normal population. Prolonged PT, PTT, or aPTT were seen most frequently; in 6/8 such patients evaluated further, there were decreased levels of factor VII or IX. However, the authors noted that use of blood products during cardiac surgery was not statistically significantly different between patients with normal or abnormal tests, and normal preoperative coagulation tests did not exclude the presence of a major bleeding diathesis

(continued on next page)

Table 3
(continued)

Type of Surgery and Reference	Age (n)	Laboratory Tests	PTT/aPTT Predictive	PT Predictive	Other Findings/Conclusions
Ferraris & Gildengorin,[27] 1989	Adult (n = 159), grouped according to packed RBC transfusion: Group I, ≤5 units (n = 139) Group II, >5 units (n = 20)	PTT, PT, BT, PC, Hct, packed RBC volume	No	No	Excessive postoperative blood transfusion was predicted by BT and RBC volume but not by PTT, PT, PC, or Hct (nor by recent use of heparin or aspirin)
Gravlee et al,[28] 1994	Adult (n = 897)	Post-CPB: ACT, aPTT, PT, TT, PC fibrinogen, fibrin/ fibrinogen degradation products, Duke's earlobe BT	No	No	Because the predictive values of the tests are so low, it does not appear sensible to screen patients routinely using these clotting tests after CPB
Williams et al,[29] 1999	Pediatric (n = 494)	PTT, PT, Hct, PC, fibrinogen, TE (before and during CPB)	Yes	No	Platelet count provided maximum sensitivity (83%) and specificity (58%) for prediction of excessive blood loss; TE was the only variable associated with total products transfused
Gynecologic					
Aghajanian & Grimes,[30] 1991	Adult (n = 1546)	PT	N/D	No	Of 25 evaluable patients with abnormal PT values, the results were not predictive in 20 cases and 5 had indications for coagulation testing based on history or physical examination. In the absence of specific indications, routine preoperative PT testing before elective gynecologic operations does not contribute to patient care and should be eliminated

Tonsillectomy/adenoidectomy

Bolger et al,[31] 1990	Adult/pediatric (n = 52)	PTT, PT, PC, BT	Yes?	Yes?	Clinical history failed to detect any previously unrecognized coagulation disorder. PT was prolonged in 5.8%, PTT in 11.5%, and BT in 9.5%. Six patients (11.5%) were considered to have important laboratory abnormalities. Laboratory screening therefore improved preoperative detection of occult hemostatic defects and allowed for appropriate alterations in perioperative care
Burk et al,[32] 1992	Pediatric (n = 1603)	CBC, aPTT, PT, BT	No	No	Laboratory abnormalities had a high specificity (0.99) and high negative predictive value (0.98) with a low sensitivity (0.03) and low positive predictive value (0.07) in predicting postoperative bleeding. The large number of false positive tests, coupled with the relative rarity of inherited and acquired coagulopathies, raises doubts about the overall value of routine screening
Close et al,[33] 1994	Adult/pediatric (n = 96)	PT, aPTT	No	No	Routine measurement of aPTT and PT in asymptomatic patients is not useful for predicting postoperative bleeding
Kang et al,[34] 1994	Pediatric (n = 1061)	PTT, PT, BT, PC	Yes	No	A coagulation profile that includes PTT and BT may be a valuable screening tool for children undergoing tonsillectomy and adenoidectomy. An initially abnormal coagulation profile may identify those more likely to bleed after surgery (22.6% vs 5.6%)
Zagólski,[35] 2010	Adult/pediatric (n = 222)	aPTT, PT/INR, PC	No	No	In healthy adults, coagulation test results are irrelevant for the course of tonsillectomy and postoperative bleeding

Abbreviations: BT, bleeding time; CBC, complete blood count; CPB, cardiopulmonary bypass; Hct, hematocrit; n, number of patients in the study; N/D, not discussed; PC, platelet count; PFA, platelet function analyzer; RBC, red blood cell; TE, thromboelastography; TT, thrombin time; vWF, von Willebrand factor.

Table 4
Retrospective studies assessing preoperative coagulation tests for predicting intraoperative and/or postoperative bleeding risk

Type of Surgery and Reference	Age (n)	Laboratory Tests	PTT/aPTT Predictive	PT Predictive	Other Findings/Conclusions
General/not specified					
Suchman & Mushlin,[36] 1986	Adult (n = 12,338)	aPTT	No	N/D	aPTT had no ability to predict the occurrence or absence of hemorrhage in patients at low clinical risk, but was a moderate predictor in high-risk patients. The data justify limiting preoperative coagulation screening to patients with active bleeding, known or suspected bleeding disorders, liver disease, malabsorption, malnutrition, or other conditions associated with acquired coagulopathies, and patients whose procedures may interfere with normal coagulation
Gewirtz et al,[37] 1996	Adult/pediatric (n = 167)	PT, PTT, BT	No	No	The value of preoperative BT was not a reliable test for assessing the risk of clinically significant perioperative bleeding. Patients with a bleeding history were more likely to have abnormal BT but there was no statistically significant association between abnormal BT and the other indicators of bleeding risk examined, or the occurrence of clinically significant perioperative bleeding

Reference	Population	Tests			Comments
Reddy et al,[38] 1999	Age not stated (n = 199): grouped according to PTT: Group 0, <23 s (n = 49) Group 1, 23-25 s (n = 50) Group 2, 28-31 s (n = 100)	PTT	Abnormally fast PTT indicated significant risk of morbidity and death	N/D	Abnormally fast PTTs, particularly if confirmed on repeat testing, indicate a significant risk of subsequent death, thrombosis, bleeding, and overall morbidity
Ng et al,[39] 2002	Age not stated (n = 828)	aPTT, PT, PC	No	No	Routine preoperative tests that are not indicated clinically should be discouraged for many reasons. They are not useful, may cause discomfort and inconvenience for the patient, may lead to more unnecessary investigations, and are costly. Use of preoperative coagulation tests in patients undergoing major noncardiac surgery should still be guided by clinical assessment
Cardiac					
Wojtkowski et al,[40] 1999	Pediatric (n = 275)	"More sensitive" aPTT and PT	No	No	An abnormal test result did not predict the need for perioperative blood products. The authors question the usefulness of preoperative coagulation screening of the pediatric cardiac surgery patient, particularly because lasting changes in physician perception regarding the clinical significance of abnormal values may lead to missed diagnoses in other settings
Craniofacial					
Genecov et al,[41] 2005	Age not stated (n = 168)	PTT, PT	Yes	No	Although the prevalence of abnormal aPTT was low (3.57%) in these patients undergoing craniofacial surgery, detection of an abnormal result required preoperative correction of coagulopathy in 4 of 5 cases (a sixth case declined surgery because of fear of surgical morbidity)

(continued on next page)

Table 4
(continued)

Type of Surgery and Reference	Age (n)	Laboratory Tests	PTT/aPTT Predictive	PT Predictive	Other Findings/Conclusions
Hernia repair/spinal anesthesia					
De Saint Blanquat et al,[42] 2002	Pediatric (former preterm infants) (n = 141)	aPTT, PT, PC	No	No	The results of coagulation tests may be impaired by reagents unsuitable for infants
Spinal					
Horlocker et al,[43] 2001	Pediatric/adult (n = 244)	aPTT, PT, INR, PC, TE	Yes	Yes	The coagulation tests with the most sensitivity and specificity for prediction of excessive surgical bleeding were INR, PT, and aPTT. TE values were of marginal use. The authors concluded that INR, PT, and aPTT may be helpful in guiding transfusion therapy in patients undergoing major spine surgery
Neurosurgical					
Schramm et al,[44] 2001	Adult (n = 1211)	aPTT, PT, PC	No	No	Prolonged aPTT was predictable on history in most patients. The authors concluded that routine screening of all preoperative neurosurgical patients is unnecessary
Tonsillectomy/adenoidectomy					
Howells et al,[45] 1997	Pediatric (n = 339)	PTT, PT	No	No	Preoperative PT/PTT provides no additional information than does a bleeding history for the general pediatric population undergoing tonsillectomy. This should only be done in selective cases where warranted by history

Manning et al,[46] 1987	Pediatric (n = 994)	PTT, PT	No	No	For patients with no history or clinical signs indicating possible bleeding disorder, preoperative PT and PTT failed to predict bleeding as an outcome. Screening PT/PTT should be reserved for patients with known or suspected coagulopathies
Zwack & Derkay,[47] 1997	Pediatric (n = 4373)	aPTT, PT	No	No	Laboratory screening has a very low predictive value in detecting occult bleeding disorders or perioperative hemorrhage, does not appear to be cost-effective, and should therefore be used selectively
Asaf et al,[48] 2001	Pediatric (n = 416)	PTT, PT, INR	No	No	Preoperative coagulation screening tests provide low sensitivity and low bleeding predictive value. Routine screening tests are not indicated unless a medical history of bleeding tendency is suspected

Abbreviations: BT, bleeding time; n, number of patients in each study; N/D, not discussed; PC, platelet count; TE, thromboelastography.

Survey of Clinical Practice

The results of a US survey published in 2009[51] indicate a discrepancy between current physician practices regarding pre-adenotonsillectomy coagulation screening compared with recommendations published in the American Academy of Otolaryngology–Head and Neck Surgery (AAO–HNS) 1999 Clinical Indicators Compendium.[52] Despite the AAO-HNS recommendation that coagulation and bleeding workup should only be performed if there was an "abnormality suspected or genetic information unavailable," 21% of physicians who responded to the survey reported that they still performed screening tests, including PT and aPTT, in patients with no known bleeding risk. The surveyed population consisted of members of the American Society of Pediatric Otolaryngology and members of the Massachusetts Society of Otolaryngology–Head and Neck Surgery. Awareness of the AAO-HNS recommendations was similar among physicians from both societies and did not affect screening practices.

Published Guidelines and Recommendations

An Australian paper published by Baker[53] in 2002 reports that laboratory testing before surgery provides assistance in assessment of bleeding tendency but that results may often be inconclusive. The author states that an adequate bleeding history is the best method for screening patients before surgical intervention. UK guidelines on preoperative tests published in 2003 by the National Institute for Clinical Excellence were actually based on expert consensus because of the paucity of data.[54] In the UK guidelines, hemostasis testing (including aPTT and PT/INR) is suggested (but not recommended) in American Society of Anesthesiologists grade 3 patients with cardiovascular disease undergoing major surgery.[54] Overall, however, such tests are not recommended because of their low predictive value, except when there is a history of abnormal bleeding.

In 2007, Kamal and colleagues[55] from the Mayo Clinic published recommendations on the interpretation and follow-up of prolonged PT, aPTT, and bleeding time in adults. The authors note that correlation of these tests with the patient's clinical and hemostatic history is critical. In 2008, the British Committee for Standards in Haematology published guidelines in which it was reported that preoperative hemostatic tests were poor predictors of bleeding risk resulting from surgery or invasive procedures.[4] In 2010, a multidisciplinary panel of experts in the United States published a "common understanding" of hemostasis in which they stated that currently available routine laboratory tests of hemostasis, including PT/INR and aPTT, do not reflect the complexity of in vivo hemostasis and can mislead the clinician.[56] Other tests, such as thromboelastography, were considered time-consuming and complex. They also highlighted the need to develop tests that can predict bleeding and complications and guide therapy if required, as well as the need for controlled trials, observational studies, and large registry and database studies to answer important clinical questions on hemostasis. In 2011, the European Society of Anaesthesiology published guidelines on the preoperative evaluation of adult patients undergoing noncardiac surgery.[57] Similar to previous guidelines and recommendations, the authors state that "routine use of coagulation tests is not recommended unless there are specific risk factors in the history."[57]

FACTORS THAT MAY PROLONG THE aPTT AND/OR PT
Drugs

As would be expected from their indications, anticoagulant therapies (warfarin, heparin, low-molecular-weight heparins) will prolong aPTT and PT test results to a varying extent, depending on the pharmacologic agent. In addition, the antibiotic daptomycin may impact aPTT reagents leading to falsely prolonged results.[58]

Test Reagents

As described above, test results may vary with the reagent used. Prolonged aPTT times have been reported with micronized silica, celite, and ellagic acid as activators.[59] Even with modern automated coagulation analyzers, discrepancies have been observed between aPTT results obtained with different evaluation modes on automated coagulation analyzers.[60]

Temperature and Time

Variations in temperature and duration of storage of blood samples before coagulation testing may influence coagulation test results. Testing of blood samples from healthy volunteers, hospitalized patients, and patients receiving oral anticoagulants or heparin showed that PT test results were stable for up to 24 hours regardless of storage conditions (with or without centrifugation, at either room temperature or 4°C).[61] aPTT results were stable in blood tested up to 8 hours after sampling, except in heparinized samples, wherein aPTT values were clinically significantly shortened in samples stored uncentrifuged at room temperature[61]; however, current guidelines and regulations mandate testing within 4 hours of specimen collection.

In blood samples left for 3, 6, and 24 hours at either room temperature or 4°C before centrifugation, aPTT was significantly prolonged compared with samples centrifuged immediately and analyzed.[62] In another study, it was shown that either plasma or whole blood samples could be accepted for PT testing up to 24 hours and for aPTT testing up to 12 hours when stored at room temperature or 4°C.[63] The INR of blood samples from patients on oral anticoagulants changed by differing amounts during storage, depending on which PT system was used.[64] Elsewhere, it was shown that the INR of centrifuged and uncentrifuged blood left at room temperature for 24 hours consistently increased by 6%, and that this could be used reliably to correct results and adjust oral anticoagulant dose accordingly.[65] However, all coagulation testing needs to be performed within 4 hours unless frozen and tested later with the exception of the PT. No laboratory should be testing on specimens greater than 4 hours old except PT. This ruling is all due to labile factors V and VIII.

One important critical factor is that both hypothermia and hyperthermia have been shown to prolong the aPTT in heparinized plasma in vitro.[66] In vivo body temperature may also affect results: hyperthermic water immersion was shown to shorten aPTT in healthy volunteers,[67] whereas mild hypothermia in patients undergoing plastic surgery resulted in longer aPTT and bleeding times.[68]

Diet

Foods containing large amounts of vitamin K (eg, beef and pork liver, green tea, broccoli, chickpeas, kale, turnip greens) may affect coagulation test results. Fasting may shorten PT and reduce levels of factors II, VII, and X.[69]

Genetically Determined and Acquired Coagulation Disorders

Table 5 summarizes a range of genetic conditions and their effects on coagulation assays and the risk of bleeding.[70–80] Acquired coagulation disorders for which abnormal test results may not predict bleeding risk include vitamin deficiency (eg,

Table 5
Effects of genetic conditions on coagulation test results and bleeding risk

Conditions in Which Abnormal Test Results Do Not Predict Bleeding Risk	Observations
Lupus anticoagulant/ antiphospholipid antibodies	—
Factor XII deficiency	Associated with prolonged aPTT but does not predispose to an increased risk in bleeding[70]
Neurofibromatosis type I	Among 30 subjects with this condition, aPTT was prolonged in 11, factor XII levels were reduced in 3, vWF levels were reduced in 4, and PFA-100 closure times were elevated in 13. However, clinically perceived bleeding risk did not appear to be correlated with laboratory test results in most cases[71]
Noonan syndrome	May be associated with prolonged aPTT and low levels of clotting factors (particularly factors XI and XII), but coagulation test results did not correlate with bruising history and may not predict bleeding risk[72]

Conditions in Which Abnormal Test Results May Predict Bleeding Risk	Observations
Factor VII deficiency	The only congenital bleeding disorder characterized by isolated PT prolongation. It is clinically heterogeneous but life-threatening bleeding may occur[73]
Prothrombin (factor II) deficiency	Typically results in prolonged PT and aPTT, with increased risk of surgical-associated or trauma-associated bleeding[74]
Factor XI deficiency	Associated with excessive bleeding following injury, surgery, or other invasive procedures, but may otherwise be asymptomatic.[75] aPTT is prolonged by more than 2 SDs above the normal mean in patients with severe factor XI deficiency, but heterozygotes may have normal or only slightly prolonged aPTT values[75]
Lupus-like anticoagulant	May cause prolonged PT and aPTT, although sensitivity varies; may sometimes be associated with impaired hemostasis[89]
Sickle cell disease	May be associated with prolonged PT but trials are needed to clarify whether abnormal coagulation tests are associated with increased risk of perioperative bleeding[76]
Rosenthal syndrome/factor XI deficiency	May be associated with prolonged PTT but PTT does not necessarily correlate with factor XI levels. Patients can be classified as low-risk or high-risk for elective surgery based on factor XI levels and prior surgical or family history[77]
Type I Gaucher disease	Prolonged PT and variable clotting factor deficiencies plus potential for increased intraoperative and postoperative bleeding risk[78]
Kasabach–Merritt syndrome	Associated with prolonged PT and aPTT, decreased hematocrit and fibrinogen levels, and severe risk of disseminated intravascular coagulation[79]

(continued on next page)

Table 5
(continued)

Conditions in Which Normal/Mildly Abnormal Test Results Do Not Exclude Bleeding Risk	Observations
vWD	PT is unaffected but aPTT may be prolonged.
Hemophilia A (factor VIII deficiency) and Hemophilia B (factor IX deficiency)	PT is unaffected but aPTT should be prolonged
Factor XIII deficiency	—
α_2-antiplasmin deficiency	—
Prekallikrein deficiency	—
High-molecular-weight kininogen deficiency	—
Passovoy factor deficiency	aPTT shows relatively mild prolongation but subjects bruise easily and have undue blood loss after procedures such as dental extraction and tonsillectomy[80]

Abbreviations: PFA, platelet function analyser; vWD, von Willebrand disease.

due to celiac disease or obstructive jaundice), liver disease, and thrombocytopenia (in which PT and aPTT are unaffected).

COAGULATION TESTS AS PREDICTORS OF PERIOPERATIVE BLEEDING
Preoperative Bleeding History and Physical Examination

A preoperative bleeding history and physical examination should be considered to potentially identify any of the bleeding risk factors summarized in **Box 1**[13] because many factors may contribute to the bleeding risk. Of paramount importance, a careful medication history should be obtained, including over-the-counter medicines that may contain aspirin and use of any anticoagulation agents or herbal supplements that may affect hemostasis such as platelet function. Particular attention should be paid to prior episodes of bleeding complications following injury, tooth extraction, pregnancy, surgery, and menstruation and to patients with a family history of bleeding issues. During physical examination, clinicians should evaluate the patient for petechiae, mucosal bleeding, ecchymoses, or mucosal bleeding that may be either acquired (ie, drug-related) or due to other platelet disorders.

Hemostatic Testing for Patients

Although multiple tests are used to assess the risk for perioperative bleeding, multiple aspects are important to consider for the interpretation of test results, including the clinical setting, underlying concomitant diseases, and applicability of the specific test used. Eckman and colleagues[13] analyzed the results from 5 observational studies in nonsurgical hospitalized patients and 12 observational studies of preoperative coagulation testing to assess coagulation testing as a diagnostic method in patients with postoperative bleeding complications. Despite the widespread use of testing, patients with a prolonged aPTT did not have a statistically significantly increased risk for postoperative complications.[13] Despite inconclusive results reported in

> **Box 1**
> **Preoperative indicators of increased bleeding risk**
>
> *Bleeding history*
> - Excessive bruising
> - Bleeding greater than 3 minutes after brushing teeth
> - Nosebleeds
> - Prolonged bleeding after cuts
> - Severe or prolonged menstruation
> - Severe bleeding after dental extraction, surgical operation, or childbirth
> - History of hemophilia or inherited familial hemorrhagic disorder
> - Personal history of liver disease, renal failure, hypersplenism, hematological disease, or collagen vascular disease
>
> *Evidence on physical examination*
> - Purpura
> - Hematoma
> - Jaundice
> - Signs of cirrhosis
>
> *Data from* Eckman MH, Erban JK, Singh SK, et al. Screening for the risk for bleeding or thrombosis. Ann Intern Med 2003;138(3):W15–24.

multiple studies, as described above, coagulation testing is extensively used in the perioperative setting. Specific considerations for diagnosis and management are reviewed in subsequent sections.

Use of Hemostatic Tests Before Dental Extractions

For the general population, routine hemostatic tests before dental extractions are not recommended. As for patients about to undergo surgery, a comprehensive medical history is the most important means of minimizing the risk of morbidity associated with invasive dentistry. For patients receiving anticoagulant or antiplatelet therapy, careful assessment of risk is warranted, including the reason for such therapy and the appropriate laboratory tests to assess coagulation levels. Based on a review of the scientific literature, it has been stated that routine discontinuation of anticoagulant therapy is unnecessary; however, INR should be used to evaluate coagulation status in warfarin anticoagulated patients before invasive dental procedures.[81]

Use of PT, aPTT, and ACT for Clinical Decision-Making—Anticoagulation Monitoring

PT and aPTT

Because aPTT reagents can vary greatly in their sensitivity to UFH, it is important first to establish a relationship between aPTT response and heparin concentration. The therapeutic aPTT range should correspond to an UFH concentration of 0.3 to 0.7 U/mL as assessed by a chromogenic anti-Xa activity assay and determined by each local laboratory based on a specific instrument and reagent combination.

Many large studies in which patients have been treated with therapeutic doses of UFH have used a simple, arbitrarily established "aPTT range," such as 1.5 to 2.5 times the upper limit of the normal reference interval. Patients treated with such heparin therapy have, in general, experienced low rates of thrombosis. In the GUSTO IIa study,[82] 2564 patients were enrolled, about half of whom received heparin. The observed low rates of both thrombosis and bleeding in this and other large contemporary studies suggest that an arbitrary aPTT reference interval for heparin may be appropriate.

A therapeutic aPTT range of 1.5 to 2.5 times control is widely accepted. It has been shown that this range corresponds to 0.2 to 0.4 IU/mL UFH by protamine titration and 0.3 to 0.7 IU/mL by anti-Xa assay.[81–85] If this type of calibration cannot be performed, the therapeutic aPTT range of 2.0 to 3.5 times normal is preferable to prevent a subtherapeutic heparin concentration.

Although preoperative coagulation testing using the PT and aPTT is widely practiced, there is no definitive evidence that performing preoperative hemostatic testing improves clinical outcomes. Despite this lack of evidence, these tests are widely used for the assessment of bleeding risk before surgery or invasive procedures in selected patients (patients with a positive bleeding history, or a clear clinical indication), or following trauma for predictive value of INR.

ACT

The ACT is a modified Lee White clotting time where an activator (usually kaolin or celite) is added to expedite the coagulation process. It has been developed as a POC test to monitor UFH in patients during cardiac surgery, on extracorporeal life support, and undergoing percutaneous invasive procedures whereby they are usually anticoagulated with heparin or bivalirudin. A normal ACT depends on the activator but is typically less than 150 s. However, for CPB, the ACT target is 350 s or greater following administration of an UFH dose of 300 to 400 IU/kg before CPB, with additional boluses given as required.[84,86] The ACT is less precise than the aPTT and lacks correlation with the aPTT or with anti-Xa levels. Moreover, the ACT is influenced by several variables that include anemia, platelet count, function, and inhibitors, temperature (hypothermia), contact activation inhibition, aprotinin, and fibrinogen levels. It is also imperative that the type of ACT cartridge used for testing correctly reflects the heparin measurement range desired.

Use of PT and aPTT for Clinical Decision-Making—Variability of Testing

For the PT and aPTT, clinicians define the "limits of erroneous results" for the comparison of the POC test results against those obtained using standard laboratory testing. Overall, the limit of erroneous results refers to the difference between 2 results from different methods that may cause harm to a patient or cause a risk to the safety of the patient. However, most laboratory-based testing has at least a 5% to 10% variability based on testing alone.

PT/INR

For the PT/INR there are clinical decision points at "normal values" and around greater than 1.5 times normal. For a PT reagent with an ISI of 1.0, a PT time of 1.5 times normal would be equivalent to an INR of 1.5. Using a POC PT test, the biological variance (interindividual and intraindividual variance) that would be considered to still provide equivalence would also be a 5% to 10% difference. Thus, for an INR of 1.5, the "gray zone" would be 1.4 to 1.6 and would lead to the same clinical decision with a POC PT test as with a laboratory test—in most cases, the decision to treat an INR of 1.4 to 1.6 would be the same.

Defining the limit of erroneous results is important because it also alters therapeutic approaches. For example, for PT, if the PT POC test is compared with a PT laboratory test with respect to plasma therapy, one should bear in mind that it is not possible to lower an INR to less than 1.5 by administering fresh frozen, thawed, or liquid plasma. For more precise anticoagulation of patients, clinicians are increasingly using chromogenic factor X assays as a guide, especially when transitioning patients from a direct thrombin inhibitor such as argatroban or bivalirudin to warfarin, because of the variability of marked increases in INR compared with actual anticoagulation. Results from these assays are used to guide interventions or other clinical decisions.

aPTT

For the aPTT, the limit of erroneous results for comparison of the aPTT POC test to an aPTT laboratory test depends on whether the test is being used for diagnostic or therapeutic purposes. The baseline aPTT value is a critical factor for monitoring anticoagulants, because anticoagulant therapy is usually directed at increasing the aPTT over a wide range, from 1.5 to 2.5 times control values. For the 5% to 10% variability, this usually has minimal impact over a 5% to 10% coefficient of variation. Also, for therapy for bleeding, the goal is to reduce the aPTT to less than 35 s, which is considered normal. Although guidelines still suggest plasma as a therapy for a prolonged aPTT, there are few data to support that practice. No randomized controlled trials have evaluated whether fresh frozen plasma administration corrects abnormal aPTT results or indeed elevated PT values and is effective in stopping bleeding.[85–88] Moreover, several uncontrolled trials have found that fresh frozen plasma does not effectively correct an abnormal PT or aPTT.[87]

SUMMARY

Coagulation testing using aPTT and PT/INR tests are not reliable predictors of excessive perioperative bleeding risk in patients without other known risk factors. Although routine preoperative use of these tests is common, the data do not support their utility for screening. However, they are used extensively for anticoagulation monitoring with many different anticoagulation agents. A thorough patient and family history, together with physical examination, is vital to identify patients at increased bleeding risk; in such cases, follow-up hemostatic testing may be appropriate.

REFERENCES

1. Halbmayer WM, Haushofer A, Schon R, et al. The prevalence of moderate and severe FXII (Hageman factor) deficiency among the normal population: evaluation of the incidence of FXII deficiency among 300 healthy blood donors. Thromb Haemost 1994;71(1):68–72.
2. Munro J, Booth A, Nicholl J. Routine preoperative testing: a systematic review of the evidence. Health Technol Assess 1997;1(12):i–iv, 1–62.
3. Reeves BC, Ascione R, Chamberlain MH, et al. Effect of body mass index on early outcomes in patients undergoing coronary artery bypass surgery. J Am Coll Cardiol 2003;42(4):668–76.
4. Chee YL, Crawford JC, Watson HG, et al. Guidelines on the assessment of bleeding risk prior to surgery or invasive procedures. British Committee for Standards in Haematology. Br J Haematol 2008;140(5):496–504.
5. Shetty S, Ghosh K, Mohanty D. Comparison of four commercially available activated partial thromboplastin time reagents using a semi-automated coagulometer. Blood Coagul Fibrinolysis 2003;14(5):493–7.
6. Clinical and Laboratory Standards Institute. Defining, establishing, and verifying reference intervals in the clinical laboratory; approved guideline.

CLSI document C28-A3. 3rd edition. Wayne (PA): Clinical and Laboratory Standards Institute; 2008.

7. Schouwers SM, Delanghe JR, Devreese KM. Lupus Anticoagulant (LAC) testing in patients with inflammatory status: does C-reactive protein interfere with LAC test results? Thromb Res 2010;125(1):102–4.

8. World Health Organization (WHO). WHO Expert Committee on Biological Standardization – Thirty-Third report. Annex 3, WHO Technical Report Series, no. 687 – Requirements for thromboplastins and plasma used to control oral anticoagulant therapy (Requirements for Biological Substances no. 30, revised 1982). 1983. Available at: http://onlinelibrary.wiley.com/doi/10.1111/j.1538-7836.2004.00775.x/pdf. Accessed December 5, 2013.

9. Sosothikul D, Seksarn P, Lusher JM. Pediatric reference values for molecular markers in hemostasis. J Pediatr Hematol Oncol 2007;29(1):19–22.

10. Preoperative routines. The Swedish Council on Technology Assessment in Health Care. Int J Technol Assess Health Care 1991;7(1):95–100.

11. Peterson P, Hayes TE, Arkin CF, et al. The preoperative bleeding time test lacks clinical benefit: College of American Pathologists' and American Society of Clinical Pathologists' position article. Arch Surg 1998;133(2):134–9.

12. Chee YL, Greaves M. Role of coagulation testing in predicting bleeding risk. Hematol J 2003;4(6):373–8.

13. Eckman MH, Erban JK, Singh SK, et al. Screening for the risk for bleeding or thrombosis. Ann Intern Med 2003;138(3):W15–24.

14. Dzik WH. Predicting hemorrhage using preoperative coagulation screening assays. Curr Hematol Rep 2004;3(5):324–30.

15. Sié P, Steib A. Central laboratory and point of care assessment of perioperative hemostasis. Can J Anaesth 2006;53(Suppl 6):S12–20.

16. Kozek-Langenecker SA. Perioperative coagulation monitoring. Best Pract Res Clin Anaesthesiol 2010;24(1):27–40.

17. Klopfenstein CE. Preoperative clinical assessment of hemostatic function in patients scheduled for a cardiac operation. Ann Thorac Surg 1996;62(6):1918–20.

18. Krishna P, Lee D. Post-tonsillectomy bleeding: a meta-analysis. Laryngoscope 2001;111(8):1358–61.

19. Eisenberg JM, Clarke JR, Sussman SA. Prothrombin and partial thromboplastin times as preoperative screening tests. Arch Surg 1982;117(1):48–51.

20. Borzotta AP, Keeling MM. Value of the preoperative history as an indicator of hemostatic disorders. Ann Surg 1984;200(5):648–52.

21. Rohrer MJ, Michelotti MC, Nahrwold DL. A prospective evaluation of the efficacy of preoperative coagulation testing. Ann Surg 1988;208(5):554–7.

22. Macpherson CR, Jacobs P, Dent DM. Abnormal peri-operative haemorrhage in asymptomatic patients is not predicted by laboratory testing. S Afr Med J 1993;83(2):106–8.

23. Houry S, Georgeac C, Hay JM, et al. A prospective multicenter evaluation of preoperative hemostatic screening tests. The French Associations for Surgical Research. Am J Surg 1995;170(1):19–23.

24. Koscielny J, Ziemer S, Radtke H, et al. A practical concept for preoperative identification of patients with impaired primary hemostasis. Clin Appl Thromb Hemost 2004;10(3):195–204.

25. Murray D, Pennell B, Olson J. Variability of prothrombin time and activated partial thromboplastin time in the diagnosis of increased surgical bleeding. Transfusion 1999;39(1):56–62.

26. Colon-Otero G, Gilchrist GS, Holcomb GR, et al. Preoperative evaluation of hemostasis in patients with congenital heart disease. Mayo Clin Proc 1987;62(5): 379–85.

27. Ferraris VA, Gildengorin V. Predictors of excessive blood use after coronary artery bypass grafting. A multivariate analysis. J Thorac Cardiovasc Surg 1989;98(4): 492–7.

28. Gravlee GP, Arora S, Lavender SW, et al. Predictive value of blood clotting tests in cardiac surgical patients. Ann Thorac Surg 1994;58(1):216–21.

29. Williams GD, Bratton SL, Riley EC, et al. Coagulation tests during cardiopulmonary bypass correlate with blood loss in children undergoing cardiac surgery. J Cardiothorac Vasc Anesth 1999;13(4):398–404.

30. Aghajanian A, Grimes DA. Routine prothrombin time determination before elective gynecologic operations. Obstet Gynecol 1991;78(5 Pt 1):837–9.

31. Bolger WE, Parsons DS, Potempa L. Preoperative hemostatic assessment of the adenotonsillectomy patient. Otolaryngol Head Neck Surg 1990;103(3):396–405.

32. Burk CD, Miller L, Handler SD, et al. Preoperative history and coagulation screening in children undergoing tonsillectomy. Pediatrics 1992;89(4 Pt 2):691–5.

33. Close HL, Kryzer TC, Nowlin JH, et al. Hemostatic assessment of patients before tonsillectomy: a prospective study. Otolaryngol Head Neck Surg 1994;111(6): 733–8.

34. Kang J, Brodsky L, Danziger I, et al. Coagulation profile as a predictor for post-tonsillectomy and adenoidectomy (T + A) hemorrhage. Int J Pediatr Otorhinolaryngol 1994;28(2–3):157–65.

35. Zagólski O. Post-tonsillectomy haemorrhage–do coagulation tests and coagulopathy history have predictive value? Acta Otorrinolaringol Esp 2010;61(4): 287–92 [in Spanish].

36. Suchman AL, Mushlin AI. How well does the activated partial thromboplastin time predict postoperative hemorrhage? JAMA 1986;256(6):750–3.

37. Gewirtz AS, Miller ML, Keys TF. The clinical usefulness of the preoperative bleeding time. Arch Pathol Lab Med 1996;120(4):353–6.

38. Reddy NM, Hall SW, MacKintosh FR. Partial thromboplastin time: prediction of adverse events and poor prognosis by low abnormal values. Arch Intern Med 1999;159(22):2706–10.

39. Ng KF, Lai KW, Tsang SF. Value of preoperative coagulation tests: reappraisal of major noncardiac surgery. World J Surg 2002;26(5):515–20.

40. Wojtkowski TA, Rutledge JC, Matthews DC. The clinical impact of increased sensitivity PT and APTT coagulation assays. Am J Clin Pathol 1999;112(2):225–32.

41. Genecov DG, Por YC, Barcelo CR, et al. Preoperative screening for coagulopathy using prothrombin time and partial thromboplastin time in patients requiring primary cranial vault remodeling. Plast Reconstr Surg 2005;116(2):389–94.

42. De Saint Blanquat L, Simon L, Laplace C, et al. Preoperative coagulation tests in former preterm infants undergoing spinal anaesthesia. Paediatr Anaesth 2002; 12(4):304–7.

43. Horlocker TT, Nuttall GA, Dekutoski MB, et al. The accuracy of coagulation tests during spinal fusion and instrumentation. Anesth Analg 2001;93(1):33–8.

44. Schramm B, Leslie K, Myles PS, et al. Coagulation studies in preoperative neurosurgical patients. Anaesth Intensive Care 2001;29(4):388–92.

45. Howells RC 2nd, Wax MK, Ramadan HH. Value of preoperative prothrombin time/partial thromboplastin time as a predictor of postoperative hemorrhage in pediatric patients undergoing tonsillectomy. Otolaryngol Head Neck Surg 1997;117(6):628–32.

46. Manning SC, Beste D, McBride T, et al. An assessment of preoperative coagulation screening for tonsillectomy and adenoidectomy. Int J Pediatr Otorhinolaryngol 1987;13(3):237–44.
47. Zwack GC, Derkay CS. The utility of preoperative hemostatic assessment in adenotonsillectomy. Int J Pediatr Otorhinolaryngol 1997;39(1):67–76.
48. Asaf T, Reuveni H, Yermiahu T, et al. The need for routine pre-operative coagulation screening tests (prothrombin time PT/partial thromboplastin time PTT) for healthy children undergoing elective tonsillectomy and/or adenoidectomy. Int J Pediatr Otorhinolaryngol 2001;61(3):217–22.
49. Jonnavithula N, Durga P, Pochiraju R, et al. Routine preoperative coagulation screening detects a rare bleeding disorder. Anesth Analg 2009; 108(1):76–8.
50. Hattersley PG. The activated coagulation time of whole blood as a routine preoperative sceening test. Calif Med 1971;114(5):15–8.
51. Wieland A, Belden L, Cunningham M. Preoperative coagulation screening for adenotonsillectomy: a review and comparison of current physician practices. Otolaryngol Head Neck Surg 2009;140(4):542–7.
52. American Academy of Otolaryngology - Head and Neck Surgery. Clinical Indicators Compendium. 2009. Available at: https://www.entnet.org/content/clinical-indicato. Accessed December 12, 2013.
53. Baker R. Pre-operative hemostatic assessment and management. Transfus Apher Sci 2002;27(1):45–53.
54. Reeves B. Clinical guideline 3. Preoperative tests. The use of routine preoperative tests for elective surgery: London: National Institute for Clinical Excellence; Available at: http://guidance.nice.org.uk/CG3/Guidance/pdf/English. Accessed December 12, 2013.
55. Kamal AH, Tefferi A, Pruthi RK. How to interpret and pursue an abnormal prothrombin time, activated partial thromboplastin time, and bleeding time in adults. Mayo Clin Proc 2007;82(7):864–73.
56. Levy JH, Dutton RP, Hemphill JC 3rd, et al. Multidisciplinary approach to the challenge of hemostasis. Anesth Analg 2010;110(2):354–64.
57. De Hert S, Imberger G, Carlisle J, et al. Preoperative evaluation of the adult patient undergoing non-cardiac surgery: guidelines from the European Society of Anaesthesiology. Eur J Anaesthesiol 2011;28(10):684–722.
58. Webster PS, Oleson FB Jr, Paterson DL, et al. Interaction of daptomycin with two recombinant thromboplastin reagents leads to falsely prolonged patient prothrombin time/International Normalized Ratio results. Blood Coagul Fibrinolysis 2008;19(1):32–8.
59. Briselli MF, Ellman L. Kaolin-correctable prolongation of the activated partial thromboplastin time. Am J Clin Pathol 1980;74(5):677–80.
60. Milos M, Herak DC, Zadro R. Discrepancies between APTT results determined with different evaluation modes on automated coagulation analyzers. Int J Lab Hematol 2010;32(1 Pt 2):33–9.
61. Adcock D, Kressin D, Marlar RA. The effect of time and temperature variables on routine coagulation tests. Blood Coagul Fibrinolysis 1998;9(6):463–70.
62. Salvagno GL, Lippi G, Montagnana M, et al. Influence of temperature and time before centrifugation of specimens for routine coagulation testing. Int J Lab Hematol 2009;31(4):462–7.
63. Rao LV, Okorodudu AO, Petersen JR, et al. Stability of prothrombin time and activated partial thromboplastin time tests under different storage conditions. Clin Chim Acta 2000;300(1–2):13–21.

64. Leeming DR, Craig S, Stevenson KJ, et al. The determination of INR in stored whole blood. J Clin Pathol 1998;51(5):360–3.

65. Froom P, Abramova D, Bar-El M, et al. Reliability of delayed prothrombin time INR determinations in a central laboratory using off-site blood sampling. Clin Lab Haematol 2001;23(3):189–92.

66. Felfernig M, Blaicher A, Kettner SC, et al. Effects of temperature on partial thromboplastin time in heparinized plasma in vitro. Eur J Anaesthesiol 2001; 18(7):467–70.

67. Boldt LH, Fraszl W, Rocker L, et al. Changes in the haemostatic system after thermoneutral and hyperthermic water immersion. Eur J Appl Physiol 2008; 102(5):547–54.

68. Cavallini M, Baruffaldi Preis FW, Casati A. Effects of mild hypothermia on blood coagulation in patients undergoing elective plastic surgery. Plast Reconstr Surg 2005;116(1):316–21 [discussion: 322–3].

69. Moriwaki Y, Sugiyama M. Effect of fasting on coagulation factors in patients who undergo major abdominal surgery. Am Surg 2010;76(2):168–71.

70. Conaglen PJ, Akowuah E, Theodore S, et al. Implications for cardiac surgery in patients with factor XII deficiency. Ann Thorac Surg 2010;89(2):625–6.

71. Favaloro EJ, Zafer M, Nair SC, et al. Evaluation of primary haemostasis in people with neurofibromatosis type 1. Clin Lab Haematol 2004;26(5):341–5.

72. Massarano AA, Wood A, Tait RC, et al. Noonan syndrome: coagulation and clinical aspects. Acta Paediatr 1996;85(10):1181–5.

73. Lapecorella M, Mariani G. Factor VII deficiency: defining the clinical picture and optimizing therapeutic options. Haemophilia 2008;14(6):1170–5.

74. Meeks SL, Abshire TC. Abnormalities of prothrombin: a review of the pathophysiology, diagnosis, and treatment. Haemophilia 2008;14(6):1159–63.

75. Seligsohn U. Factor XI deficiency in humans. J Thromb Haemost 2009; 7(Suppl 1):84–7.

76. Raffini LJ, Niebanck AE, Hrusovsky J, et al. Prolongation of the prothrombin time and activated partial thromboplastin time in children with sickle cell disease. Pediatr Blood Cancer 2006;47(5):589–93.

77. Borud LJ, Matarasso A, Spaccavento CM, et al. Factor XI deficiency: implications for management of patients undergoing aesthetic surgery. Plast Reconstr Surg 1999;104(6):1907–13.

78. Katz K, Tamary H, Lahav J, et al. Increased operative bleeding during orthopaedic surgery in patients with type I Gaucher disease and bone involvement. Bull Hosp Jt Dis 1999;58(4):188–90.

79. Menendez LR, Thommen VD. Kasabach-Merritt syndrome complicating treatment of a closed femoral fracture. Clin Orthop Relat Res 1995;(316):185–8.

80. Jackson JM, Marshall LR, Herrmann RP. Passovoy factor deficiency in five Western Australian kindreds. Pathology 1981;13(3):517–24.

81. Jeske AH, Suchko GD. Lack of a scientific basis for routine discontinuation of oral anticoagulation therapy before dental treatment. J Am Dent Assoc 2003; 134(11):1492–7.

82. Randomized trial of intravenous heparin versus recombinant hirudin for acute coronary syndromes. The Global Use of Strategies to Open Occluded Coronary Arteries (GUSTO) IIa Investigators. Circulation 1994;90(4):1631–7.

83. Douketis JD, Spyropoulos AC, Spencer FA, et al. Perioperative management of antithrombotic therapy: antithrombotic therapy and prevention of thrombosis, 9th ed: American College of Chest Physicians evidence-based clinical practice guidelines. Chest 2012;141(Suppl 2):e326S–50S.

84. Garcia DA, Baglin TP, Weitz JI, et al. Parenteral anticoagulants: antithrombotic therapy and prevention of thrombosis, 9th ed: American College of Chest Physicians evidence-based clinical practice guidelines. Chest 2012;141(Suppl 2): e24S–43S.

85. Kearon C, Akl EA, Comerota AJ, et al. Antithrombotic therapy for VTE disease: antithrombotic therapy and prevention of thrombosis, 9th ed: American College of Chest Physicians evidence-based clinical practice guidelines. Chest 2012; 141(Suppl 2):e419S–94S.

86. Despotis GJ, Levine V, Goodnough LT. Relationship between leukocyte count and patient risk for excessive blood loss after cardiac surgery. Crit Care Med 1997;25(8):1338–46.

87. Puetz J. Fresh frozen plasma: the most commonly prescribed hemostatic agent. J Thromb Haemost 2013;11(10):1794–9.

88. Rosendaal FR, Reitsma PH. Is administering blood as useless as blood letting? J Thromb Haemost 2013;11(10):1793.

89. Mannucci PM, Canciani MT, Mari D, et al. The varied sensitivity of partial thromboplastin and prothrombin time reagents in the demonstration of the lupus-like anticoagulant. Scand J Haematol 1979;22(5):423–32.

Measurement of Dabigatran in Standardly Used Clinical Assays, Whole Blood Viscoelastic Coagulation, and Thrombin Generation Assays

CrossMark

Joanne van Ryn, PhD[a],*, Oliver Grottke, MD, PhD[b], Henri Spronk, PhD[c]

KEYWORDS

- Anticoagulation • Dabigatran • Measurement • Thrombin generation
- Thromboelastometry

KEY POINTS

- Dabigatran, an oral direct thrombin inhibitor, does not require routine monitoring; however, it is readily measured by many available coagulation assays.
- The partial thromboplastin time gives an approximation of dabigatran activity but is not linear over dabigatran concentrations used clinically.
- The prothrombin time should not be used to determine dabigatran concentrations because it is insensitive to its effects.
- The thrombin time (TT) is overly sensitive for dabigatran but useful to identify low levels of the drug.
- The diluted thrombin time (dTT) is a sensitive method to measure the anticoagulation effect of dabigatran and is increasingly used to determine its effect when needed.

Continued

Conflicts of Interest: J. van Ryn is an employee of Boehringer Ingelheim. O. Grottke has received research funding from Boehringer Ingelheim, Biotest, CSL Behring, Novo Nordisk, and Nycomed and honoraria for consultancy and/or travel support from Bayer Healthcare, Boehringer Ingelheim, and CSL Behring. H. Spronk has received research funding from Boehringer Ingelheim and honoraria for consultancy and/or travel support from Bayer Healthcare and Boehringer Ingelheim.

[a] Department of CardioMetabolic Disease Research, Boehringer Ingelheim Pharma GmbH & Co KG, Birkendorfer Street 65, Biberach 88397, Germany; [b] Department of Anesthesiology, RWTH Aachen University Hospital, Pauwelsstrasse 30, Aachen 52074, Germany; [c] Laboratory for Clinical Thrombosis and Haemostasis, Department of Internal Medicine, Cardiovascular Research Institute Maastricht, Maastricht University Medical Center, PO Box 616, Maastricht 6200 MD, The Netherlands
* Corresponding author.
E-mail address: joanne.vanryn@boehringer-ingelheim.com

Clin Lab Med 34 (2014) 479–501
http://dx.doi.org/10.1016/j.cll.2014.06.008
0272-2712/14/$ – see front matter © 2014 Elsevier Inc. All rights reserved.

labmed.theclinics.com

Continued

- Viscoelastic coagulation tests may be useful in the detection of coagulopathy associated with dabigatran and in monitoring the effects of reversal therapy.
- Thrombin generation assays can be used to measure direct thrombin inhibitors, but the lack of standardization of these assays makes comparability of data difficult.

INTRODUCTION

New oral anticoagulants have become widely used in recent years as an alternative therapy to vitamin K antagonists (VKAs), such as warfarin, in patients with atrial fibrillation (AF).[1] In large clinical trials, the efficacy and safety profiles of these agents have been shown to be similar or superior to that of anticoagulation with VKAs or low-molecular-weight heparin (LMWH) in indications that include prevention of thrombosis in orthopedic settings, treatment and secondary prevention of established thrombosis in patients with venous thromboembolism (VTE), and prevention of stroke in patients with AF.[2–6] Compared with VKAs and with parenteral anticoagulants such as heparins, these new oral anticoagulants present several advantages, including fewer drug-drug interactions, efficacy and safety profiles that do not depend on variation of food intake, and no requirement for the routine monitoring that is characteristic of VKA therapy.[7] However, despite the lack of required monitoring of the new oral anticoagulants, routine and/or specialized assays are used to measure their activity in situations in which this is required, such as emergencies or surgery.[8,9]

This review focuses on the new oral anticoagulant dabigatran and summarizes the assays that are available to measure its activity, discussing the relative sensitivity of these assays for this agent. It focuses not only on plasma-based clotting tests but also on assays more commonly used in surgical/emergency settings, such as activated clotting time (ACT) and thromboelastometry/thromboelastography (TEM/TEG). In addition, this review discusses the use of thrombin generation, a test that has received much attention in recent years as a method to determine the capacity of a patient to produce thrombin and thus determine if the patient is at elevated risk of thrombosis or bleeding. Most of these assays have been in use for many years and were developed for purposes other than the measurement of new oral anticoagulants activity. They were developed and standardized for the measurement of heparin- or VKA-induced anticoagulation or to determine coagulopathies in the absence of anticoagulation (eg, assays such as TEM or thrombin generation). Thus, the sensitivity of these assays for measuring dabigatran-induced anticoagulation differs from test to test and even between manufacturers of the same test.

PLASMA-BASED CLOTTING ASSAYS
Historical Perspectives

Two of the most commonly used assays are for clinically monitoring VKAs and unfractionated heparin (UFH). Owing to the variability of anticoagulation responses associated with these drugs and their small therapeutic window, monitoring these agents is important clinically.[9,10] The first of these assays is the international normalized ratio (INR), which is described by the equation INR = [patient PT/normal PT]^{ISI}, where PT is the prothrombin time and ISI is the international sensitivity index. Normal PT is the mean assay result obtained from healthy adult populations not given anticoagulants; this equation is then normalized for the PT reagent used as follows. The PT assay is initiated by adding tissue factor (TF) and phospholipids (PL) (this mixture is known as tissue thromboplastin) and calcium. The INR was introduced to standardize the PT internationally because tissue thromboplastin used in the PT assay is produced by different manufacturers and is variable in origin. Each manufacturer of thromboplastin reagents compares its reagent to an international standard, and a calculation factor (ISI) is provided by each manufacturer so that the INR calculated as described earlier is manufacturer-independent and comparable across laboratories. The PT assay is sensitive to the presence of factor (F) X, IX, VII, prothrombin (FII), and fibrinogen (**Fig. 1**). When PT is measured in FVII-depleted plasma, it is prolonged greater than 5-fold over control levels (**Fig. 2**). Anticoagulants that inhibit any of these factors influence the INR to some extent, but the predominance of vitamin K–dependent coagulation factors that are sensitive to the PT assay illustrates why VKAs can be monitored so sensitively via this method.

A second assay that is frequently used clinically is the activated partial thromboplastin time (aPTT). aPTT is more sensitive to intrinsic clotting factor inhibition; coagulation factors sensitive to the aPTT include FXII, FXI, FIX, FVIII, FV, FII, and fibrinogen (see **Fig. 1**). Thus, anticoagulants that inhibit any of these factors also affect the aPTT to some extent, either in a linear or nonlinear manner. UFH prolongs the aPTT in a concentration-dependent, linear manner over the therapeutic clinical range. The aPTT is only slightly influenced by VKAs owing to its insensitivity to the presence of FVII (see **Fig. 1**). There is no prolongation of the aPTT when using FVII-depleted plasma (see **Fig. 2**). Conversely, the INR response to VKAs is linear across the therapeutic range, whereas the INR is only mildly affected by heparin.

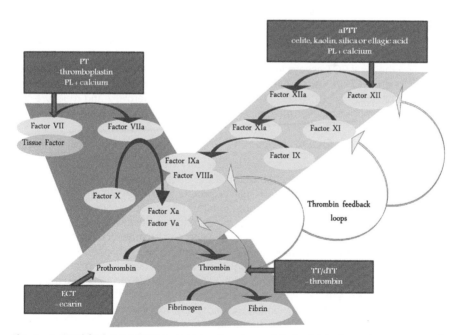

Fig. 1. A simplified coagulation cascade, showing extrinsic, intrinsic, and common pathways, site of principal activators for each coagulation assay, and the principal pathway influenced. aPTT, activated partial thromboplastin time; ECT, ecarin clotting time. (*Adapted from* Favaloro EJ, Lippi G. The new oral anticoagulants and the future of haemostasis laboratory testing. Biochem Med (Zagreb) 2012;22:329–41.)

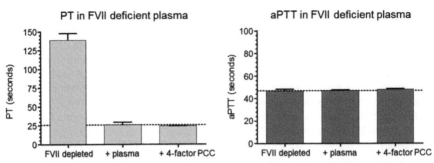

Fig. 2. Effect of FVII depletion on PT and aPTT. There was no effect of FVII depletion on the aPTT, but the PT was prolonged greater than 5-fold. Addition of normal plasma or 4-factor PCC (Kcentra) reversed the prolonged PT to control levels. Assays were performed with FVII-depleted human plasma, addition of human plasma or 4-factor PCC ($n = 3$ per assay); the dotted line in each graph represents control human plasma. aPTT, activated partial thromboplastin time; PCC, prothrombin complex concentrate.

In addition to these frequently used clinical tests, there exist supplemental tests that are not as widely used but are available in many laboratories. These include TT, ecarin clotting time (ECT), and ecarin chromogenic assay (ECA-T; for thrombin inhibitors). The TT assay is performed by adding thrombin to the plasma being tested; human or bovine thrombin can be used. This test is also sensitive to fibrinogen levels (see **Fig. 1**) and is prolonged by UFH.

The ECT assay involves the direct activation of prothrombin, resulting in the formation of meizothrombin, a proteolytically active thrombin intermediate.[11,12] Ecarin is a purified metalloprotease from the venom of the *Echis carinatus* snake.[12] There is no commercially available ECT kit; thus, cross-laboratory validations somewhat depend on the local ECT assays in use. Meizothrombin is inhibited by direct thrombin inhibitors such as hirudin or bivalirudin; therefore, the ECT is used primarily for direct thrombin inhibitors.[11,12] ECA-T assays are available commercially and measure the amount of chromogenic substrate conversion by meizothrombin generation.[13]

Laboratory Assays to Measure Dabigatran

Dabigatran is the active principle, that is, the direct thrombin inhibitor, present in plasma after oral ingestion and absorption of the double prodrug, dabigatran etexilate.[8,14] Dabigatran is predominantly renally excreted, with a half-life of 13 to 17 hours in elderly human volunteers, and is approximately 30% plasma protein bound.[15,16] Approximately 20% of the circulating active dabigatran is glucuronidated in humans; this metabolite is also pharmacologically active and can be measured using coagulation assays but is not always measurable when using liquid chromatography–mass spectrometry/mass spectrometry (LC-MS/MS) methods (see later discussion). In patients with AF, dabigatran etexilate is administered in doses of 110 or 150 mg twice daily, resulting in an approximate 2:1 peak to trough ratio with 12-hour dosing intervals.[14–16] Thus, when measuring anticoagulation, it is important to take into account when blood was sampled in relation to the last dose taken.

Liquid chromatography with tandem mass spectrometry

LC-MS/MS measurements are considered the gold standard for measuring dabigatran plasma levels and were used extensively during phase I, II, and III testing in patients.[17] This assay is limited in its availability, is complex and costly, and has a long turnaround time, making it unsuitable as a routinely available assay in the clinic, although it is available in some institutions.

This test is an analytical assay that can determine total dabigatran in blood, including all plasma protein-bound dabigatran, as well as levels of dabigatran metabolites. The methodology requires that plasma undergoes extraction, to remove dabigatran from plasma proteins, and complete alkaline cleavage of glucuronidated dabigatran (also pharmacologically active) to release nonconjugated dabigatran. Without this step, conjugated dabigatran does not elute at the same peak as active dabigatran using LC-MS/MS. Although this step is not necessary when dabigatran concentrations are measured in spiked human plasma, it is important when the method is used to determine dabigatran levels in the plasma of patients, where approximately 20% of active dabigatran is present in the glucuronidated form. Thus, even though this method is considered the gold standard for dabigatran measurement, with incorrect methodology, it underestimates the amount of active dabigatran present in patient samples as compared with clotting assays.[18]

Clinical coagulation tests and dabigatran measurement

There have been many studies published highlighting the sensitivity of different clinical tests to dabigatran.[8,14,19–25] The findings of all these studies are consistent and show that the PT is a poor test for dabigatran, as it is insensitive to direct thrombin inhibition by dabigatran until high concentrations of dabigatran are achieved.

The aPTT gives an approximation of dabigatran activity. This test is not linear over the range of dabigatran concentrations measured clinically and plateaus at high dabigatran concentrations.[8,14] However, if the aPTT is prolonged in a patient taking dabigatran, then it can be assumed there are measurable levels present. Studies have shown that a normal aPTT can often, but not always, exclude the presence of dabigatran, and thus a test more sensitive to lower levels of dabigatran may be of additional benefit.[24] In addition, studies have shown that different aPTT reagents react differently to dabigatran, with some being more sensitive than others.[19–24] In the clinical trial program performed with dabigatran, the aPTT reagent used for all measurements was originally obtained from Boehringer Mannheim (Mannheim, Germany), which was then distributed by Roche (Mannheim, Germany), and is today commercially available as CK Prest (Stago, Asnieres sur Seine, France). These differences in responses of dabigatran to different aPTT reagents illustrate that these commercial reagents were historically standardized for UFH measurement. The composition of the activators differs among manufacturers, resulting in the different sensitivities obtained with different agents.

Studies have also consistently shown that the TT is overly sensitive for dabigatran.[8,19–24] This test is sensitive for thrombin inhibitors, including UFH, and clotting is initiated by adding a standard amount of thrombin to patient plasma. Even very low concentrations of dabigatran can result in a prolonged TT. There may also be differences in responses to dabigatran depending on whether human or bovine thrombin is used as the initiating stimulus. Dabigatran is a more potent inhibitor of human than bovine thrombin; thus, cross-laboratory comparisons may also need to take different TT assays and thrombin sources into account (**Fig. 3**). Therefore, the clinical usefulness of this test is limited to identifying low levels of dabigatran.

The ECT is also a test traditionally used for measuring direct thrombin inhibitors and is linear over a large range of dabigatran concentrations.[8,19–24] Thus, this test is useful for measuring dabigatran; however, it is not available as a commercial kit. The ECA-T test also uses ecarin to activate coagulation, and outcome is measured chromogenically.[13] The readout is independent of patient prothrombin levels, as it requires dilution

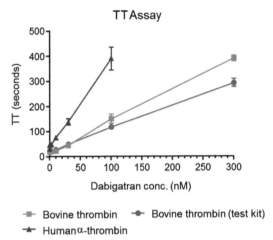

Fig. 3. Effect of different thrombin sources on clotting in the TT assay in human plasma in the presence of dabigatran. Purified bovine and human thrombin was obtained from Sigma (Steinheim, Germany); bovine thrombin included in thrombin time kit from Siemens Healthcare (Marburg, Germany) was also used. Data represented as mean ± SE, $n = 6$ determinations. SE, standard error.

of the plasma in a 1:5 ratio with a buffer containing prothrombin.[13] The specificity of the ECA-T for thrombin inhibitors can be seen in **Fig. 4**, and, although the response is not linear with increasing concentrations of dabigatran, there is a good dose response over a large dabigatran concentration range. At present, there is no commercial ECA-T kit available with dabigatran standards and controls, although commercial tests are in development.

Diluted thrombin time

The dTT was developed as a direct thrombin inhibitor test for parenteral inhibitors such as hirudin and bivalirudin. However, the kit has been modified to include both

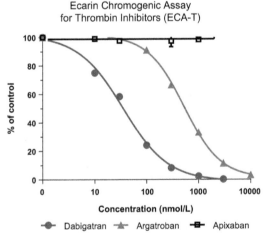

Fig. 4. Effect of increasing concentrations of argatroban, dabigatran, and apixaban on ECA-T in human plasma. Data represent the mean of duplicate determinations; ECA-T provided by Stago (Asnieres sur Seine, France).

calibrators and controls with dabigatran active substance dissolved in human plasma. Thus, the assay can be validated locally in laboratories to measure dabigatran anticoagulation[26] and allows cross-laboratory comparisons.[20,25,27]

The assay response to dabigatran is linear over a large concentration range and is useful for determining dabigatran plasma levels based on clotting times. The assay is simple to perform: patient plasma is diluted 1:8 in the buffer provided and then pooled human plasma, which is included in the kit, is added back to the diluted patient plasma (two-thirds pooled plasma and one-third diluted 1:8 patient sample). Thus, any coagulopathies present in the original patient plasma, such as low fibrinogen levels or hemodilution, which could influence undiluted plasma-based assays like aPTT, would have little effect on measurement of dabigatran using the dTT. As with TT, the stimulus for clotting is thrombin, which is also provided in the dTT kit (see **Fig. 1**); this avoids variation due to different sources of thrombin being used in different laboratories.

Whole Blood Clotting Tests

There is less information available regarding whole blood clotting tests. Dabigatran has been shown to prolong the PT in one whole blood point-of-care assay (given as an INR test value); however, this is not necessarily generalizable to all point-of-care INR tests. In addition, the results were not comparable to the plasma-based INR, which was much lower.[28–30] This result illustrates again that these tests were historically standardized for VKAs and results with dabigatran can be reagent and manufacturer specific.

Activated clotting time

ACT is used predominantly to monitor levels of heparinization during surgery.[31] Dabigatran prolongs the ACT in a manner similar to that of the aPTT. The kaolin ACT (Hemochron Response) test has been shown to approximate dabigatran levels but plateaus at high concentrations, and a normal clotting time does not necessarily indicate the absence of dabigatran.[8,21] More studies are required to understand the relationship between dabigatran concentrations and prolongation of ACT for clinical applications. Most of the current data have been obtained from experiments using dabigatran-spiked whole blood. However, when comparing potential additive effects of dabigatran and heparin in vitro with spiked human blood, it could be shown that the effect of the combination of dabigatran and heparin on the ACT was additive when compared with that of each treatment alone (**Table 1**).

Table 1				
Measurement of anticoagulation using ACT in the presence of increasing concentrations of dabigatran, heparin, or a combination of both in citrated human whole blood				
Dabigatran (nM)	0	250	500	1000
ACT (s)	123	187	245	364
Heparin (U/mL)		0.5	1	2
ACT (s)		146	195	286
Dabigatran (nM) + Heparin (U/mL)		250 + 0.5	500 + 1.0	1000 + 2.0
ACT (s)		265	417	733

Blood was tested in Hemochron Signature Elite test system (ITC, Edison, NJ, USA) with kaolin activator; data shown as mean, $n = 3$.

THROMBOELASTOGRAPHY/ROTATION THROMBOELASTOMETRY
Historical Perspective

Hartert first described TEG in 1948 as a method to assess global hemostatic function from a single blood sample.[32] In the earlier literature, the terms thromboelastography, thromboelastograph, and TEG were used generically. However, in 1996, thromboelastograph and TEG became registered trademarks of the Hemoscope Corporation (Hemoscope, Niles, IL, USA). Since then, these terms have been used by some researchers to describe the assay performed on Hemoscope instrumentation only, whereas others still use them as a general term for viscoelastic testing of blood samples. Another manufacturer, TEM International (ROTEM, TEM Innovations, Munich, Germany) markets a modified instrumentation using the terminology rotation thromboelastometry (ROTEM) or TEM. Although TEM and TEG offer similar types of tests with closely related clotting measurements, they are not interchangeable owing to differences in types of reagents and blood samples (**Table 2**).[33]

Methodological Considerations

Both viscoelastic coagulation tests measure the coagulation status under static conditions in a cuvette. Whole blood is added to a heated cuvette at 37°C. A pin is suspended within the cuvette and connected to a detector system. The TEG system uses a torsion wire, and the TEM device uses an optical detector. The cuvette and pin move relative to each other at an angle of 4°45′. The movement is initiated from either the cuvette (TEG) or the pin (TEM).[34,35] Fibrin strands form between the cuvette and pin as the blood clots, and rotation of the cuvette is either transmitted to the pin (TEG) or impedes the rotation of the pin (ROTEM). This rotation is detected, and a trace is generated accordingly (**Fig. 5**). Both TEG and TEM commonly use citrated whole blood that is recalcified to initiate coagulation. It is also common to use an activator, as this standardizes the test and also speeds up the rate at which clotting takes place and hence the rate at which a result is generated. The TEG and TEM devices have

Table 2
Nomenclature of selected TEG and TEM variables

Variable	TEM	TEG
Time from start to when the waveform reaches 2 mm above baseline (s)	CT	R
Time from 2 mm above baseline to 20 mm above baseline (s)	CFT	K
Alpha angle (°)	α (angle of tangent at 2 mm amplitude)	α (slope between R and K)
Maximum strength (mm)	MCF	MA
Time to maximum strength (s)	MCF-t	—
Amplitude at a specific time (mm)	A5, A10	A30, A60
Clot elasticity (X)	MCE	G
Maximum lysis (X)	CLF	—
Clot lysis at a specific time (min)	LY30, LY45, LY60	CL30, CL60
Time to lysis	CLT (10% difference from MCF)	2 mm from MA

Abbreviations: A, amplitude; CFT, clot formation time; CL, clot lysis; CLT, clot lysis time; CT, clotting time; K, kinetics; LY, lysis; MA, maximum amplitude; MCF, maximum clot firmness; R, reaction time.

ROTEM® Parameters

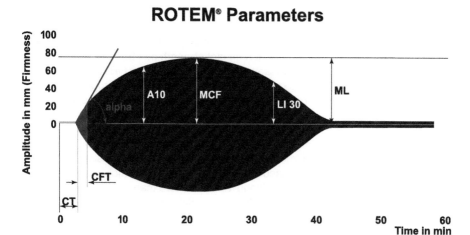

CT (clotting time): **time from start of measurement until initiation of clotting**
→ initiation of clotting, thrombin formation, start of clot polymerisation

CFT (clot formation time): **time from initiation of clotting until a clot firmness of 20mm is detected**
→ fibrin polymerisation, stabilisation of the clot with thrombocytes and F XIII

MCF (maximum clot firmness): **firmness of the clot**
→ increasing stabilisation of the clot by the polymerised fibrin, thrombocytes as well as F XIII

ML (maximum lysis) reduction of the clot firmness after MCF in relation to MCF
→ stability of the clot (ML < 15%) or fibrinolysis (ML > 15% within 1 h)

Fig. 5. Typical trace of viscoelastic point-of-care coagulation device ROTEM. A5, amplitude 5 min after CT; A10, amplitude 10 min after CT; CFT, clot formation time; CT, clotting time; LI30, lysis 30 min after CT; MCF, maximum clot firmness; ML, maximum lysis; α-angle, slope of tangent at 2 mm amplitude. (*Courtesy of* TEM Systems, Inc. (ROTEM®), Durham, NC. Available at: www.rotem-usa.com.)

several separate channels allowing several samples to be run simultaneously or sequentially. Local reference ranges should be used according to specific patient populations (adults or children), ethnicity, and underlying diseases.

Long turnaround times may be considered as the overriding drawback of conventional plasma-based coagulation tests. In contrast, TEG or TEM can be performed at the bedside and blood does not have to be processed (eg, centrifugation) in the central laboratory. Thus, faster turnaround times are feasible, which can allow prompt decision making on coagulation therapy. Severely bleeding patients require treatment without delay, raising the prospect, in clinical practice, of administering empirical therapy before test results become available. The coagulation status changes rapidly in bleeding patients; thus, test results may not reflect the patient's actual status when they become available.[36] Another consideration is that in recent years, the classic coagulation cascade has been challenged by the cell-based model.[37] According to the cell-based model, both TF and platelets have a major role in establishing hemostasis. Owing to the assessment of whole blood in TEG or TEM, useful information regarding in vivo coagulation, including system interactions with platelets and red blood cells, is provided.

The clot development, including clot initiation (CT), clot strength, and lysis, can be visually displayed in real time (see **Fig. 5**). However, clotting times are not specific for any one factor and are influenced by changes in any of the coagulation factors to a varying degree. Viscoelastic signals therefore depend on sufficient thrombin generation, fibrin polymerization, and fibrin interactions with platelet glycoprotein IIb/IIIa receptors.[38] For instance, decreased levels of clot strength may indicate insufficient concentrations of fibrinogen or platelets. By blocking platelet function through cytochalasin in TEM, the impact of fibrinogen on clot strength can be measured (FIBTEM assay). Combined with the EXTEM assay (stimulated with TF), the FIBTEM assay allows the discrimination of hypofibrinogenemia and isolated thrombocytopenia. Furthermore, studies indicate a correlation between FIBTEM-derived fibrin polymerization and plasma fibrinogen levels.[39–41] Therefore, TEM is often used clinically to guide therapy with fibrinogen concentrates. However, because hematocrit influences clot strength in whole blood, the hematocrit must be taken into account when interpreting fibrinogen levels.[42,43] Finally, hyperfibrinolysis may be detected by using the APTEM assay, as described later in the discussion. Generally, hyperfibrinolysis is suspected when the decrease in the amplitude during 1 hour is more than 15% of the maximum amplitude on TEG or TEM. After the addition of aprotinin (APTEM assay), hyperfibrinolysis can be confirmed; this has been shown to be associated with increased mortality in trauma patients.[44,45] However, mild forms of hyperfibrinolysis may not be detectable by TEM.[46]

Clinical Studies with TEG or TEM

The use of either TEG or TEM may enable clinicians to use a more individualized hemostatic therapy. Results from both animal studies and clinical studies performed in various clinical settings indicate that this approach might be associated with decreased need for plasma transfusion.[47–55] However, with regard to the application of prothrombin complex concentrate (PCC) in trauma-associated coagulopathy, the authors have shown that TEM variables can only serve as a surrogate of thrombin generation.[56,57] In addition, viscoelastic coagulation tests measure hemostasis in a cuvette and not in an endothelialized blood vessel. Thus, information on primary hemostasis is not provided. Finally, randomized prospective studies investigating the concept of targeted therapy versus conventional hemostatic therapy with regard to clinically relevant end points are largely missing, and the use of TEM-based algorithms in severely injured patients needs further investigation.[58–60]

Anticoagulation with Dabigatran on TEG or TEM

In principle, the ideal laboratory diagnostic for dabigatran should (1) show a correlation between increasing plasma concentrations of dabigatran and the degree of anticoagulation (eg, prolongation of CT) and (2) allow measurement of the effect of hemostatic therapy (eg, coagulation factor therapy with activated and nonactivated PCCs). There have been few preclinical or clinical studies of the potential of viscoelastic coagulation tests to monitor anticoagulation with dabigatran. In a study in healthy volunteers, blood samples were spiked ex vivo with dabigatran. At therapeutic plasma concentrations of dabigatran, a significant prolongation of CT both in the INTEM and EXTEM assay (ROTEM) was observed.[29] Consistent with this study, Davis and colleagues[61] showed that the TEG reaction time (R-value) may serve as a sensitive measure of the degree of anticoagulation due to dabigatran. Xu and colleagues[62] investigated the effect of several representative thrombin inhibitors, including dabigatran, on thrombin generation and TEG variables. At low dabigatran concentrations, there was primarily an effect on the clotting time (R). The addition of higher dabigatran concentrations also began to affect clot strength. In addition, dabigatran had the strongest potentiating effect on tPA-induced fibrinolytic activity ex vivo. This effect might be attributed to the inhibition of clot-bound thrombin by dabigatran. The inhibition of clot-bound thrombin may enhance fibrinolysis by reducing platelet activation and via associated reductions in plasminogen activator inhibitor-1 and thrombin activatable fibrinolysis inhibitor levels.[63] In line with the aforementioned studies, a strong dose-dependent correlation between the direct thrombin inhibitor argatroban and the CT in TEM analysis has been reported.[64]

To study the effect of dabigatran on TEM, the authors investigated the anticoagulant effects of dabigatran in combination with trauma-induced bleeding in an experimental porcine model.[65] Dabigatran etexilate (30 mg/kg) was given orally for 3 days to achieve plasma levels of 380 ± 106 ng/mL, and then dabigatran (active substance) was infused before surgery to achieve supratherapeutic plasma concentrations of dabigatran of 1423 ± 432 ng/mL. The effect of dabigatran was evaluated at several time points on TEM parameters (**Figs. 6** and **7**). After oral intake, only a substantial prolongation of CT in EXTEM was measured. However, no effect of oral administration of dabigatran etexilate on clot formation time and on clot strength (maximum clot firmness) was observed. After the infusion of dabigatran, a further prolongation of CT and an alteration of clot formation was measured. These changes in coagulation parameters, including a significant reduction of clot strength, were compounded by blood loss after trauma. However, decreased clot strength was reversed after the ex vivo addition of activated and nonactivated PCC.[65] Thus, the decrease in clot strength observed after dabigatran infusion was mainly attributable to a decrease in the amount of thrombin available for the conversion of fibrinogen to fibrin, as opposed to insufficient clot substrate (fibrinogen, platelets). Once sufficient thrombin becomes available through the addition of activated and nonactivated PCC, transformation of fibrinogen to fibrin is restored and clot formation is no longer impaired.

Overall, viscoelastic coagulation tests may be useful in the detection of coagulopathy associated with dabigatran and in monitoring the effects of reversal therapy. However, at present, there is a lack of studies investigating TEG and TEM to monitor coagulation therapy in patients receiving new oral anticoagulants such as dabigatran. Thus, clinical studies are warranted to investigate further the benefits and limitations of viscoelastic coagulation tests in this clinical setting.

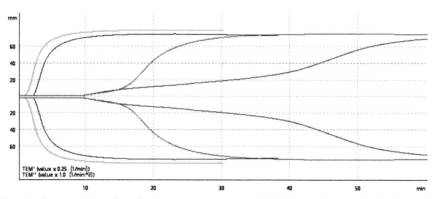

Fig. 6. Characteristic thromboelastometry curves (EXTEM: extrinsic activation) under different plasma concentrations of dabigatran using porcine blood and 60 min after trauma. Green line, baseline (0 ng/mL dabigatran); blue line, 236 ng/mL dabigatran; purple line, 850 ng/mL dabigatran; brown line, 60 min after trauma (677 ng/mL dabigatran). (*Data from* Grottke O, van Ryn J, Spronk H, et al. Prothrombin complex concentrates and a specific antidote (aDabi-Fab) are effective ex-vivo in reversing the effects of dabigatran in an anticoagulation/liver trauma experimental model. Crit Care 2014;18(1):R27.)

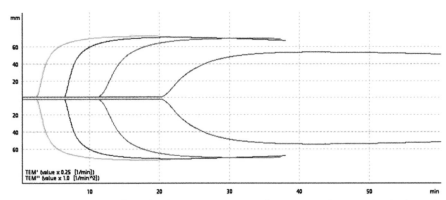

Fig. 7. Characteristic thromboelastometry curves (INTEM: intrinsic activation) under different plasma concentrations of dabigatran using porcine blood and 60 min after trauma. Green line, baseline (0 ng/mL dabigatran); blue line, 236 ng/mL dabigatran; purple line, 850 ng/mL dabigatran; brown line, 60 min after trauma (677 ng/mL dabigatran). (*Data from* Grottke O, van Ryn J, Spronk H, et al. Prothrombin complex concentrates and a specific antidote (aDabi-Fab) are effective ex-vivo in reversing the effects of dabigatran in an anticoagulation/liver trauma experimental model. Crit Care 2014;18(1):R27.)

THROMBIN GENERATION
Historical Perspective

Classically, thrombin generation is assessed through activation markers such as thrombin-antithrombin complex levels, prothrombin fragment 1.2, and D-dimer levels. Although these markers reflect ongoing or previous thrombin formation, they cannot be directly correlated with actual thrombin generation. For instance, D-dimer is a direct marker of fibrinolysis, and because fibrinolysis most likely does not occur without previous thrombin formation and subsequent fibrin clot formation, D-dimers are used as an indirect marker of active coagulation. However, formation of fibrin degradation products independently of previous thrombin generation has been suggested to occur in atherosclerotic lesions, in which D-dimers are generated without detectable coagulation activity.[66,67] In addition, fibrin degradation products do not provide information about the time between coagulation and fibrinolysis. Finally, the clearance and half-life of the marker, as well as the time between actual thrombin formation and sample drawing, might also influence the association; therefore, interpretation of data should be done with care.

Classic coagulation assays such as the PT and aPTT are based on the formation of the initial fibrin clot. Only a small portion of prothrombin needs to be converted into thrombin to generate minimum amounts of fibrin. Most (up to 95%) of the thrombin is generated after formation of the fibrin needed to assess PT or aPTT.[68] Although thrombin activation markers such as the thrombin-antithrombin complex reflect, at best, ongoing coagulation, clotting times are mostly applicable in the assessment of bleeding disorders. However, these assays are insensitive to mild bleeding disorders, completely lack sensitivity for increased coagulability (eg, hypercoagulability), and need to be adapted to be useful in the desired diagnostic field. To overcome the complications with the classic clotting times and thrombin activation markers, thrombin generation assays that assess the in vitro coagulation potential in a plasma sample may be used.

Methodological Considerations

In the past, thrombin generation assays were performed manually in (mostly defibrinated) plasma. Béguin and colleagues,[69] among others, mainly focused their efforts on the modification of an assay with cumbersome and laborious subsampling methods toward a more automated continuous measurement of thrombin generation. Initially, their work focused on the mode of action of heparins, and thrombin generation assays were used to solve the question of why LMWHs weakly enhance the binding of thrombin to antithrombin. The discovery that a thrombin substrate with high affinity and fast conversion could be replaced by one with poor binding to and low consumption by thrombin marked the transition toward the methods used today.[70] The search for such a substrate and the subsequent development of a fluorogenic substrate not only made assessment of thrombin generation possible in plasma containing fibrinogen/fibrin but also allowed for semiautomated monitoring of thrombin generation in multiple plasmas simultaneously. Although various different methods have been developed, they are based on the same principle of applying a substrate that binds loosely to and is slowly converted by thrombin.

The Calibrated Automated Thrombogram (CAT) (Thrombinoscope BV, Maastricht, the Netherlands) as developed by Hemker and colleagues[71] has important monitoring capabilities compared with other methods. The CAT uses a fluorogenic substrate and, through the simultaneous measurement of a calibrator, the resulting fluorescent signal is converted into the concentration of thrombin formed versus time. Thrombin bound to α_2-macroglobulin is applied as a calibrator, and the known fixed amount of thrombin is used to derive the actual thrombin concentration from the electronic signal. Furthermore, the use of a calibrator made it possible to correct for 3 problems associated with the measurement of fluorescence in plasma. First, constant fluorescent product formation is not linear with the fluorescence intensity, causing a decreasing velocity of fluorescence increase (inner-filter effect). Second, the consumption of substrate is higher at the beginning of the reaction and declines as substrate is consumed. Third, the fluorescent signal depends on the color of the plasma. The fluorescent signal is corrected by parallel assessment of thrombin generation in plasma and in the same plasma supplemented with calibrator. Thus, with the development of a software package, Hemker and colleagues[71] made it possible to compare both signals and derive the actual thrombin generation curve.

Several parameters can be derived from a typical thrombin generation curve (**Fig. 8**). The lag time (minutes) is the initiation phase in which thrombin generation has just started. Classically, the lag time is calculated as the time required to reach 10 nM thrombin or one-sixth of the peak height. After the initial phase, the production of thrombin increases quickly until it reaches a maximum that is represented by the peak height (nanomoles of thrombin) and the time to peak (minutes). The maximum slope of the initial part of the curve is translated into a velocity index (nanomoles per minute), reflecting the speed at which thrombin is generated. Thrombin is not only produced but also inhibited by anticoagulant proteins such as antithrombin and activated protein C (APC). After the peak, deactivation exceeds thrombin formation and the thrombin level declines until the curve reaches baseline. The first derivative of the original measurement curve does not decline to baseline owing to the buildup of α_2-macroglobulin–thrombin complex during the course of the experiment. After correction for this phenomenon,[72] the time to tail (minutes) at which thrombin generation has declined to zero can be calculated. The area under the curve is known as the endogenous thrombin potential (ETP; nanomoles minute), which reflects the potential amount of thrombin that can be generated in a plasma sample on stimulation with a given trigger.

High trigger levels are used in the classic PT and aPTT clotting time assays, whereas thrombin generation assays are activated by much lower levels of TF or activators of the contact pathway. Thrombin generation assays are highly sensitive to preanalytical

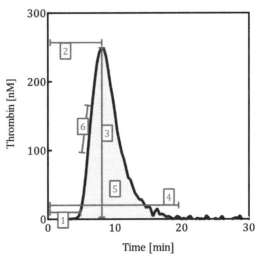

Fig. 8. Parameters derived from a typical thrombin generation curve. (1) Lag time in minutes defined as one-sixth of the peak height or the time to reach 10 nM thrombin generation; (2) time to peak in minutes; (3) peak height in nanomoles thrombin; (4) time to tail in minutes; (5) the area under the curve known as the endogenous thrombin potential (in nanomole minutes); (6) velocity index in nanomoles per minute.

variables that are known to cause activation of FXII, particularly at low TF levels (ie, <1 pM final concentration).[73] These preanalytical variables include the type of needle and tube used for blood collection, centrifugation times and speeds, and incubation of plasma at room temperature or even at 37°C. Therefore, thrombin generation assays are preferably performed according to a standardized procedure.[73] Typical thrombin generation experiments in platelet-poor plasma by means of the CAT method are conducted in 80 μL human plasma, with a total reaction volume of 120 μL including trigger and calcium.[74] Standard trigger reagents are 4 μM PL alone at 20:20:60 mol% phosphatidylserine: phosphatidylethanolamine: phosphatidylcholine, 1 pM TF with 4 μM PL or 5 pM TF with 4 μM PL (all final reaction concentrations). The trigger (20 μL) is added to the plasma, and after 10 min of preheating at 37°C in the fluorometer, the low affinity substrate (Z-Gly-Gly-Arg-AMC) is added together with calcium (20 μL) to start the reaction. In parallel, and to correct for inner-filter effects and substrate consumption, each thrombin generation measurement is calibrated against the fluorescence curve obtained in a sample from the same plasma (80 μL), to which has been added a fixed amount of α_2-macroglobulin–thrombin complex (20 μL Thrombin Calibrator, Thrombinoscope BV), 20 μL substrate, and calcium. Finally, thrombin generation curves are calculated from the initial fluorescence signal.

Correlation of Thrombin Generation with Thrombosis and Bleeding Outcomes

Analysis of the potential to generate thrombin suggests a correlation between increased thrombin generation parameters and increased risk of developing thrombosis or between a low potential to form thrombin and increased bleeding risk. Indeed, thrombin generation assays have been applied to both venous and arterial thrombosis, as well as to assess bleeding risk. To include the protein C pathway, a known contributor to venous thrombosis, both APC and thrombomodulin can be added to the assay, thereby increasing sensitivity for genetic and acquired thrombophilia, such as

FV Leiden thrombophilia and thrombophilia caused by oral contraceptives, respectively.[75] Two separate studies showed an increased risk for VTE in subjects with enhanced thrombin generation (peak height)[76] and a clear association between VTE risk and ETP.[77] However, including thrombin generation analysis in the workup of individual patients requires both standardization of the method and definition of reference values. The predictive value of thrombin generation for recurrent VTE has been demonstrated in several studies. One of the first studies showed a low risk of recurrent VTE in patients with a thrombin generation value less than a certain cutoff level.[78] Although a clear association between increased thrombin generation and an increased risk of recurrent VTE was demonstrated in 2 studies,[79,80] another study did not confirm this and showed only a risk association between thrombin generation and first VTE.[81] The hypercoagulable state in patients after a first VTE is apparent, as thrombin generation remains elevated during 24 months after developing VTE, with a diminished response to thrombomodulin.[82] The obvious next question is whether assessment of thrombin generation can be used to predict recurrence of VTE. This point remains to be evaluated and should include the applicability of each parameter derived from thrombin generation. One study showed association of the ETP, peak height, and lag time with VTE,[79] whereas others reported that only the ETP was associated with the risk of VTE.[80,81]

Although common genetic thrombophilic traits have less influence on the risk of acute arterial thrombosis,[83] coagulation activity and enhanced thrombin generation potential have been associated with atherosclerosis.[84,85] Moreover, both thrombin-antithrombin complexes and plasma thrombin generation are positively associated with the severity of computed tomographic scan-based coronary calcification.[86] The thrombin generating potential is increased after an acute myocardial infarction,[87–89] whereas a lower rather than higher thrombin generation profile was associated with recurrent atherothrombosis, despite a positive association of D-dimer levels with recurrent thrombosis.[87] A clear explanation for this paradoxic finding cannot be given, although the contribution of TF pathway inhibitor cannot be ruled out.[90]

For the profiling of bleeding risk, thrombin generation assays might have potential benefits. Not only is thrombin generation affected by coagulation factor deficiencies[91] but this method may also have the potential to monitor bypassing therapy in patients with coagulation factor inhibitors[92] and procoagulant treatment on trauma-induced coagulopathy.[57] The applicability of thrombin generation assays to monitor anticoagulant therapy, however, is not clear yet. Although many anticoagulants diminish thrombin generation, their overall influence on the different thrombin generation parameters cannot easily be derived from the literature. A variety of assays has been applied, including both platelet-poor and platelet-rich plasma, commercial and homemade reagents, and laboratory protocols. With focus on the direct thrombin and FXa inhibitors, Wong and colleagues[93] showed comparable prolongation of the lag time and time to peak on addition of apixaban, rivaroxaban, and dabigatran to platelet-poor plasma and thrombin generation triggered with 5 pM TF. The peak height and velocity index were sensitive for the direct FXa inhibitors, whereas the ETP proved to be the least sensitive parameter for all 3 anticoagulants. In contrast, in an in vitro study by Samama and colleagues,[94] the peak height and velocity index, and not the lag time and time to peak, were the most reduced on addition of rivaroxaban. In a study applying platelet-rich plasma, as opposed to platelet-poor plasma, which was used in the previous 2 studies, thrombin generation was inhibited at lower concentrations of rivaroxaban (nanomole range) and the dose of rivaroxaban needed to reduce the ETP by 50% was 3.5-fold higher than that required to double the lag time.[95] In line with these findings, a study comparing neonatal with adult plasma showed that rivaroxaban had a greater effect on the lag time, time to peak, and peak height than on the ETP.[96] Thus, different new oral anticoagulants have different effects on the thrombin generation curve, and direct comparisons using only ETP do not reflect these differences.

The effects of dabigatran on thrombin generation in platelet-poor plasma reported by Wong and colleagues[93] were comparable to those reported by Wienen and colleagues,[97] with the highest sensitivity on lag time and time to peak. In both studies, approximately 1 μM ($\sim$500 ng/mL) dabigatran effectively abolished plasma thrombin generation. However, spiking plasma from patients with cardiovascular disease with dabigatran required almost 0.5 mM ($\sim$250,000 ng/mL) to double the lag time and reduce the peak height from 450 to 350 nM.[98] One explanation for the required higher concentration might come from the variety in thrombin generation conditions used. The latter study applied commercial plasma reagent dissolved in 2 mL water, whereas the normal recommended procedure is preparation with 1 mL water. Doubling the volume dilutes not only the final TF trigger from 5 to 2.5 pM but also the PL (from 4 to 2 μM). The recommended 4 μM PL in the reaction provides an optimized level of procoagulant surface, and decreasing the concentration not only attenuates coagulation but also makes the method sensitive for platelet remnants and microparticles present in plasma. The study also applied 3.8% (w/v) sodium citrated blood, whereas the calcium concentration in the reaction was optimized for 3.2% (w/v) citrated plasma. Overall, differences in these technical details add to biased interpretation of the presented data and again emphasize the need for standardized procedures and conditions. As an example, added TF contributes to the sensitivity of the thrombin generation assay for dabigatran in plasma (**Fig. 9**, unpublished data). Thrombin generation triggered with 1 pM TF is almost not sensitive to dabigatran levels; however, the sensitivity of the assay for dabigatran increased with higher TF triggers, especially at 20 pM TF.

At low concentrations of direct thrombin inhibitors, the thrombin generation peak height increases compared with baseline and declines at higher levels of anticoagulant,[62,99,100] an effect also observed in vivo.[101] Potential mechanisms explaining this paradoxic effect are the anticoagulant inhibition of APC[99] and the presence of α_2-macroglobulin.[100] The reasons behind attributing this effect to APC stem from thrombin generation experiments in the presence of thrombomodulin or in protein C–deficient plasma. Furugohri and colleagues[99] performed thrombin generation assays triggered with 2.5 pM TF and observed increased peak height on spiking plasma with the direct thrombin inhibitor melagatran. The investigators diluted the commercial plasma reagent (5 pM TF) to obtain 2.5 pM TF as trigger but state that the PL concentration remained unchanged at 4 μM (should be 2 μM on dilution). Thrombin bound to thrombomodulin is more potently inhibited by direct thrombin inhibitors,[102] and activation of protein C is even further diminished under conditions of limited procoagulant surface. As described earlier, the CAT method corrects for the α_2-macroglobulin–thrombin complex generated during thrombin generation. Wagenvoord and colleagues[100] suggest that direct thrombin inhibitors decrease free functional thrombin and transiently increase free α_2-macroglobulin–thrombin complex with nonfunctional thrombin. Both free inhibited thrombin and inhibited thrombin in the α_2-macroglobulin–thrombin complex can still hydrolyze the fluorogenic substrate. The software algorithm subtracts the α_2-macroglobulin–thrombin activity from the total amidolytic activity, in which the transient increase in complex is not subtracted. The final result is an artificial increase in thrombin generation. It was proposed to use the half-ETP value to correct for this technical error.[100]

Another technical limitation in performing thrombin generation assays by means of the CAT in plasma containing a direct thrombin inhibitor is the inhibition of the

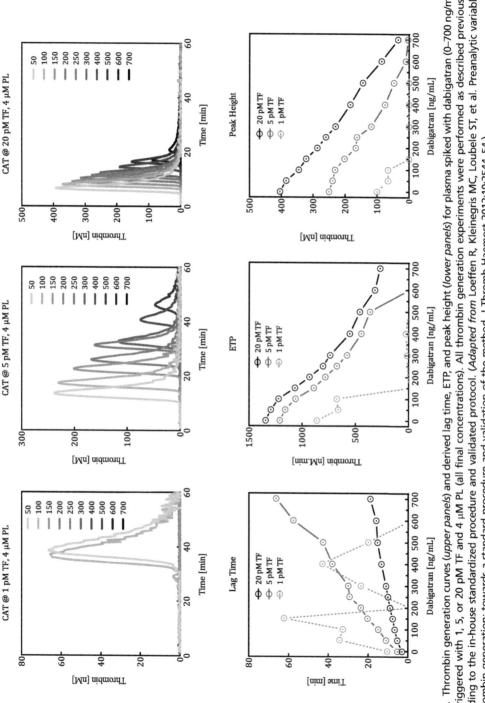

Fig. 9. Thrombin generation curves (*upper panels*) and derived lag time, ETP, and peak height (*lower panels*) for plasma spiked with dabigatran (0–700 ng/mL) and triggered with 1, 5, or 20 pM TF and 4 μM PL (all final concentrations). All thrombin generation experiments were performed as described previously, according to the in-house standardized procedure and validated protocol. (*Adapted from* Loeffen R, Kleinegris MC, Loubele ST, et al. Preanalytic variables of thrombin generation: towards a standard procedure and validation of the method. J Thromb Haemost 2012;10:2544–54.)

calibrator. This limitation is not a problem for in vitro experiments in which the inhibitor is added but the assay is calibrated using the nonspiked plasma. However, assessing thrombin generation in plasma from patients treated with a direct thrombin inhibitor cannot be calibrated. The direct thrombin inhibitor will bind to the α_2-macroglobulin–thrombin complex, thereby lowering the activity of the calibrator. The software package will convert the lower activity to the defined activity, causing an overestimation of the actual thrombin generation in the measured plasma sample.

Overall, in vitro plasma thrombin generation is a sensitive tool to assess both hypocoagulability and hypercoagulability, although standardization of the applied conditions is extremely important for it to become a routine clinical application; this is true not only for assessment of genetic bleeding or thrombosis risk but also for the anticoagulant-induced acquired bleeding risk. With the introduction of new direct coagulation factor inhibitors, it becomes even more important to standardize the methodology, to state clear descriptions of the applied conditions and presentation of the derived parameters.

REFERENCES

1. Hankey GJ, Eikelboom JW. Dabigatran etexilate: a new oral thrombin inhibitor. Circulation 2011;123:1436–50.
2. Connolly SJ, Ezekowitz MD, Yusuf S, et al. Dabigatran versus warfarin in patients with atrial fibrillation. N Engl J Med 2009;361:1139–51.
3. Connolly SJ, Ezekowitz M, Yusuf S, et al. Newly identified events in the RE-LY trial. N Engl J Med 2010;363:1875–6.
4. Patel MR, Mahaffey KW, Garg J, et al. Rivaroxaban versus warfarin in nonvalvular atrial fibrillation. N Engl J Med 2011;365:883–91.
5. Granger CB, Alexander JH, McMurray JJ, et al. Apixaban versus warfarin in patients with atrial fibrillation. N Engl J Med 2011;365:981–92.
6. Giugliano RP, Ruff CT, Braunwald E, et al. Edoxaban versus warfarin in patients with atrial fibrillation. N Engl J Med 2013;369:2093–104.
7. Hylek EM. The need for new oral anticoagulants in clinical practice. J Cardiovasc Med 2009;10:605–9.
8. van Ryn J, Stangier J, Haertter S, et al. Dabigatran etexilate – a novel, reversible, oral direct thrombin inhibitor: interpretation of coagulation assays and reversal of anticoagulant activity. Thromb Haemost 2010;103:1116–27.
9. Mani H, Kasper A, Lindhoff-Last E. Measuring the anticoagulant effects of target specific oral anticoagulants – reasons, methods and current limitations. J Thromb Thrombolysis 2013;36:187–94.
10. Favaloro EJ, Lippi G. The new oral anticoagulants and the future of haemostasis laboratory testing. Biochem Med (Zagreb) 2012;22:329–41.
11. Greinacher A, Warkentin TE. The direct thrombin inhibitor hirudin. Thromb Haemost 2008;99:819–29.
12. Nowak G. The ecarin clotting time, a universal method to quantify direct thrombin inhibitors. Pathophysiol Haemost Thromb 2003;33:173–83.
13. Haemosys Ecarin Chromogenic Assay. ECA-T Kit for quantitative determination of direct synthetic thrombin inhibitors in plasma [package Insert]. JenAffin GmbH, Jena, Germany; 2010.
14. Huisman MV, Lip GY, Diener HC, et al. Dabigatran etexilate for stroke prevention in patients with atrial fibrillation: resolving uncertainties in routine practice. Thromb Haemost 2012;107:838–47.

15. Stangier J, Stahle H, Rathgen K, et al. Pharmacokinetics and pharmacodynamics of the direct oral thrombin inhibitor dabigatran in healthy elderly subjects. Clin Pharmacokinet 2008;47:47–59.
16. Stangier J, Rathgen K, Staehle H, et al. Influence of renal impairment on the pharmacokinetics and pharmacodynamics of oral dabigatran etexilate: an open label, parallel group, single-centre study. Clin Pharmacokinet 2010;49: 259–68.
17. Stangier J, Rathgen K, Stahle H, et al. The pharmacokinetics, pharmacodynamics and tolerability of dabigatran etexilate, a new oral direct thrombin inhibitor, in healthy male subjects. Br J Clin Pharmacol 2007;64:292–303.
18. Douxfils J, Dogné JM, Mullier F, et al. Comparison of calibrated dilute thrombin time and aPTT tests with LC-MS/MS for the therapeutic monitoring of patients treated with dabigatran etexilate. Thromb Haemost 2013;110:543–9.
19. Dager WE, Gosselin RC, Kitchen S, et al. Dabigatran effects on the international normalized ratio, activated partial thromboplastin time, thrombin time, and fibrinogen: a multicenter, in vitro study. Ann Pharmacother 2012;46:1627–36.
20. Gosselin R, Hawes E, Moll S, et al. Performance on various laboratory assays in the measurement of dabigatran in patients receiving therapeutic doses. Am J Clin Pathol 2014;141:262–7.
21. Douxfils J, Mullier F, Robert S, et al. Impact of dabigatran on a large panel of routine or specific coagulation assays. Laboratory recommendations for monitoring of dabigatran etexilate. Thromb Haemost 2012;107:985–97.
22. Harenberg J, Giese C, Marx S, et al. Determination of dabigatran in human plasma samples. Semin Thromb Hemost 2012;38:16–22.
23. Lindahl TL, Baghaei F, Blixter IF, et al. Effects of the oral, direct thrombin inhibitor dabigatran on five common coagulation assays. Thromb Haemost 2011;105: 371–8.
24. Hawes EM, Deal AM, Funk-Adcock D, et al. Performance of coagulation tests in patients on therapeutic doses of dabigatran: a cross-sectional pharmacodynamic study based on peak and trough plasma levels. J Thromb Haemost 2013;11:1495–502.
25. Hapgood G, Butler J, Malan E, et al. The effect of dabigatran on the activated partial thromboplastin time and thrombin time as determined by the hemoclot thrombin inhibitor assay in patient plasma samples. Thromb Haemost 2013; 110:308–15.
26. Stangier J, Feuring M. Using the HEMOCLOT direct thrombin inhibitor assay to determine plasma concentrations of dabigatran. Blood Coagul Fibrinolysis 2012;23:138–43.
27. Avecilla ST, Ferrell C, Chandler WL, et al. Plasma-diluted thrombin time to measure dabigatran concentrations during dabigatran etexilate therapy. Am J Clin Pathol 2012;137:572–4.
28. Baruch L, Sherman O. Potential inaccuracy of point-of-care INR in dabigatran-treated patients. Ann Pharmacother 2011;45(7–8):e40.
29. Deremer CE, Gujral JS, Thornton JW, et al. Dabigatran falsely elevates point of care international normalized ratio results. Am J Med 2011;124(9):e5–6.
30. van Ryn J, Baruch L, Clemens A. Interpretation of point-of-care INR in patients treated with dabigatran. Am J Med 2012;125:417–20.
31. Lefemine AA, Lewis M. Activated clotting time for control of anticoagulation during surgery. Am Surg 1985;51:274–8.
32. Hartert H. Blutgerinnungstudien mit der Thrombelastographie, einem neuen Untersuchungsverfahren. Klin Wochenschr 1948;26:557–83.

33. Bolliger D, Seeberger MD, Tanaka KA. Principles and practice of thromboelastography in clinical coagulation management and transfusion practice. Transfus Med Rev 2012;26:1–13.

34. Available at: http://www.rotem.de. Accessed January 21, 2014.

35. Available at: http://www.haemonetics.com/en/. Accessed January 21, 2014.

36. Grottke O. Coagulation management. Curr Opin Crit Care 2012;18:641–6.

37. Hoffman M, Monroe DM 3rd. A cell-based model of hemostasis. Thromb Haemost 2001;85:958–65.

38. Ganter MT, Hofer CK. Coagulation monitoring: current techniques and clinical use of viscoelastic point-of-care coagulation devices. Anesth Analg 2008;106:1366–75.

39. Rugeri L, Levrat A, David JS, et al. Diagnosis of early coagulation abnormalities in trauma patients by rotation thromboelastography. J Thromb Haemost 2007;5:289–95.

40. Roullet S, Pillot J, Freyburger G, et al. Rotation thromboelastometry detects thrombocytopenia and hypofibrinogenaemia during orthotopic liver transplantation. Br J Anaesth 2010;104:422–8.

41. Ogawa S, Szlam F, Chen EP, et al. A comparative evaluation of rotation thromboelastometry and standard coagulation tests in hemodilution induced coagulation changes after cardiac surgery. Transfusion 2012;52:14–22.

42. Amukele TK, Ferrell C, Chandler WL. Comparison of plasma with whole blood prothrombin time and fibrinogen on the same instrument. Am J Clin Pathol 2010;133:550–6.

43. Ogawa S, Szlam F, Bolliger D, et al. The impact of hematocrit on fibrin clot formation assessed by rotational thromboelastometry. Anesth Analg 2012;115:16–21.

44. Kashuk JL, Moore EE, Sawyer M, et al. Primary fibrinolysis is integral in the pathogenesis of the acute coagulopathy of trauma. Ann Surg 2010;252:434–42.

45. Theusinger OM, Wanner GA, Emmert MY, et al. Hyperfibrinolysis diagnosed by rotational thromboelastometry (ROTEM) is associated with higher mortality in patients with severe trauma. Anesth Analg 2011;113:1003–12.

46. Raza I, Davenport R, Rourke C, et al. The incidence and magnitude of fibrinolytic activation in trauma patients. J Thromb Haemost 2013;11(2):307–14.

47. Fries D, Haas T, Klingler A, et al. Efficacy of fibrinogen and prothrombin complex concentrate used to reverse dilutional coagulopathy – a porcine model. Br J Anaesth 2006;97:460–7.

48. Grottke O, Braunschweig T, Henzler D, et al. Effects of different fibrinogen concentrations on blood loss and coagulation parameters in a pig model of coagulopathy with blunt liver injury. Crit Care 2010;14(2):R62.

49. Weber CF, Gorlinger K, Meininger D, et al. Point-of-care testing: a prospective, randomized clinical trial of efficacy in coagulopathic cardiac surgery patients. Anesthesiology 2012;117:531–47.

50. Gorlinger K, Fries D, Dirkmann D, et al. Reduction of fresh frozen plasma requirements by perioperative point-of-care coagulation management with early calculated goal-directed therapy. Transfus Med Hemother 2012;39:104–13.

51. Rourke C, Curry N, Khan S, et al. Fibrinogen levels during trauma hemorrhage, response to replacement therapy, and association with patient outcomes. J Thromb Haemost 2012;10:1342–51.

52. Rahe-Meyer N, Solomon C, Hanke A, et al. Effects of fibrinogen concentrate as first-line therapy during major aortic replacement surgery: a randomized, placebo-controlled trial. Anesthesiology 2013;118:40–50.

53. Schoechl H, Nienaber U, Maegele M, et al. Transfusion in trauma: thromboelastometry-guided coagulation factor concentrate-based therapy versus standard fresh frozen plasma-based therapy. Crit Care 2011;15:R83.
54. Schoechl H, Forster L, Woidke R, et al. Use of rotation thromboelastometry (RO-TEM) to achieve successful treatment of polytrauma with fibrinogen concentrate and prothrombin complex concentrate. Anaesthesia 2010;65:199–203.
55. Fassl J, Matt P, Eckstein F, et al. Transfusion of allogeneic blood products in proximal aortic surgery with hyopthermic circulatory arrest: effects of thromboelastometry-guided transfusion management. J Cardiothorac Vasc Anesth 2013;27:1181–8.
56. Honickel M, Rieg A, Rossaint R, et al. Prothrombin complex concentrate re-duces blood loss and enhances thrombin generation in a pig model with blunt liver injury under severe hypothermia. Thromb Haemost 2011;106:724–33.
57. Grottke O, Braunschweig T, Spronk HM, et al. Increasing concentrations of pro-thrombin complex concentrate induce disseminated intravascular coagulation in a pig model of coagulopathy with blunt liver injury. Blood 2011;118:1943–51.
58. Afshari A, Wikkelsø A, Brok J, et al. Thrombelastography (TEG) or thromboelas-tometry (ROTEM) to monitor haemotherapy versus usual care in patients with massive transfusion. Cochrane Database Syst Rev 2011;(3):CD007871.
59. Wikkelsoe AJ, Afshari A, Wetterslev J, et al. Monitoring patients at risk of massive transfusion with thromboelastography or thromboelastometry: a sys-tematic review. Acta Anaesthesiol Scand 2011;55:1174–89.
60. Eller T, Busse J, Dittrich M, et al. Dabigatran, rivaroxaban, apixaban, argatroban and fondaparinux and their effects on coagulation POC and platelet function tests. Clin Chem Lab Med 2014;9:1–10.
61. Davis PK, Musunuru H, Walsh M, et al. The ex vivo reversibility of dabigatran-induced whole-blood coagulopathy as monitored by thromboelastography: mechanistic implications for clinical medicine. Thromb Haemost 2012;108:586–8.
62. Xu Y, Wu W, Wang L, et al. Differential profiles of thrombin inhibitors (heparin, hirudin, bivalirudin, and dabigatran) in the thrombin generation assay and thromboelastography in vitro. Blood Coagul Fibrinolysis 2013;24:332–8.
63. Mosnier LO, Buijtenhuijs P, Marx PF, et al. Identification of thrombin activatable fibrinolysis inhibitor (TAFI) in human platelets. Blood 2003;101:4844–6.
64. Engström M, Rundgren M, Schött U. An evaluation of monitoring possibilities of argatroban using rotational thromboelastometry and activated partial thrombo-plastin time. Acta Anaesthesiol Scand 2010;54:86–9.
65. Grottke O, van Ryn J, Spronk H, et al. Prothrombin complex concentrates and a specific antidote (aDabi-Fab) are effective ex-vivo in reversing the effects of da-bigatran in an anticoagulation/liver trauma experimental model. Crit Care 2014;18(1):R27.
66. Spronk HM, van der Voort D, ten Cate H. Blood coagulation and the risk of athe-rothrombosis: a complex relationship. Thromb J 2004;2:12.
67. Loeffen R, Spronk HM, ten Cate H. The impact of blood coagulability on athero-sclerosis and cardiovascular disease. J Thromb Haemost 2012;10:1207–16.
68. Hemker HC, Dieri al R, de Smedt E, et al. Thrombin generation, a function test of the haemostatic-thrombotic system. Thromb Haemost 2006;96:553–61.
69. Béguin S, Lindhout T, Hemker HC. The mode of action of heparin in plasma. Thromb Haemost 1988;60:457–62.
70. Hemker HC. Recollections on thrombin generation. J Thromb Haemost 2008;6:219–26.

71. Hemker HC, Giesen P, AlDieri R, et al. The calibrated automated thrombogram (CAT): a universal routine test for hyper- and hypocoagulability. Pathophysiol Haemost Thromb 2002;32:249–53.

72. Hemker HC, Béguin S. Thrombin generation in plasma: its assessment via the endogenous thrombin potential. Thromb Haemost 1995;74:134–8.

73. Loeffen R, Kleinegris MC, Loubele ST, et al. Preanalytic variables of thrombin generation: towards a standard procedure and validation of the method. J Thromb Haemost 2012;10:2544–54.

74. Spronk HM, Dielis AW, de Smedt E, et al. Assessment of thrombin generation II: validation of the calibrated automated thrombogram in platelet-poor plasma in a clinical laboratory. Thromb Haemost 2008;100:362–4.

75. Castoldi E, Castoldi E, Rosing J, et al. Thrombin generation tests. Thromb Res 2011;127:S21–5.

76. Lutsey PL, Folsom AR, Heckbert SR, et al. Peak thrombin generation and subsequent venous thromboembolism: the Longitudinal Investigation of Thromboembolism Etiology (LITE) study. J Thromb Haemost 2009;7: 1639–48.

77. Tripodi A, Martinelli I, Chantarangkul V, et al. The endogenous thrombin potential and the risk of venous thromboembolism. Thromb Res 2007;121:353–9.

78. Hron G, Kollars M, Binder BR, et al. Identification of patients at low risk for recurrent venous thromboembolism by measuring thrombin generation. JAMA 2006; 296:397–402.

79. Tripodi A, Legnani C, Chantarangkul V, et al. High thrombin generation measured in the presence of thrombomodulin is associated with an increased risk of recurrent venous thromboembolism. J Thromb Haemost 2008;6:1327–33.

80. Besser M, Baglin C, Luddington R, et al. High rate of unprovoked recurrent venous thrombosis is associated with high thrombin-generating potential in a prospective cohort study. J Thromb Haemost 2008;6:1720–5.

81. van Hylckama Vlieg A, Christiansen SC, Luddington R, et al. Elevated endogenous thrombin potential is associated with an increased risk of a first deep venous thrombosis but not with the risk of recurrence. Br J Haematol 2007; 138:769–74.

82. Cate-Hoek ten AJ, Dielis AW, Spronk HM, et al. Thrombin generation in patients after acute deep-vein thrombosis. Thromb Haemost 2008;100:240–5.

83. ten Cate H. Thrombin generation in clinical conditions. Thromb Res 2012;129: 367–70.

84. Páramo JA, Orbe J, Beloqui O, et al. Prothrombin fragment 1+2 is associated with carotid intima-media thickness in subjects free of clinical cardiovascular disease. Stroke 2004;35:1085–9.

85. With Notø AT, Mathiesen EB, Østerud B, et al. Increased thrombin generation in persons with echogenic carotid plaques. Thromb Haemost 2008;99:602–8.

86. Borissoff JI, Joosen IA, Versteylen MO, et al. Accelerated in vivo thrombin formation independently predicts the presence and severity of CT angiographic coronary atherosclerosis. JACC Cardiovasc Imaging 2012;5:1201–10.

87. Smid M, Dielis AW, Winkens M, et al. Thrombin generation in patients with a first acute myocardial infarction. J Thromb Haemost 2011;9:450–6.

88. Smid M, Dielis AW, Spronk HM, et al. Thrombin generation in the Glasgow Myocardial Infarction Study. PLoS One 2013;8:e66977.

89. Orbe J, Zudaire M, Serrano R, et al. Increased thrombin generation after acute versus chronic coronary disease as assessed by the thrombin generation test. Thromb Haemost 2008;99:382–7.

90. Winckers K, Siegerink B, Duckers C, et al. Increased tissue factor pathway inhibitor activity is associated with myocardial infarction in young women: results from the RATIO study. J Thromb Haemost 2011;9:2243–50.
91. Nair SC, Dargaud Y, Chitlur M, et al. Tests of global haemostasis and their applications in bleeding disorders. Haemophilia 2010;16(Suppl 5):85–92.
92. Dargaud Y, Lienhart A, Negrier C. Prospective assessment of thrombin generation test for dose monitoring of bypassing therapy in hemophilia patients with inhibitors undergoing elective surgery. Blood 2010;116:5734–7.
93. Wong PC, White A, Luettgen J. Inhibitory effect of apixaban compared with rivaroxaban and dabigatran on thrombin generation assay. Hosp Pract (1995) 2013; 41:19–25.
94. Samama MM, Martinoli JL, LeFlem L, et al. Assessment of laboratory assays to measure rivaroxaban – an oral, direct factor Xa inhibitor. Thromb Haemost 2010; 103:815–25.
95. Gerotziafas GT, Elalamy I, Depasse F, et al. In vitro inhibition of thrombin generation, after tissue factor pathway activation, by the oral, direct factor Xa inhibitor rivaroxaban. J Thromb Haemost 2007;5:886–8.
96. Novak M, Schlagenhauf A, Bernhard H, et al. Effect of rivaroxaban, in contrast to heparin, is similar in neonatal and adult plasma. Blood Coagul Fibrinolysis 2011; 22:588–92.
97. Wienen W, Stassen JM, Priepke H, et al. In-vitro profile and ex-vivo anticoagulant activity of the direct thrombin inhibitor dabigatran and its orally active prodrug, dabigatran etexilate. Thromb Haemost 2007;98:155–62.
98. Serebruany V, Sani Y, Lynch D, et al. Effects of dabigatran in vitro on thrombin biomarkers by calibrated automated thrombography in patients after ischemic stroke. J Thromb Thrombolysis 2012;33:22–7.
99. Furugohri T, Sugiyama N, Morishima Y, et al. Antithrombin-independent thrombin inhibitors, but not direct factor Xa inhibitors, enhance thrombin generation in plasma through inhibition of thrombin-thrombomodulin-protein C system. Thromb Haemost 2011;106:1076–83.
100. Wagenvoord RJ, Deinum J, Elg M, et al. The paradoxical stimulation by a reversible thrombin inhibitor of thrombin generation in plasma measured with thrombinography is caused by alpha-macroglobulin-thrombin. J Thromb Haemost 2010;8:1281–9.
101. Furugohri T, Shiozaki Y, Muramatsu S, et al. Different antithrombotic properties of factor Xa inhibitor and thrombin inhibitor in rat thrombosis models. Eur J Pharmacol 2005;514:35–42.
102. Mattsson C, Menschik-Lundin A, Nylander S, et al. Effect of different types of thrombin inhibitors on thrombin/thrombomodulin modulated activation of protein C in vitro. Thromb Res 2001;104:475–86.

Pharmacology and Laboratory Testing of the Oral Xa Inhibitors

Meyer Michel Samama, MD, PharmD[a,b], Sadia Meddahi, PharmD[a,b],
Charles Marc Samama, MD, PhD[c],*

KEYWORDS

- Rivaroxaban • Apixaban • Edoxaban • Betrixaban • Bleeding • Monitoring

KEY POINTS

- Among the new oral anticoagulants, the use of factor Xa inhibitors is increasing.
- Rivaroxaban, apixaban, and edoxaban have already been licensed in some countries. The clinical development of betrixaban is less advanced.
- Although the mechanism of action of these agents is similar, their pharmacodynamic and pharmacokinetic characteristics vary.
- These inhibitors have been investigated for prophylaxis of venous thromboembolism in major orthopedic surgery, treatment of initial and recurrent deep vein thrombosis and pulmonary embolism, prevention of thrombotic events in nonvalvular atrial fibrillation, and prevention of cardiac events in patients with acute coronary syndrome, with varying results.
- No routine coagulation monitoring is required, but evidence is accumulating in support of using certain reliable, readily available tests in specific clinical circumstances.

INTRODUCTION

During previous decades, anticoagulants for the prevention and treatment of venous thromboembolism (VTE) or arterial occlusive events were limited to parenteral

Disclosure: M.M. Samama has received research grants, consulting fees as a member of advisory boards, and speaker and/or investigator fees from Bayer, Boehringer Ingelheim, Bristol-Myers Squibb (BMS), Daiichi Sankyo, GlaxoSmithKline (GSK), Pfizer, Rovi, and Sanofi. S. Meddahi discloses no conflict of interest. C.M. Samama has received research grants, consulting fees as a member of advisory boards, and speaker and/or investigator fees from Abbott, AstraZeneca, Baxter, Bayer, Boehringer Ingelheim, Bristol-Myers Squibb (BMS), CSL Behring, Daiichi Sankyo, Fresenius-Kabi, GlaxoSmithKline (GSK), Haemonetics, Laboratoire Français du Fractionnement et des Biotechnologies (LFB), Lilly, Novo Nordisk, Pfizer, Rovi, and Sanofi.
[a] Department of Biological Hematology, Cochin Hôtel-Dieu University Hospitals, 27 rue du Faubourg St-Jacques, Paris 75014, France; [b] BIOMNIS Laboratories, 78 Avenue de Verdun, Ivry-sur-Seine 94200, France; [c] Department of Anesthesia and Intensive Care Medicine, Cochin Hôtel-Dieu University Hospitals, 27 rue du Faubourg St-Jacques, Paris 75014, France
* Corresponding author.
E-mail address: marc.samama@cch.aphp.fr

Clin Lab Med 34 (2014) 503–517
http://dx.doi.org/10.1016/j.cll.2014.06.009
0272-2712/14/$ – see front matter © 2014 Elsevier Inc. All rights reserved.

administration of heparins, fondaparinux, and oral administration of vitamin K antagonists (VKAs). The discovery of heparin by Jay McLean in 1916 aided the development of cardiac surgery and the treatment and prevention of venous and arterial thrombosis.[1] Warfarin was subsequently discovered by Karl Paul Link in 1933 and has been used for 60 years.[2] However, several factor Xa inhibitors are now available or under development, giving clinicians further options for anticoagulation. Factor Xa inhibitors were first used for the prevention of VTE in orthopedic surgery; however, they have recently been approved for new indications including prevention of stroke in patients with atrial fibrillation and treatment of VTE. The 3 direct factor Xa inhibitors that are currently licensed are rivaroxaban (Bay 59–7939), apixaban (BMS 52247-01), and edoxaban (DU-176b). Other direct factor Xa inhibitors at varying stages of development include betrixaban (PRT054021), LY517717, erixaban (PD0348292), and FXV 573.[3] This article discusses the pharmacologic and pharmacokinetic properties of some of these new oral anticoagulants, namely rivaroxaban, apixaban, edoxaban, and betrixaban, to summarize results from respective clinical studies that showed their effectiveness and safety profiles, and to discusses the role of coagulation tests in emergency or critical situations in which the anticoagulation effect needs to be monitored.

Rivaroxaban

Pharmacologic characteristics
Rivaroxaban (Xarelto) is a direct competitive and reversible inhibitor of factor Xa that inhibits the intrinsic and extrinsic coagulation pathways (**Fig. 1**), and prolongs prothrombin time (PT) and activated partial thromboplastin time (aPTT). Rivaroxaban is available as 10-mg, 15-mg, and 20-mg tablets. It has a molecular weight of 439.9 Da and a bioavailability of approximately 80%, which decreases for the higher doses. Its binding to plasma albumin is high (more than 80%) and precludes its removal by dialysis.[4] Peak plasma concentration is reached after about 2 hours,

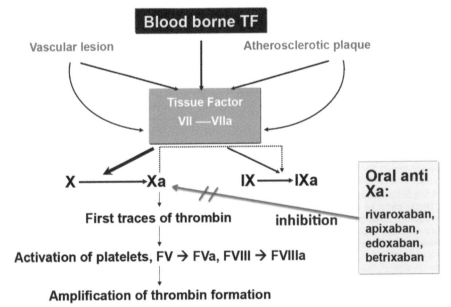

Fig. 1. Mechanism of action of the new oral factor Xa inhibitors. TF, tissue factor.

and the half-life is 9 to 13 hours (**Table 1**). Rivaroxaban is excreted primarily by the kidney ($\sim$65%) (see **Table 1**).[3,4] Its metabolism also depends on the cytochrome P34A (CYP34A) system and it is a substrate of P-glycoprotein (P-gp). Therefore, the anticoagulant activity of rivaroxaban can be affected by ketonazole, amiodarone, and rifampicin, as well as protease inhibitors used for treatment of human immunodeficiency virus (HIV). In addition, certain medicines such as St John's Wort (prescribed in depression), phenytoin, carbamazepine, and phenobarbital reduce the plasma concentration of rivaroxaban and should be used with caution. Aspirin does not alter the activity of rivaroxaban, as shown in a study in healthy volunteers,[5] and in a study of major orthopedic surgery the addition of aspirin did not result in increased bleeding.[6] However, an increase in bleeding events associated with comedication with aspirin has been observed in another study.[7] In addition, hepatic dysfunction alters the pharmacodynamic and pharmacokinetic characteristics of rivaroxaban.[8]

Clinical studies

Total hip and knee replacement in adults Rivaroxaban is effective in the prophylaxis of thromboembolic events in patients undergoing major orthopedic surgery such as total hip and knee replacement, as reported in the RECORD (Regulation of Coagulation in Orthopedic Surgery to Prevent Deep Venous Thrombosis and Pulmonary Embolism) 1, 2, 3, and 4 studies.[9–12] In these phase 3 studies, patients received rivaroxaban 10 mg once daily, or enoxaparin 40 mg once daily or 30 mg twice daily, in the European protocol and North American protocols, respectively. The first dose of rivaroxaban was administered 8 hours after surgery. Enoxaparin was started 12 hours before surgery in the 40-mg group and after surgery in the 30-mg twice-daily group. These 4 studies

Table 1
Comparison of the new oral direct factor Xa inhibitors

	Rivaroxaban	Apixaban	Edoxaban	Betrixaban
Target	Factor Xa	Factor Xa	Factor Xa	Factor Xa
Brand name	Xarelto	Eliquis	Lixiana	NA
Route of administration	Oral	Oral	Oral	Oral
Frequency of administration	Once daily	Twice daily	Once daily	Once daily
Bioavailability (%)	80	51–85	50	35
T_{max} (h)	2–4	3	0.5–2	3–4
Half-life (h)	9–13	10–14	8–10	36
Renal excretion (%)	60–66 (half inactive)	25	35	10
Interferences with P-gp and cytochromes	P-gp + Cyt3A4 + Cyt2J2	P-gp + Cyt3A4	P-gp + Cyt3A4	P-gp + Cyt450
Specific antidote	No	No	No	No

Abbreviations: Cyt, cytochrome; NA, not applicable; P-gp, P-glycoprotein; T_{max}, Time to maximal plasma concentration.

Data from Weitz JI, Eikelboom JW, Samama MM, American College of Chest Physicians. New antithrombotic drugs: antithrombotic therapy and prevention of thrombosis, 9th ed: American College of Chest Physicians evidence-based clinical practice guidelines. Chest 2012;141 Suppl 2:e120S–51S; and Connolly SJ, Eikelboom J, Dorian P, et al. Betrixaban compared with warfarin in patients with atrial fibrillation: results of a phase 2 randomized dose-ranging study (EXPLORE-Xa). Eur Heart J 2013;34:1498–505.

included more than 13,000 patients and showed that rivaroxaban was more effective than enoxaparin. However, a slight increase in bleeding was also observed in the rivaroxaban group, although major bleeding events were rare.[9–12]

Nonvalvular atrial fibrillation In the ROCKET-AF (Rivaroxaban Once Daily Oral Direct Factor Xa Inhibition Compared with Vitamin K Antagonism for Prevention of Stroke and Embolism Trial in Atrial Fibrillation) study, 14,264 patients with nonvalvular atrial fibrillation (AF) were randomized to rivaroxaban 20 mg once daily or warfarin (target International Normalized Ratio [INR], 2.5 [2.0–3.0]). Rivaroxaban was as effective as warfarin and was not associated with any increase in bleeding events. The intracranial hemorrhage (ICH) rate was significantly decreased with rivaroxaban compared with warfarin (**Table 2**). In contrast, mucosal bleeding, particularly gastrointestinal, was more common with rivaroxaban than with warfarin.[13,14] Overall, rivaroxaban showed efficacy in a population at high risk of thrombosis.

Acute VTE For the treatment of proximal deep vein thrombosis (DVT) and the prevention of recurrence after treatment cessation, rivaroxaban was compared with warfarin in the EINSTEIN-DVT study,[15] and with placebo in the EINSTEIN-Extension study.[16] The efficacy and safety of rivaroxaban and warfarin in the acute phase of venous thrombosis were comparable, but rivaroxaban was more effective than placebo for the prevention of DVT recurrence.[16]

The EINSTEIN-PE study showed a comparable efficacy of rivaroxaban and warfarin in patients treated for pulmonary embolism (PE), with a reduction in major bleeding observed in the rivaroxaban group (**Table 3**).[17] The doses of rivaroxaban were 15 mg twice daily for 3 weeks and 20 mg once daily during the remainder of treatment, as in the EINSTEIN-DVT study (see **Table 3**). In the EINSTEIN-Extension study, the dose was 20 mg once a day. These three studies included 3449, 1197, and 4832 patients, respectively.

Patients at risk of VTE hospitalized with severe acute illness Rivaroxaban has also been studied in patients hospitalized for acute medical issues and/or infection with increased risk factors for VTE (MAGELLAN [Multicenter, Randomized, Parallel Group

Table 2
Use of rivaroxaban, apixaban, and edoxaban in patients with AF: study results

Trials (Factor Xa Inhibitor)	ROCKET-AF (Rivaroxaban)[13,14]	ARISTOTLE (Apixaban)[25]	ENGAGE-AF (Edoxaban)[32]
N	14,264	18,201	21,105
Design	Double blind	Double blind	Double blind
Dose (mg)	20 qd	5 bid	60 qd/30 qd
Control	Warfarin	Warfarin	Warfarin
Efficacy (%)	1.70 (R) vs 2.20 (W), noninferiority	1.27 (A) vs 1.60 (W), superiority	1.18 (E60) vs 1.50 (W) vs 1.61 (E30), noninferiority
Intracranial bleeding (%)	0.50 (R) vs 0.70 (W)	0.24 (A) vs 0.47 (W), (hemorrhagic stroke)	0.26 (E30) vs 0.39 (E60) vs 0.85 (W)
Major bleeding (%)	3.40 (W) vs 3.60 (R)	2.13 (A) vs 3.09 (W)	1.62 (E30) vs 2.75 (E60) vs 3.43 (W)

Abbreviations: A, apixaban; bid, twice daily; E, edoxaban; qd, once daily; R, rivaroxaban; W, warfarin.

Table 3
Use of rivaroxaban, apixaban, and edoxaban in patients with acute VTE: study results

Trials	EINSTEIN-DVT (Rivaroxaban)[15]	EINSTEIN-PE (Rivaroxaban)[17]	AMPLIFY (Apixaban)[26]	HOKUSAI-VTE (Edoxaban)[33]
N	3449	4832	5395	8240
Treatment	Rivaroxaban 15 mg bid for 21 d, then 20 mg qd	Rivaroxaban 15 mg bid for 21 d, then 20 mg qd	Apixaban 10 mg bid for 7 d, then 5 mg bid	Enoxaparin or UFH for ≥5 d then edoxaban 60 mg qd or 30 mg qd if CrCl 30–50 mL/min, or body weight <60 kg, or inhib P-gp
Control	Enoxaparin then warfarin	Enoxaparin then warfarin	Enoxaparin then warfarin	Enoxaparin or UFH for ≥5 d then warfarin
Primary efficacy end point	Symptomatic, recurrent VTE, defined as the composite of DVT or nonfatal or fatal PE	Symptomatic recurrent VTE, defined as the composite of fatal or nonfatal PE or DVT	Incidence of the adjudicated composite of recurrent symptomatic VTE or death related to VTE	Incidence of adjudicated symptomatic recurrent VTE, defined as a composite of DVT or nonfatal or fatal PE
Efficacy (%)	2.1 (R) vs 3 (W), noninferiority	2.1 (R) vs 1.8 (W), noninferiority	2.3 (A) vs 2.7 (W), noninferiority	3.2 (E) vs 3.5 (W), noninferiority
Clinically relevant bleeding (%)	8.1 (R) vs 8.1 (W)	10.3 (R) vs 11.4 (W)	4.3 (A) vs 9.7 (W)	8.5 (E) vs 10.3 (W), superiority
Major bleeding (%)	0.8 (R) vs 1.2 (W)	1.1 (R) vs 2.2 (W)	0.6 (A) vs 1.8 (W), superiority	1.4 (E) vs 1.6 (W), superiority

Abbreviations: CrCl, creatinine clearance; inhib, inhibitors; UFH, unfractionated heparin.

Efficacy and Safety Study for the Prevention of Venous Thromboembolism in Hospitalized Acutely Ill Medical Patients Comparing Rivaroxaban with Enoxaparin] study).[18] In these patients, a 10-mg dose of rivaroxaban once daily for 35 days was compared with a once-daily preventive dose of enoxaparin (40 mg) for only 10 days. The efficacy of rivaroxaban was noninferior to that of enoxaparin, but the frequency of bleeding was significantly higher in the rivaroxaban group (4.1% vs 1.7%; $P<.0001$).

Acute coronary syndrome The ATLAS-TIMI 51 (Anti-Xa Therapy to Lower Cardiovascular Events in Addition to Standard Therapy in Subjects with Acute Coronary Syndrome–Thrombolysis in Myocardial Infarction 51 [ATLAS ACS 2–TIMI 51]) trial was a randomized, double-blind study in patients with acute coronary syndrome (ACS). Patients received antiplatelet therapy chosen by their cardiologist in addition to rivaroxaban, either 2.5 or 5 mg twice daily, or placebo.[19] The efficacy end point was incidence of cardiovascular death, myocardial infarction (MI), or ischemic stroke. Compared with placebo, patients receiving either dose of rivaroxaban had a reduced frequency of these events. Moreover, the lower dose of rivaroxaban (2.5 mg twice daily) was also associated with a reduction in cardiovascular mortality and all-cause mortality. Treatment with the twice-daily 2.5-mg dose resulted in fewer fatal bleeding events than the twice-daily 5-mg dose (0.1% vs 0.4%; $P = .04$).

To date, rivaroxaban is approved for use in the different indications in the studies described earlier, such as prophylaxis of VTE in major orthopedic surgery; treatment of DVT and PE, and recurrent DVT or PE; prevention of thrombotic events in non-valvular AF; and prevention of cardiac events in patients with ACS. However, the preventive indication in connection with the MAGELLAN study has not yet been approved by the US and European health authorities.

Apixaban

Pharmacologic characteristics
Apixaban (Eliquis) is another direct and reversible oral factor Xa inhibitor. It is available as 2.5-mg and 5-mg tablets, which are administered twice daily. Approximately 58% is absorbed and peak plasma concentrations occur in 3 to 4 hours.[3,4] In addition, the affinity for free factor Xa is similar for apixaban and rivaroxaban, which have binding affinities (K_i) of 0.08 nM and 0.04 nM, respectively. The half-life of apixaban is 10 to 14 hours (see **Table 1**), and it is eliminated via both renal (25%) and intestinal (55%) routes. Its metabolism depends on the CYP34A system and it is a substrate of P-gp.[20] Therefore, coadministration of apixaban with P-gp inhibitors or inhibitors of this cytochrome, such as antifungals, antibiotics such as rifampicin, and some other inhibitors used in the treatment of HIV, should be avoided.

Populations and special situations
Apixaban dosage does not need to be adjusted for age, weight, or gender. Given the lack of clinical experience in patients with renal failure who have a creatinine clearance less than or equal to 15 mL/min, or in those undergoing dialysis, apixaban is not recommended in these patient populations owing to an increased risk of bleeding. It is also contraindicated in patients with hepatic disease associated with coagulopathy and clinically relevant bleeding risk.

Clinical studies
Total hip and knee replacement in adults Apixaban is approved for the prevention of VTE after total hip replacement (THR) or total knee replacement (TKR) in adults. The phase 3 North American controlled clinical trial ADVANCE 1 (The Apixaban Dosed Orally Versus Anticoagulation with Injectable Enoxaparin to Prevent Venous Thromboembolism) compared the efficacy and safety of thromboprophylaxis with apixaban 2.5 mg given orally twice a day with enoxaparin 30 mg administered subcutaneously (SC) twice a day after TKR. In this study, the prespecified clinical end point of noninferiority was not met, even though results in both groups were similar. However, the incidence of major and clinically relevant nonmajor bleeding events was significantly lower in the apixaban group.[21]

The licensing of apixaban in Europe is primarily based on the results of 2 double-blind clinical studies, ADVANCE 2 and 3. ADVANCE 2 enrolled 3195 patients undergoing TKR,[22] and ADVANCE 3 included 3866 patients undergoing THR.[23] These studies showed the noninferiority of apixaban 2.5 mg twice daily to enoxaparin 40 mg SC once daily, with a similar frequency of adverse events.[22,23] The recommended dose of apixaban is 2.5 mg orally twice daily, with the initial dose administered 12 to 24 hours after orthopedic surgery; physicians should determine the appropriate timing of the first dose within this window according to potential benefits of VTE prophylaxis and the individual risk of postsurgical bleeding from anticoagulant therapy.

Nonvalvular AF
AVERROES The AVERROES (Apixaban Versus Acetylsalicylic Acid [ASA] to Prevent Stroke in Atrial Fibrillation Patients Who Have Failed or Are Unsuitable for Vitamin K

Antagonist Treatment) study compared apixaban at a dose of 5 mg twice daily with aspirin 81 to 324 mg once daily in 5599 patients with AF for the prevention of stroke and systemic embolism.[24] Apixaban was shown to be superior to aspirin and therefore the trial was ended prematurely. The results show that for every 1000 patients treated with apixaban instead of aspirin for 1 year, 18 strokes could be prevented in addition to 10 deaths, 31 hospitalizations, and 2 major bleeding events.[24] There was no difference in major bleeding or clinically relevant bleeding events, but, more importantly, no major or fatal ICH was observed in the apixaban arm, even though other bleeding events were more common with apixaban than with aspirin.[24]

ARISTOTLE The ARISTOTLE (Apixaban for Reduction in Stroke and Other Thromboembolic Events in Atrial Fibrillation) study compared apixaban 5 mg twice daily with warfarin (target INR of 2.5) for a minimum of 12 months for the prevention of stroke and systemic embolism in 18,201 patients with nonvalvular AF and at least 1 additional risk factor for stroke.[25] A subset of patients with 2 of the following 3 criteria received apixaban 2.5 mg twice daily: age more than 80 years, body weight less than 60 kg, creatinine greater than 15 mg/L. The risk of stroke (CHADS$_2$ [congestive heart failure; hypertension; age; diabetes; prior stroke, transient ischemic attack] score) of the patients included in the ARISTOTLE study was similar to that of the RE-LY (Randomized Evaluation of Long-Term Anticoagulation Therapy) trial, but weaker than in the ROCKET-AF study. The duration of treatment was between 12 and 39 months with an average duration of 1.8 years.[25] Systemic embolism or stroke occurred significantly less frequently with apixaban than with warfarin (1.27% vs 1.60%, respectively; P<.01) (see **Table 2**). All-cause mortality was also lower for apixaban (P = .04). However, the incidence of MI was not significantly lower in the apixaban group, but the frequency of bleeding events was significantly lower with apixaban than with warfarin, especially for ICH (0.24% vs 0.47%). Thus, apixaban was superior to warfarin in patients with nonvalvular AF and at least 1 additional risk factor.[25]

Acute VTE AMPLIFY (Apixaban for the Initial Management of Pulmonary Embolism and Deep-Vein Thrombosis as First-Line Therapy) was a randomized, double-blind study that compared apixaban (10 mg twice daily for 7 days, followed by 5 mg twice daily for 6 months) with conventional therapy (SC enoxaparin, followed by warfarin) in 5395 patients with VTE.[26] The primary efficacy outcome (recurrent symptomatic VTE or death related to VTE) occurred in 59 of 2609 patients (2.3%) in the apixaban group compared with 71 of 2635 (2.7%) in the conventional-therapy group (relative risk [RR], 0.84). Major bleeding occurred in 0.6% of patients receiving apixaban and in 1.8% of those receiving conventional therapy (RR, 0.31; P<.001 for superiority). The composite outcome of major bleeding and clinically relevant nonmajor bleeding occurred in 4.3% of patients in the apixaban group, compared with 9.7% of those in the conventional-therapy group (RR, 0.44; P<.001) (see **Table 3**).[26]

This study was followed by AMPLIFY-Extension, in which, after discontinuation of the initial treatment, patients were randomized to apixaban or placebo. The frequency of relapses was reduced without a significant increase in bleeding events in the apixaban group.[27] The frequency of PE, cardiovascular mortality, and all-cause mortality was statistically similar in both groups, with an RR of 1.00 (P = .064).

Patients hospitalized for severe acute illness with a risk factor for VTE In a randomized pilot study of 125 patients with metastatic cancer requiring chemotherapy, in which patients received apixaban 5, 10, or 20 mg daily or placebo for 12 weeks, no thromboembolic events occurred in the apixaban groups. In addition, apixaban was well tolerated.[28]

In another study (ADOPT [Apixaban Dosing to Optimize Protection from Thrombosis]), apixaban was given at a dose of 2.5 mg twice daily for 30 days and was compared with an enoxaparin regimen of 40 mg daily for 6 to 14 days in hospitalized patients with a risk factor for thrombosis. Apixaban was as effective as enoxaparin in preventing VTE; however, an increase in bleeding episodes was observed in the apixaban group.[29]

ACS Compared with the positive results observed with rivaroxaban in patients with ACS,[19] the results of the APRAISE-2 (Apixaban for Prevention of Acute Ischemic and Safety Event) study, in which patients received apixaban 5 mg twice daily in combination with an antiplatelet regimen or a standard dual antiplatelet regimen, were not so encouraging: apixaban plus antiplatelet therapy was associated with an increase in major bleeding events and fatal intracranial bleedings, without any significant reduction in recurrences of coronary incidents.[30]

At present, apixaban is approved for use in prophylaxis of VTE in major orthopedic surgery and for the prevention of thrombotic events in nonvalvular AF.

Edoxaban

Pharmacologic characteristics
Edoxaban (DU-176b, Lixiana) is a direct factor Xa inhibitor, approved in Japan for the prevention of VTE following lower-limb orthopedic surgery. Edoxaban is an oral agent with a K_i of 0.56 nM for factor Xa. The maximal concentration occurs within 30 to 120 minutes after oral administration, and the half-life (8 to 10 hours) is similar to that of rivaroxaban (see **Table 1**), but the protein binding is lower than that of rivaroxaban. Edoxaban's bioavailability is ~50% and it undergoes both renal (35%) and fecal (65%) elimination.[3,31] Its metabolism also depends on the CYP34A system and it is a substrate of P-gp.

Clinical studies
Nonvalvular AF ENGAGE-AF (Effective Anticoagulation with Factor Xa Next Generation in Atrial Fibrillation–Thrombolysis in Myocardial Infarction 48 [ENGAGE AF-TIMI 48]) was a randomized trial comparing 2 once-daily regimens of edoxaban (60 mg and 30 mg) with warfarin in 21,105 patients with a moderate-risk to high-risk AF (median follow-up, 2.8 years).[32] The annualized rate of the primary efficacy end point (stroke or systemic embolism) was 1.50% with warfarin (median time in the therapeutic range, 68.4%), compared with 1.18% with high-dose edoxaban ($P<.001$ for noninferiority) and 1.61% with low-dose edoxaban ($P = .005$ for noninferiority) (see **Table 2**). In the intention-to-treat analysis, there was a trend favoring high-dose edoxaban versus warfarin and an unfavorable trend with low-dose edoxaban versus warfarin. The annualized rate of major bleeding was 3.43% with warfarin versus 2.75% with high-dose edoxaban ($P<.001$) and 1.62% with low-dose edoxaban ($P<.001$) (see **Table 2**). The corresponding annualized rates of death from cardiovascular causes were 3.17% versus 2.74% ($P = .01$), and 2.71% ($P = .008$).[32]

Acute VTE The HOKUSAI-VTE study was a randomized, noninferiority study that enrolled 8240 patients with an acute VTE who had initially received heparin to receive either edoxaban 60 mg once daily (30 mg once daily for the subset of patients with creatinine clearance of 30 to 50 mL/min or a body weight <60 kg) or warfarin for 3 to 12 months.[33] A total of 4921 patients presented with DVT, and 3319 with PE. Edoxaban was noninferior to warfarin with respect to the primary efficacy outcome (recurrent symptomatic VTE), which occurred in 130 patients in the edoxaban group (3.2%) and 146 patients in the warfarin group (3.5%) ($P<.001$ for noninferiority). The safety outcome (major or clinically relevant nonmajor bleeding) occurred in 349 patients (8.5%) in the edoxaban group and 423 patients (10.3%) in the warfarin group (*P* = .004 for superiority) (see **Table 3**).

Betrixaban

Pharmacologic characteristics

Betrixaban (PRT 054021), is a factor Xa inhibitor from the anthranilamides class. It inhibits factor Xa both in free form and in the presence of prothrombinase. Interindividual variability is moderate.[34] After oral administration, the maximum concentration is reached within 3 to 4 hours and the terminal half-life is ~36 hours (see **Table 1**). The K$_i$ is 0.12 nM, its metabolism depends on the cytochrome P450 system, and it is a substrate of P-gp. Betrixaban has a lower bioavailability than the other factor Xa inhibitors discussed in this article, at approximately 35%, and elimination is primarily via the biliary route, with renal elimination of less than 10% (see **Table 1**).

Clinical studies

Major orthopedic surgery The phase 2 EXPERT randomized study, including 215 patients undergoing knee surgery, compared betrixaban at a dose of 15 or 40 mg twice daily with enoxaparin 30 mg every 12 hours for 10 to 14 days. Efficacy was assessed on the unilateral venography (operated limb) and the frequency of symptomatic forms of DVT or PE observed during the treatment period.[35] The frequency of thrombotic events was 20%, 15.4%, and 10% for the groups receiving betrixaban 15 mg twice daily, betrixaban 40 mg twice daily, and enoxaparin, respectively. A single episode of PE was diagnosed in each of the two betrixaban groups.

Nonvalvular AF EXPLORE-Xa was a phase 2 safety study evaluating escalating doses of betrixaban (40, 60, or 80 mg once daily) in 508 patients with nonvalvular AF.[36] The duration of treatment was 12 to 50 weeks. The frequency of ischemic stroke with betrixaban was the same as that of the control group receiving warfarin.[36] The dose of 40 mg was associated with a lower frequency of bleeding events than in the warfarin group, whereas doses of 60 mg and 80 mg were associated with a higher frequency of bleeding events than both the betrixaban 40 mg and warfarin groups. Overall, results of this phase 2 study showed a reduced incidence of ischemic and bleeding events with the 40-mg dose of betrixaban compared with warfarin.[36]

Phase 3 studies are ongoing. At present, the biliary elimination of betrixaban is almost exclusive to this class of oral direct Xa inhibitors, and could be of importance in patients with renal insufficiency.

Coagulation monitoring and new anticoagulants

In general, there is no need to regularly monitor the impact of new anticoagulants on coagulation. However, there are specific clinical circumstances in which the study of coagulation may be useful, in particular:

- Need for emergency invasive procedures or surgery
- Occurrence of thrombosis or severe hemorrhage
- Occurrence of a stroke, especially if a thrombolytic treatment is proposed
- Suspicion of poor adherence to treatment
- Doubt about a possible influence of comedication
- Control of the biological activity of a prohemostatic treatment

In circumstances in which monitoring is required, blood should be drawn, when possible, either before taking the next dose (lowest anticoagulant concentration), or 2 to 4 hours after having taken a new dose (highest concentration).

In these cases, which test(s) can be used?

However, all coagulation tests may be biased and inaccurate in the presence of these newer oral anticoagulant agents.[37–41] For instance, false-positives for lupus anticoagulant can be caused by the interference with the factor Xa inhibitor. A laboratory technique in which the factor Xa inhibitor does not interfere with testing should be considered. For instance, measuring antithrombin using methods that use thrombin as a target is not appropriate for patients treated with dabigatran, whereas a method targeting factor Xa is appropriate in these patients. In contrast, for a factor Xa inhibitor–treated patient, methods that use thrombin as a target are more appropriate. In addition, INR cannot be used, because it was developed only for VKAs, which have a different mechanism of action from that of the newer anticoagulants. However, a modified INR for rivaroxaban has been determined by Tripodi and colleagues.[42] No further studies investigating this method have been conducted.

PT and aPTT are not specific tests, and results may vary depending on the reagent used.[37,40,43] The PT is generally increased in response to factor Xa inhibitor treatment, but its sensitivity is much higher for rivaroxaban than for apixaban.[41] The aPTT is also less sensitive to the action of apixaban than that of rivaroxaban.[37,39,41] However, these tests can provide information on the possible drug accumulation. For instance, the PT expressed in patient/control ratio or percentage may be informative in patients receiving rivaroxaban when the ratio for the patient is at least twice that of the control, especially on blood taken just before the next dose (lowest drug concentration). In contrast with VKAs, test results may vary according to the time between drug intake and blood sampling. It is possible to estimate the maximum concentration (C_{max}) 2 to 4 hours after oral administration, or the minimum concentration (C_{min}; C_{trough}) in blood taken just before the next dose intake. Also, there is a potential for high interindividual variability among patients,[44–47] suggesting a potential need for biological measurements (specific anti–factor Xa test).

For all direct factor Xa inhibitors, the specific test is the determination of the anti–factor Xa activity. However, this test is not routinely available in all laboratories, and is the same test that is used for measuring low-molecular-weight heparins (LMWHs), but the technique must be slightly modified when used for the new oral anticoagulants. In addition, this test is influenced by heparin and the results should not be expressed in anti–factor Xa units, but in nanograms per milliliter of the given plasma drug. Calibrated plasmas are commercially available for rivaroxaban (**Fig. 2**) and will soon be available for apixaban. The expected concentrations depend on the drug and the dosage used and have already been published.[46–48] These calibrated plasmas make it easier to evaluate patients' responses and whether they are hyporesponders, normal responders, or hyper-responders. However, the same amount of anticoagulant can induce a variable degree of anticoagulation in different patients, and therefore anti–factor Xa measurements must be interpreted with this limitation in mind. Our working group has developed a method for measuring the anti–factor Xa activity, which is also specific to direct inhibitors but is not influenced by indirect inhibitors, such as heparins and fondaparinux.[49]

Guidelines for treatment initiation with new oral anticoagulants

Direct factor Xa inhibitors are registered for different indications in different countries. Therefore, available agents should be used according to the local label. It is critical to evaluate the patients' hepatic and renal function, as well as ensuring the availability of the correct blood type for hospitalized patients, the absence of anemia or thrombocytopenia, and, if possible, checking that both PT and aPTT are normal before initiating any new treatment.

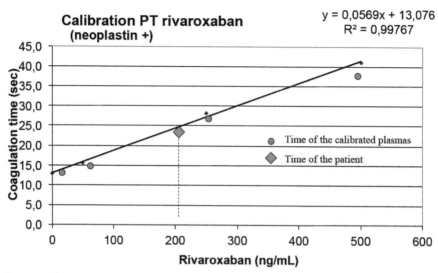

Fig. 2. Calibration with rivaroxaban calibrators and coagulation time of the patient indicating corresponding rivaroxaban concentration in plasma.

For patients who are already receiving treatment with a VKA, treatment should first be discontinued, with a daily monitoring of INR; treatment with a new oral factor Xa inhibitor should only be initiated when the INR is less than 3 for the treatment of AF and less than 2.5 for VTE.[50] The switch to a new oral factor Xa inhibitor from LMWH does not require any particular consideration; the LMWH parenteral injection is replaced by taking the first tablet of the selected new anticoagulant 0 to 2 hours before the next LMWH dose is due.[50] If a new oral factor Xa inhibitor needs to be switched to a VKA, both anticoagulants are administered simultaneously, the factor Xa inhibitor is stopped when the INR reaches or exceeds 2, and the VKA is continued with regular monitoring of INR.[50]

Discussion

The approval of the direct factor Xa inhibitors is a therapeutic revolution. Rivaroxaban, apixaban, edoxaban, and betrixaban seem at least as effective as traditional anticoagulants (eg, LMWH or warfarin), depending on the indication.

At present, rivaroxaban is approved in European and North American markets for several indications outside the hospital (eg, preventing DVT-PE in patients at high risk), whereas edoxaban is only approved in Japan for orthopedic surgery.[51] The approval of edoxaban in nonvalvular AF and acute thromboembolism is awaited in Europe. Promising results have been obtained for apixaban, which was approved in Europe for the prevention of venous thrombosis after THR and TKR in adults, as well as in patients with nonvalvular AF. The results of recent trials in indications other than major orthopedic surgery will introduce the long-term use of anticoagulant treatment, and therefore increased vigilance from the medical community to further characterize the long-term safety profiles of these drugs may be needed.

The absence of a requirement for regular monitoring of blood coagulation should not prevent clinicians monitoring patients on a regular basis. Moreover, clinical pathologists and biologists must be kept appraised of new drug developments and be able to measure their biological activity, often in an emergency situation. In addition, to date, no specific antidotes are available. Some proposals regarding reversal are discussed in Dickneite elsewhere in this issue. The physician's practical experience with these new drugs as well as physician and patient education are also essential. It is especially important to know the influence of these new molecules on traditional coagulation tests. In addition, improved availability of new techniques for the determination of anticoagulant activity (ie, the measurement of anti–factor Xa activity with expression of results in plasma concentration of the drug) is essential to ensure that clinicians are not limited to using PT or aPTT tests, which have limitations with regard to their use in monitoring the effects of new oral anticoagulants.

At present, when severe bleeding events occur in patients treated with a new anti–factor Xa agent, clinicians must take into account the elimination half-life to determine the duration of treatment interruption while accounting for the patient's renal function (Cockroft-Gault formula), which influences the rate of elimination of the drug.[52] Further clinical and laboratory studies are currently underway to define the threshold below which these drugs are no longer effective, and the threshold above which the risk of bleeding remains high; these data will provide important information for managing these patients. In addition, there is a risk of bleeding with all these factor Xa inhibitors.[53] It might be useful to investigate the impact of lower doses of the new anti–factor Xa agents than those currently used in comparison with LMWH; these lower doses could reduce bleeding while retaining comparable efficacy with LMWH. Furthermore, the development of biological studies could allow an adjustment of doses in patients in order to find an effective dose, but with a lower risk of bleeding. It may be also be possible to use oral anticoagulants instead of heparin in patients developing heparin-induced thrombocytopenia, as reported in an observation in the literature in which dabigatran use was suggested.[54,55]

SUMMARY

The new oral anticoagulants are convenient to use, but there is still limited experience of the management of patients treated with these new agents in real-world clinical practice. From the clinical trials performed to date, they are noninferior or superior to the older anticoagulants. The study of renal function and monitoring plays an important role in the tolerance of new anticoagulants. Biological monitoring of coagulation is only indicated in special circumstances with the new anticoagulants. In contrast with VKAs, comedications have little influence on their activity, but patients who are not required to attend regular anticoagulant clinic monitoring may run the risk of neglecting to meet their physicians on a regular basis if not educated about potential risks of their anticoagulant treatment with the new factor Xa inhibitors. As a result, compliance of the patient with the instructions in drug labeling, dosages, and patient education are essential to avoid jeopardizing therapeutic progress. These new molecules constitute a true therapeutic progression that could be greatly beneficial to many patients, providing they are used as per the approved indications.

REFERENCES

1. Jay McLean (1890-1957), discoverer of heparin. JAMA 1967;201(10):770.
2. Link KP. The discovery of dicumarol and its sequels. Circulation 1959;19: 97–107.
3. Weitz JI, Eikelboom JW, Samama MM. American College of Chest Physicians. New antithrombotic drugs: antithrombotic therapy and prevention of thrombosis, 9th edition: American College of Chest Physicians evidence-based clinical practice guidelines. Chest 2012;141(Suppl 2):e120S–51S.

4. Samama MM, Conard J, Flaujac C, et al. Hétérogénéité pharmacologique des nouveaux anticoagulants. J Mal Vasc 2011;36(Suppl 1):S10–5.
5. Kubitza D, Becka M, Mueck W, et al. Safety, tolerability, pharmacodynamics, and pharmacokinetics of rivaroxaban – an oral, direct factor Xa inhibitor – are not affected by aspirin. J Clin Pharmacol 2006;46:981–90.
6. Ericksson BI, Rosencher N, Friedman RJ, et al. Concomitant use of medication with antiplatelet effects in patients receiving either rivaroxaban or enoxaparin after total hip of knee arthroplasty. Thromb Res 2011;130:147–51.
7. Mega JL, Braunwald E, Mohanavelu S, et al. Rivaroxaban versus placebo in patients with acute coronary syndromes (ATLAS ACS-TIMI 46): a randomized, double-blind, phase II trial. Lancet 2009;374:29–38.
8. Halabi A, Kubitza D, Zuehlsdorf M, et al. Effect of hepatic impairment on the pharmacodynamics and tolerability of rivaroxaban – an oral, direct factor Xa inhibitor. J Thromb Haemost 2007;5(Suppl 2):635.
9. Eriksson BI, Borris LC, Friedman RJ, et al. Rivaroxaban versus enoxaparin for thromboprophylaxis after hip arthroplasty. N Engl J Med 2008;358:2765–75.
10. Kakkar AK, Brenner B, Dahl OE, et al. Extended duration rivaroxaban versus short term enoxaparin for the prevention of venous thromboembolism after total hip arthroplasty: a double blind, randomised controlled trial. Lancet 2008;372:31–9.
11. Lassen MR, Agneo W, Borris LC, et al. Rivaroxaban versus enoxaparin for thromboprophylaxis after total knee arthroplasty. N Engl J Med 2008;358: 2776–86.
12. Turpie AG, Lassen MR, Davidson BL, et al. Rivaroxaban versus enoxaparin for thromboprophylaxis after total knee arthroplasty: a randomised trial. Lancet 2009;373:1673–80.
13. Patel MR, Mahaffey KW, Garg J, et al. Rivaroxaban versus warfarin in non-valvular atrial fibrillation. N Engl J Med 2011;365:883–91.
14. ROCKET AF Study Investigators. Rivaroxaban – once daily, oral, direct factor Xa inhibition compared with vitamin K antagonism for prevention of stroke and embolism trial in atrial fibrillation: rationale and design of the ROCKET AF study. Am Heart J 2010;159:340–7.
15. Buller HR, Lensing AW, Prins MH, et al. A dose-ranging study evaluating once daily oral administration of the factor Xa inhibitor rivaroxaban in the treatment of patients with acute symptomatic deep vein thrombosis: the Einstein-DVT Dose-Ranging Study. Blood 2008;112:2242–7.
16. Romualdi E, Donadini MP, Ageno W. Oral rivaroxaban after symptomatic venous thromboembolism: the continued treatment study (Einstein-extension study). Expert Rev Cardiovasc Ther 2011;9:841–4.
17. EINSTEIN–PE Investigators, Büller HR, Prins MH, et al. Oral rivaroxaban for the treatment of symptomatic pulmonary embolism. N Engl J Med 2012;366: 1287–97.
18. Cohen AT, Spiro TE, Spyropoulos AC. MAGELLAN Steering Committee. Rivaroxaban for thromboprophylaxis in acutely ill medical patients. N Engl J Med 2013; 368:1945–6.
19. Mega JL, Braunwald E, Wiviott SD, et al. Rivaroxaban in patients with a recent acute coronary syndrome. N Engl J Med 2012;366:9–19.
20. Wang L, Zhang D, Raghavan N, et al. *In vitro* assessment of metabolic drug-drug interaction potential of apixaban through cytochrome P450 phenotyping, inhibition and induction studies. Drug Metab Dispos 2009;38:448–58.
21. Lassen MR, Raskob GE, Gallus A, et al. Apixaban or enoxaparin for thromboprophylaxis after knee replacement. N Engl J Med 2009;361:504–604.

22. Lassen MR, Raskob GE, Gallus A, et al, ADVANCE-2 Investigators. Apixaban versus enoxaparin for thromboprophylaxis after knee replacement (ADVANCE-2): a randomized double-blind trial. Lancet 2010;375:807–15.

23. Lassen MR, Gallus A, Raskob GE, et al. Apixaban versus enoxaparin for thromboprophylaxis after hip replacement. N Engl J Med 2010;363:2487–98.

24. Connolly SJ, Eikelboom J, Joyner C, et al. Apixaban in patients with atrial fibrillation (AVERROES Study). N Engl J Med 2011;364:806–17.

25. Granger CB, Alexander JH, McMurray JJ, et al. Apixaban versus warfarin in patients with atrial fibrillation. N Engl J Med 2011;365:981–92.

26. Agnelli G, Büller HR, Cohen A, et al. Oral apixaban for the treatment of acute venous thromboembolism. New Engl J Med 2013;369:799–808.

27. Agnelli G, Buller HR, Cohen A, et al, AMPLIFY-EXT Investigators. Apixaban for extended treatment of venous thromboembolism. N Engl J Med 2013;368: 699–708.

28. Levine MN, Gu C, Liebman HA, et al. A randomized phase II trial of apixaban for the prevention of thromboembolism in patients with metastatic cancer. J Thromb Haemost 2012;10:807–14.

29. Goldhaber SZ, Leizorovicz A, Kakkar AK, et al. Apixaban versus enoxaparin for thromboprophylaxis in medically ill patients. N Engl J Med 2011;365:2167–77.

30. Alexander JH, Lopes RD, James S, et al. Apixaban with antiplatelet therapy after acute coronary syndrome. N Engl J Med 2011;365:699–708.

31. Camm AJ, Bounameaux H. Edoxaban: a new oral direct factor Xa inhibitor. Drugs 2011;71:1503–26.

32. Giugliano RP, Ruff CT, Braunwald E, et al. Edoxaban versus warfarin in patients with atrial fibrillation. New Engl J Med 2013;369:2093–104.

33. The Hokusai-VTE Investigators. Edoxaban versus warfarin for the treatment of symptomatic venous thromboembolism. New Engl J Med 2013;369:1406–15.

34. Zhang P, Huang W, Wang L, et al. Discovery of betrixaban (PRT054021), N-(5-chloropyridin-2-yl)-2-(4-(N,N-dimethylcarbamimidoyl)benzamido)-5-methoxy benzamide, a highly potent, selective, and orally efficacious factor Xa inhibitors. Bioorg Med Chem Lett 2009;19:2179–85.

35. Turpie AG, Bauer KA, Davidson BL, et al. A randomized evaluation of betrixaban an oral factor Xa inhibitor for prevention of thromboembolism events after total knee replacement (EXPERT). Thromb Haemost 2009;101:68–76.

36. Connolly SJ, Eikelboom J, Dorian P, et al. Betrixaban compared with warfarin in patients with atrial fibrillation: results of a phase 2 randomized dose-ranging study (EXPLORE-Xa). Eur Heart J 2013;34:1498–505.

37. Samama MM, Guinet C. Laboratory assessment of new anticoagulants. Clin Chem Lab Med 2011;49:761–72.

38. Samama MM, Guinet C, Le Flem L. Deux nouveaux anticoagulants: dabigatran et Rivaroxaban. Leur impact sur les examens de laboratoire. Biotribune 2011; 38:16–21.

39. Gouin-Thibault I, Mismetti P, Flaujac C, et al. Nouveaux anticoagulants par voie orale: quelle place pour les analyses de biologie médicale? Sang Thrombose Vaisseaux 2011;23:8–17.

40. Gerotziafas GT, Baccouche H, Sassi M, et al. Optimisation of the assays for the measurement of clotting factor activity in the presence of rivaroxaban. Thromb Res 2012;129:101–3.

41. Douxfils J, Chatelain C, Chatelain B. Impact of apixaban on routine and specific coagulation assays: a practical laboratory guide. Thromb Haemost 2013;110: 283–94.

42. Tripodi A, Chantarangkul V, Guinet C, et al. The International Normalized Ratio calibrated for rivaroxaban has the potential to normalize prothrombin time results for rivaroxaban-treated patients: results of an in vitro study. J Thromb Haemost 2011;9:226–8.
43. Samama MM, Martinoli JL, Le Flem L, et al. Assessment of laboratory assays to measure rivaroxaban – an oral, direct factor Xa inhibitor. Thromb Haemost 2010; 103:815–25.
44. Freyburger G, Macouillard G, Labrouche S, et al. Coagulation parameters in patients receiving dabigatran etexilate or rivaroxaban: two observational studies in patients undergoing total hip or total knee replacement. Thromb Res 2011;127: 457–65.
45. Samama MM, Guinet C, Le Flem L, et al. Measurement of dabigatran and rivaroxaban in primary prevention of venous thromboembolism in 106 patients, who have undergone major orthopedic surgery: an observational study. J Thromb Thrombolysis 2013;35:140–6.
46. Samama MM, Contant G, Spiro TE, et al. Evaluation of the prothrombin time for measuring rivaroxaban plasma concentrations using calibrators and controls: results of a multicenter field trial. Clin Appl Thromb Hemost 2012;18:150–8.
47. Samama MM, Contant G, Spiro TE, et al. Evaluation of the anti-Xa chromogenic assay for the measurement of rivaroxaban plasma concentrations using calibrators and controls. Thromb Haemost 2012;107:379–87.
48. Gouin-Thibault I, Flaujac C, Delavenne X, et al. Assessment of apixaban plasma levels by laboratory tests: suitability of three anti-Xa assays. A multicentre French GEHT study. Thromb Haemost 2014;111(2):240–8.
49. Samama MM, Amiral J, Guinet C, et al. An optimised, rapid chromogenic assay, specific for measuring direct factor Xa inhibitors (rivaroxaban) in plasma. Thromb Haemost 2010;104:1078–9.
50. Pernod G, Elias A, Gouin I, et al. Questions-réponses sur l'utilisation du rivaroxaban dans le traitement de la maladie thromboembolique veineuse. J Mal Vasc 2012;37:300–10.
51. Rohatagi S, Mendell J, Kastrissios H, et al. Characterisation of exposure versus response of edoxaban in patients undergoing total hip replacement surgery. Thromb Haemost 2012;108:887–95.
52. Sié P, Samama CM, Godier A, et al. Surgery and invasive procedures in patients on long-term treatment with oral direct thrombin or factor Xa inhibitors. Ann Fr Anesth Reanim 2011;30:645–50.
53. Samama MM, Conard J, Lillo-Le Louët A. Accidents hémorragiques des nouveaux anticoagulants. J Mal Vasc 2013;38:259–70.
54. Mirdamadi A. Dabigatran, a direct thrombin inhibitor, can be a life-saving treatment in heparin-induced thrombocytopenia. ARYA Atheroscler 2013;9:112–4.
55. Bhatt VR, Aryal MR, Armitage JO. Nonheparin anticoagulants for heparin-induced thrombocytopenia. N Engl J Med 2013;368:2333–4.

Treatment and Long-Term Management of Venous Thromboembolism

Ahmed Al-Badri, MD[a],*, Alex C. Spyropoulos, MD, FRCPC[b]

KEYWORDS

- Venous thromboembolism • Bridge therapy • Switch therapy
- Outpatient venous thromboembolism treatment • New oral anticoagulants

KEY POINTS

- An increased emphasis on risk stratification and standardization may provide a rationale for inpatient versus outpatient treatment of PE and DVT.
- Three options are available when treating patients with new onset VTE: monotherapy, bridging therapy, and switch therapy.
- For provoked VTE, anticoagulation treatment for 3 months is usually considered to be sufficient.
- For unprovoked VTE, treatment for 3 to 6 months should be considered. After that time, patients should be evaluated for the need for extended anticoagulation treatment.
- Newer oral anticoagulants have been developed to overcome the drawbacks of other anticoagulation agents, improve patient care, and simplify and improve VTE management.
- Evidence from several phase III trials suggests that NOACs are effective for secondary prevention of VTE in patients who have completed standard anticoagulation therapy.

INTRODUCTION

The term "venous thromboembolism" (VTE) covers a range of conditions from deep vein thrombosis (DVT) to pulmonary embolism (PE), all of which can be life-threatening. Thrombi that form in lower-extremity veins can embolize, leading to occlusion of the pulmonary vasculature. As a reflection of this pathophysiologic relationship, most patients with symptomatic PE have DVT and many patients with DVT

Disclosure: Dr A. Al-Badri has no relevant financial or non-financial relationships to disclose; Dr A.C. Spyropoulos is a consultant for Daiichi-Sankyo, Boehringer-Ingelheim, Janssen, Bayer, Bristol-Myers Squibb, Pfizer and Sanofi.
[a] Department of Medicine, Lenox Hill Hospital, NSLIJHS, 130 East 77th Street, 6th Floor, Black Hall Building, New York, NY 10075, USA; [b] Department of Medicine, Lenox Hill Hospital, NSLIJHS, 130 East 77th Street, 5th Floor, Achilles Building, New York, NY 10075, USA
* Corresponding author.
E-mail address: aalbadri@nshs.edu

Clin Lab Med 34 (2014) 519–536
http://dx.doi.org/10.1016/j.cll.2014.06.011
0272-2712/14/$ – see front matter © 2014 Elsevier Inc. All rights reserved.

labmed.theclinics.com

have asymptomatic PE.[1] The aims of treatment are to alleviate symptoms, to minimize acute morbidity and mortality by preventing the extension or potentially fatal embolization of the initial thrombus, and to avoid postthrombotic syndrome. The anticoagulants heparin and dicumarol were discovered serendipitously in 1916 and 1939, respectively, and heparin has been commercially available to treat blood clots since 1940. In the 1970s, three different research groups in Stockholm, London, and Ontario began work on low-molecular-weight heparin (LMWH) and by the mid-1980s, LMWH preparations were being tested in clinical trials. LMWH first became commercially available in 1993, and was followed by the introduction of fondaparinux and bivalirudin. Because of the advantages of LMWHs compared with unfractionated heparin (UFH) (Box 1), LMWHs have now replaced heparin for most indications. However, their parenteral administration and their restricted use in patients with renal failure limit their use. In the 2010s, a new era of oral anticoagulation has started (Fig. 1).

PHASES OF ANTICOAGULATION

Anticoagulant therapy, the mainstay of treatment of VTE, has two goals. First, anticoagulant therapy treats or "turns off" the acute episode of thrombosis, which improves acute symptoms, prevents thrombus extension, and reduces the risk of early PE. Second, anticoagulant therapy prevents new episodes of VTE that do not arise directly from the acute episode of thrombosis.[2] There are two main phases during anticoagulation therapy: the acute (ie, active treatment) and chronic phases (ie, secondary prevention) (Fig. 2).

Acute Phase

In the acute phase, the risk of thrombus extension and PE is high, but the initiation of treatment rapidly reduces this risk.[3,4] Therefore, it is critical that anticoagulant therapy is started as soon as possible when VTE is diagnosed (or is highly suspected).[3] Moreover, because there is a high risk of VTE progression in the acute phase, the use of a higher-intensity anticoagulant therapy at the start of treatment is recommended.[2,5-7] Furthermore, if anticoagulant therapy is stopped before treatment of the acute episode of thrombosis has been completed, there may be reactivation of the initial thrombosis with a further increase in the risk of recurrent VTE.[2,5-7] Four observations support duration for anticoagulant therapy for approximately 3 months for active (acute) treatment of VTE.[2,5-7] These reports suggest that treatment for 3 months is associated with the same risk of recurrent VTE as treatment for 6 months or longer, suggesting that 3 months is adequate therapy.[2]

Box 1
Advantages of LMWH compared with UFH

- Less binding to plasma proteins so more predictable dosing response
- Lower incidence of HIT
- Less or no monitoring needed
- Less osteopenia
- Does not cross the placental barrier
- Fixed, weight-based dose

Abbreviations: HIT, heparin-induced thrombocytopenia; LMWH, low-molecular-weight heparin; UFH, unfractionated heparin.

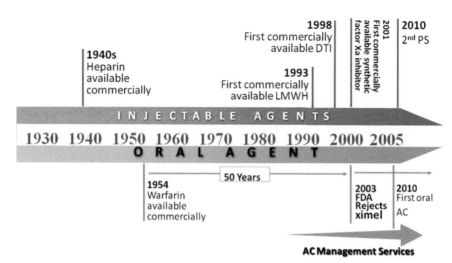

Fig. 1. Advances in anticoagulation therapy for venous thromboembolism treatment. AC, anticoagulant; DTI, direct thrombin inhibitor; FDA, Food and Drug Administration; LMWH, low-molecular-weight heparin; PS, pentasaccharide (idraparinux, idrabiotapinarux).

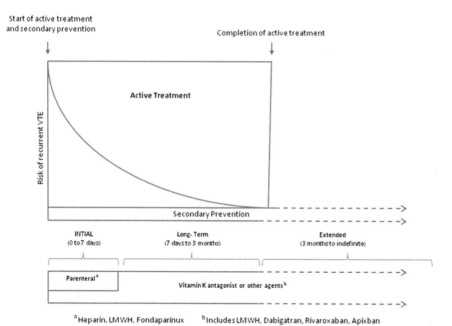

Fig. 2. Phases of anticoagulation and the risk of recurrent venous thromboembolism. LMWH, low-molecular-weight heparin; VTE, venous thromboembolism. (*Data from* Kearon C, Akl EA, Comerota AJ, et al. Antithrombotic therapy for VTE disease: antithrombotic therapy and prevention of thrombosis, 9th ed: American College of Chest Physicians Evidence-Based Clinical Practice Guidelines. Chest 2012;141(Suppl 2):e419S–94S; and Kearon C. A conceptual framework for two phases of anticoagulant treatment of venous thromboembolism. J Thromb Haemost 2012;10:507–11.)

Chronic Phase

Once the initial thrombosis (ie, the acute phase) has been adequately treated, further anticoagulation serves as secondary prevention of new, unrelated, episodes of thrombosis (ie, the chronic phase). The treatment of VTE can be continued indefinitely as "secondary prevention" if the risk of recurrence remains unacceptably high having completed treatment during the acute phase. The risk of recurrent VTE after finishing the acute phase of treatment depends on the patient's intrinsic risk. If a patient's intrinsic risk of recurrent VTE is not high enough to justify indefinite anticoagulant therapy, it is important to be able to identify when acute treatment has been completed so that anticoagulants can be stopped at that time (ie, absence of VTE-related symptoms).[4-7] Primary factors for estimating the risk of recurrence are the presence of a reversible provoking risk factor, unprovoked VTE, or the presence of active cancer,[8] which are the most relevant factors that influence risk of recurrent VTE after stopping anticoagulation. Provoking risk factors include recent surgery, estrogen therapy, pregnancy, leg injury, and flights longer than 8 hours in duration.[8] Other factors that should be considered in deciding the duration of treatment are whether the DVT is confined to the distal veins, which is estimated to be associated with about half of all recurrences of proximal DVT or PE,[9-12] and whether the VTE is a second or subsequent episode of VTE, which is estimated to be associated with about a 50% higher risk of recurrence compared with a first VTE (**Table 1**).[13,14]

OUTPATIENT VTE TREATMENT

Validated protocols have been used to identify patients who meet clinical or psychosocial criteria for outpatient DVT treatment with LMWH (**Box 2**).[15-17] One such protocol, the Lovelace Health Systems protocol, defines absolute and relative clinical criteria that stratify patients as high, moderate, or low risk for outpatient DVT treatment and individualizes treatment based on risk category (**Box 3**).[17] These treatment protocols could potentially identify patients for whom outpatient management of DVT with new oral anticoagulants (NOACs) optimizes the risk/benefit ratio. Using these

Table 1				
Duration of anticoagulation treatment				
		Provoked (eg, Recent Surgery, Estrogen Therapy, Pregnancy, Leg Injury, Flight of >8 h)	Unprovoked	
			First Episode	Recurrent
VTE Location	Proximal	3 mo	Extended anticoagulation therapy[a]	Extended anticoagulation therapy[a]
	Distal	3 mo[b]	3 mo[b]	3 mo[b]
	PE	3 mo	Extended anticoagulation therapy[a]	Extended anticoagulation therapy[a]

[a] If patient has a low or moderate risk of bleeding. In patients with a high risk of bleeding, 3 months of anticoagulation therapy is acceptable.
[b] Patients in whom a decision has been made to treat with anticoagulation, however not all patients with distal DVT are prescribed anticoagulation.
Data from Kearon C, Akl EA, Comerota AJ, et al. Antithrombotic therapy for VTE disease: antithrombotic therapy and prevention of thrombosis, 9th ed: American College of Chest Physicians Evidence-Based Clinical Practice Guidelines. Chest 2012;141(Suppl 2):e419-94S.

Box 2
Exclusionary risk factors for outpatient treatment of DVT

Absolute exclusionary risk factors

- Platelet count less than 100,000/μL
- Active hemorrhage
- Gastrointestinal bleed within 6 months
- Heparin sensitivity
- Underlying liver disorder
- Familial bleeding disorder
- Hypertensive: SBP greater than 220 and DBP greater than 120 mm Hg
- Catheter-associated DVT
- Recent surgery
- Morbid obesity greater than 130% ideal body weight
- Congenital/acquired hypercoagulable state
- Iliofemoral thrombosis
- Comorbid illness

Relative exclusionary risk factors

- Age greater than 75 years
- Pregnancy
- PE (clinically unstable or massive PE is absolute exclusionary criterion)
- Renal insufficiency (CrCl <30 mL/min or dialysis-dependent patient is absolute exclusionary criterion)
- Other factors increasing risk of home treatment (eg, comorbidity, insurance compliance)
- History of noncompliance with medicines
- History of substance abuse
- Language barrier
- Inability to pay for LMWH
- Inaccessibility to clinic or telephone
- Unstable home environment
- Incompetence to assume responsibility of self-care or inability of family/friend/nurse to administer care

Abbreviations: CrCl, creatinine clearance; DBP, diastolic blood pressure; DVT, deep vein thrombosis; LMWH, low-molecular-weight heparin; PE, pulmonary embolism; SBP, systolic blood pressure.
 Data from Agnelli G, Buller HR, Cohen A, et al. Apixaban for extended treatment of venous thromboembolism. N Engl J Med 2013;368:699–708.

---

protocols, clinical indicators and severity indices to standardize risk stratification and guide treatment with NOACs may also help to differentiate a subset of high-risk patients (particularly those with PE) who may require hospitalization, from low-risk patients who can be treated in an outpatient setting, likely with a monotherapy approach.

The Pulmonary Embolism Severity Index (PESI) is a prognostic–predictive tool for patients with PE. Developed in 2005, it describes 11 clinical elements that can be

Box 3
Risk stratification for outpatient treatment of DVT (Lovelace Health Systems Protocol)

High risk

One absolute or two or more relative exclusionary risk factors

- Administer inpatient intravenous UFH

Moderate risk

One relative exclusionary risk factor and home health issues or third-party payer issues

- Treat in hospital short-term with LMWH, then restratify and treat accordingly

Low risk

No exclusionary risk factors

- Outpatient LMWH treatment or no hospitalization

Absolute exclusionary risk factors

Platelet count less than 100,000/μL

Active hemorrhage

Gastrointestinal bleed within 6 months

Heparin sensitivity

Underlying liver disorder

Familial bleeding disorder

SBP greater than 220 mm Hg and DBP greater than 120 mm Hg

Catheter-associated DVT

Recent surgery

Morbid obesity greater than 130% ideal body weight

Comorbid illness

Iliofemoral thrombosis

Congenital/acquired hypercoagulable state

Relative exclusionary risk factors

Age greater than 75 years

Pregnancy

PE (clinically unstable or massive PE is absolute exclusionary criteria)

Renal insufficiency (CrCl <30 mL/min or dialysis-dependence is absolute exclusionary criteria)

Other factors increasing risk of home treatment (eg, comorbidity, insurance compliance)

History of noncompliance with medicines

History of substance abuse

Language barrier

Inability to pay for LMWH

Inaccessibility to clinic or telephone

Unstable home environment

Incompetence to assume responsibility of self-care or inability of family/friend/nurse to administer care

Abbreviations: CrCl, creatinine clearance; DBP, diastolic blood pressure; DVT, deep vein thrombosis; LMWH, low-molecular-weight heparin; PE, pulmonary embolism; SBP, systolic blood pressure; UFH, unfractionated heparin.

Data from Spyropoulos A, Kardos J, Wigal P. Outcomes analyses of the outpatient treatment of venous thromboembolic disease using the low-molecular-weight heparin enoxaparin in a managed care organization. J Manag Care Pharm 2000;6(4):298–306.

used to stratify patients into five risk classes (**Table 2**).[18] These 11 elements are individually weighted and the overall PESI score relies on mathematical calculations. The simplified PESI (sPESI) was developed to introduce a less complex risk-stratification tool[19]; it uses six clinical indications to classify patients as low or high risk for death within 30 days of disease presentation (see **Table 2**). The predictive–prognostic reliability of the sPESI is comparable with PESI.[19] Another prognostic model for acute PE is the Geneva score, which comprises six predictive elements (see **Table 2**); however, PESI is a more accurate prognostic indicator because it contains more variables.[20]

Additionally, some prognostic tools have been developed that incorporate measures of right ventricular (RV) dysfunction to guide outpatient management of PE, and these have been shown to offer improved accuracy in predicting risk over prognostic tools that use only clinical elements. The first such tool is produced by the European Society of Cardiology: it stratifies patients into three risk categories (low, intermediate, and high) through the use of clinical findings (ie, shock or

Table 2
Pulmonary embolism severity clinical assessment tools

	Points Assigned	Risk Stratification
Pulmonary embolism severity index[18]		
Age, years	Equal to age	Class I ≤65 points,
Male	+10	very low risk
History of cancer	+30	
History of heart failure	+10	Class II 66–85 points,
History of chronic lung disease	+10	low risk
Pulse ≥110/min	+20	
SBP <100 mm Hg	+30	Class III 86–105 points,
Respiratory rate ≥30/min	+20	intermediate risk
Temperature <36°C	+20	Class IV 106–125 points,
Altered mental status	+60	high risk
Arterial oxygen saturation <90%	+20	Class V >125 points,
		very high risk
Simplified pulmonary embolism severity index[19]		
Age >80 y	+1	0 points, low risk
History of cancer	+1	
History of chronic cardiopulmonary disease	+1	
Pulse ≥110/min	+1	≥1 points, high risk
SBP <100 mm Hg	+1	
Arterial oxygen saturation <90%	+1	
Geneva[20]		
History of cancer	+2	≤2 points, low risk
History of heart failure	+1	
History of DVT	+1	
SBP <100 mm Hg	+2	≥3 points, high risk
Arterial oxygen saturation <8 kPa	+1	
DVT shown by ultrasound	+1	

Abbreviations: DVT, deep vein thrombosis; SBP, systolic blood pressure.
Adapted from Spyropoulos AC, Turpie A. Venous thromboembolism management: where do novel anticoagulants fit? Curr Med Res Opin 2013;29:783–90.

hypotension), markers of RV dysfunction (RV dilatation, hypokinesis or pressure overload on echocardiography, RV dilatation on spiral computed tomography, B-type natriuretic peptide [BNP] or N-terminal–probrain natriuretic peptide [NT-pro-BNP] elevation, and elevated right heart pressure at right heart catheterization) and markers of cardiac injury (ie, cardiac troponin T or I).[21] Research indicates that the use of markers of RV dysfunction in conjunction with PESI is more accurate than the use of PESI alone and that the European Society of Cardiology criteria offer improved predictive accuracy compared with both the PESI and sPESI.[22,23] The serum levels of NT-pro-BNP, a measure of cardiac wall expansion, have demonstrated utility in risk stratification. Patients with a low or normal NT-pro-BNP level (<500 pg/mL) have been successfully treated for PE as outpatients.[24] Furthermore, the low-risk PE decision rule (**Box 4**) incorporates clinical assessments and markers of cardiac stress into a formula used to determine 30-day mortality, and it has been demonstrated to be superior to the PESI and Geneva criteria in terms of predictive accuracy.[25] Therefore, appropriate use of these tools, with an increased emphasis placed on risk stratification and standardization, may help clinicians determine the most appropriate treatment setting (inpatient vs outpatient) for patients with PE. Patients with acute PE who meet the following criteria seem to be suitable for outpatient treatment[8]:

1. Clinically stable with good cardiopulmonary reserve (eg, PESI score of <85[26] or simplified PESI score of 0[19]) and the absence of hypoxia, recent bleeding, severe chest pain, PE while on anticoagulant therapy, and severe liver or renal disease, with systolic blood pressure less than 100 mm Hg, and platelet count less than 70,000/μL
2. Good social support with ready access to medical care
3. Expected to be compliant with follow-up

MANAGEMENT

Treatment decisions should be modified according to the predisposition for VTE (provoked or unprovoked), the site and extent of thrombus, the presence or absence of symptomatic embolism, and the patient's bleeding risk. It is therefore essential that each patient's management is individualized.

Box 4
Low-Risk Pulmonary Embolism Decision Rule variables to predict 1-month all-cause mortality in patients with acute pulmonary embolism

- Age
- Chronic heart failure
- Atrial fibrillation at admission
- Troponin I
- Creatinine
- Glycemia
- C-reactive protein

Data from Barra S, Paiva L, Providência R, et al. LR-PED rule: low risk pulmonary embolism decision rule. A new decision score for low risk pulmonary embolism. Thromb Res 2012;130:327–33.

Acute-Phase Treatment

Thrombolytics and surgical embolectomy

Thrombolytic therapy is more effective than heparin in achieving early lysis of VTE and can reduce mortality in clinically unstable patients (ie, hypotension, tachycardia, elevated jugular venous pressure, and evidence of decreased tissue perfusion).[21] Although systemic thrombolysis is used in patients with massive PE and in some patients with proximal DVT, controversy persists with respect to the appropriate patient selection for this intervention.[27] Additionally, the role of thrombolytic therapy in the treatment of DVT is uncertain. Systemic thrombolytic therapy increases lysis of DVT, and may reduce the risk of developing the postthrombotic syndrome; however, it increases the frequency of major bleeding, including intracranial hemorrhage. If thrombolytic therapy is contraindicated, surgical embolectomy should be considered.[1,8,21] Thromboendarterectomy is effective in selected cases of chronic thromboembolic pulmonary hypertension caused by proximal pulmonary arterial obstruction.[8,28]

Anticoagulation

Anticoagulation with conventional therapy includes the use of heparins, fondaparinux, and vitamin K antagonists (VKAs), primarily warfarin. However, VTE management with these agents is complex. Heparin administration is parenteral, which limits its use in chronic disease management, and some heparin products can induce clinically significant thrombocytopenia. Warfarin has unpredictable pharmacokinetics and is susceptible to numerous drug–drug and food–drug interactions, and use of warfarin therefore requires routine monitoring.[1] Newer oral anticoagulants, such as direct thrombin inhibitors (eg, dabigatran etexilate) and direct factor Xa inhibitors (eg, rivaroxaban, apixaban, and edoxaban), have been developed to overcome the drawbacks of traditional anticoagulation agents, improve patient care, and simplify and improve DVT and PE management. Each agent has its own pharmacokinetic features, with many benefits over warfarin, such as a rapid onset and offset of action and limited interactions with food or drugs (**Table 3**). Phase III clinical trials have been conducted to evaluate the efficacy of NOACs in the treatment of acute VTE (**Table 4**).

Three different anticoagulation approaches can be used in the treatment of VTE (**Fig. 3**):

- Bridge therapy or the conventional therapy approach: VKAs should be initiated on the same day as VTE diagnosis, along with parenteral anticoagulation (ie, UFH, LMWH, or fondaparinux); parenteral anticoagulation should be continued for a minimum of 5 days and until INR is ≥2.0 for at least 24 hours.
- Switch therapy: UFH or LMWH should be initiated for 6 days, after which therapy should be switched to either a direct thrombin inhibitor (dabigatran twice daily) or direct factor Xa inhibitors (edoxaban once daily).[29,30]
- Monotherapy: Rivaroxaban or apixaban (direct factor Xa inhibitors) can be started once VTE is diagnosed or highly suspected. Higher doses of anticoagulation should be used in the early phase of treatment (eg, rivaroxaban, 15 mg twice daily for the first 3 weeks, followed by 20 mg once daily thereafter). If apixaban is used, 10 mg twice daily for 7 days followed by 5 mg twice daily, is recommended.[31,32]

Mechanical

Inferior vena cava filters are generally used only if anticoagulant therapy has failed or is contraindicated because of the risk of serious hemorrhage.[8] Retrievable inferior vena

Table 3
Comparison of pharmacokinetic features of warfarin, dabigatran, rivaroxaban, apixaban, and edoxaban

	Warfarin	Dabigatran[45]	Rivaroxaban[46]	Apixaban[47]	Edoxaban[48,49]
Mechanism of action	VKOR inhibitor	Direct thrombin inhibitor (reversible)	Factor Xa inhibitor (reversible)	Factor Xa inhibitor (reversible)	Factor Xa inhibitor (reversible)
Onset of action	24–72 h	Rapid	Rapid	Rapid	Rapid
Offset of action	Long	Short	Short	Short	Short
Absorption	Rapid	Rapid	Rapid	Rapid	Rapid
Bioavailability (%)	100	6.5	80	50	62
t_{max} (h)	2.0–4.0	1.0–3.0	2.5–4.0	1.0–3.0	1.0–2.0
V_d (L)	10	60–70	50–55	21	—
Protein binding (%)	99	35	95	87	55
$t\frac{1}{2}$ (h)	40	12–17	5–9 (young individuals) 11–13 (elderly)	8–15	8–10
Renal excretion	None	80	33	27	35
Fecal excretion	None	20	28	50–70	62
Food effect	No effect on absorption; vitamin K influences pharmacodynamics characteristics	Delayed absorption with food with no influence on bioavailability	Delayed absorption with food with increased bioavailability	None	None
Drug transporter	None	P-gp	P-gp, BCRP	P-gp, BCRP	P-gp
Monitoring	INR	No need for monitoring	No need for monitoring	No need for monitoring	No need for monitoring

Abbreviations: BCRP, breast cancer resistance protein; INR, international normalized ratio; p-gp, p-glycoprotein; t½, terminal half-life; t_{max}, time to maximum plasma concentration; V_d, volume of distribution; VKOR, vitamin K epoxide reductase enzyme.

Table 4
Summary of phase III trials of the new oral anticoagulant agents in the treatment of acute VTE

Study (Patients)	Design	Treatment Duration	Treatment		Outcome	Safety	
			Group 1 (No. of Patients)	Group 2 (No. of Patients)	Recurrent VTE or VTE-Related Death (Group 1/Group 2)	Major Bleeding (Group 1/Group 2)	Clinically Relevant Non-Major Bleeding (Group 1/Group 2)
Amplify[31] (VTE)	Randomized, double-blind trial	6 mo	Apixaban, 10 mg twice daily for 7 d then 5 mg twice daily (2691)	LMWH with warfarin (2635)	59/71	15/49	103/215
EINSTEIN-DVT[32] (DVT)	Open-label, randomized, noninferiority trial	3–12 mo	Rivaroxaban, 15 mg twice daily for 3 wk then 20 mg once daily (1731)	LMWH followed by warfarin (1718)	36/51	14/20	129/119
EINSTEIN-PE[50] (PE)	Open-label, randomized, noninferiority trial	3–6 mo	Rivaroxaban, 15 mg twice daily for 3 wk then 20 mg once daily (2419)	LMWH followed by warfarin (2413)	50/44	26/52	223/222
RECOVER[29] (VTE)	Randomized, double-blind, noninferiority trial	6 mo	UFH or LMWH for 6 d then dabigatran twice daily (1274)	UFH or LMWH for 6 d then warfarin (1265)	30/27	20/24	71/111
Recover II[51] (VTE)	Randomized, double-blind, noninferiority trial	6 mo	UFH or LMWH for 6 d then dabigatran twice daily (1279)	UFH or LMWH for 6 d then warfarin (1289)	30/28	15/22	64/102
HOKUSAI-VTE[30] (VTE)	Randomized, double-blind, noninferiority trial	3–12 mo	UFH or LMWH for 6 d then edoxaban daily (4118)	UFH or LMWH for 6 d then warfarin (4122)	130/146	56/66	298/368

Abbreviations: DVT, deep venous thrombosis; LMWH, low-molecular-weight heparin; PE, pulmonary embolism; UFH, unfractionated heparin; VTE, venous thromboembolism.

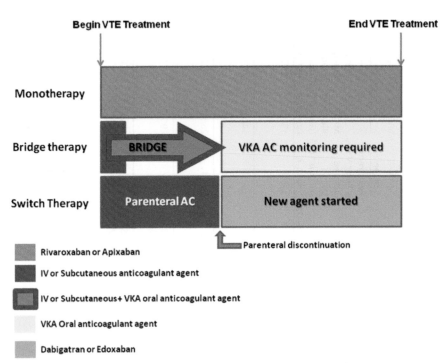

Fig. 3. Venous thromboembolism treatment paradigms. AC, anticoagulant; IV, intravenous.

cava filters are an option in patients with an expected temporary contraindication to anticoagulants (eg, acute VTE <2 weeks before major surgery). Familiarity with potential complications of inferior vena cava filter placement is critical when weighing the risks and benefits of this treatment option (**Box 5**).

Box 5
Complications of inferior vena cava filters

Procedural complication

- Venous access site complication: bleeding, hematoma, inadvertent arterial puncture, and infection
- Malposition of the device
- Defective filter deployment

Delayed complications

- Migration
- Thrombosis
- Filter fracture
- Inferior vena cava perforation
- Pulmonary embolism
- Device infection

Data from Van Ha T. Complications of inferior vena caval filters. Semin Intervent Radiol 2006;23:150–5.

Extended Therapy

Although it is well established that anticoagulation is the foundation of treatment of VTE, the optimal duration of therapy is still under debate. Prandoni and colleagues[33] found that after discontinuation of anticoagulation, the cumulative incidence of recurrent VTE was 18% after 2 years of follow-up, 25% after 5 years, and 30% after 8 years, which suggests that VTE is a chronic illness. Patients with an unprovoked DVT should be treated with anticoagulation therapy for at least 3 months. After 3 months of treatment, patients should be evaluated for the risk/benefit ratio of extended therapy (ie, the risk of bleeding vs the avoidance of recurrent VTE). In general, in patients with a recurrent unprovoked VTE, extended anticoagulation therapy (ie, >3 months) is recommended and the continuing use of treatment should be reassessed annually.[8] Oral anticoagulants (VKAs, rivaroxaban, apixaban, and dabigatran) and antiplatelet agents (acetylsalicylic acid [aspirin]) have been evaluated for long-term secondary prevention of recurrent VTE in patients at high risk of recurrence.

Aspirin

Because patients who have had a first episode of unprovoked VTE have a high risk of recurrence after anticoagulants are discontinued (ie, after treatment for 3–6 months), the effect of aspirin in preventing a recurrence of VTE was investigated in the ASPIRE and WARFASA trials (**Table 5**). In the ASPIRE trial, aspirin was associated with a nonsignificant trend toward fewer recurrent VTE events and fewer cardiovascular events than placebo.[34] The WARFASA trial[35] showed aspirin was associated with fewer VTE recurrences than placebo, with no statistically significant differences in cardiovascular events or major bleeding. The discordance between the results of the two studies may be explained by the fact that only about two-thirds of ASPIRE patients received at least 6 months of anticoagulation before the initiation of aspirin, whereas all patients in WARFASA received at least 6 months of anticoagulation.[33,34] Despite these positive results, there are no major guidelines that recommend the use of aspirin for the secondary prevention of VTE.

Warfarin

The effect of warfarin in patients with idiopathic VTE who had received full-dose anticoagulation therapy for at least 6 months was studied in the PREVENT trial.[36] The trial was terminated early because of the highly significant 64% reduction in recurrent VTE among patients who received warfarin compared with those receiving placebo (see **Table 5**). There was no significant difference in the rate of bleeding between the two groups. Another trial, ELATE, compared low-intensity warfarin therapy (target INR of 1.5–1.9) with conventional-intensity warfarin therapy (target INR of 2.0–3.0) for long-term prevention of recurrent VTE. The trial showed that conventional-intensity warfarin therapy is more effective than low-intensity warfarin therapy for the long-term prevention of recurrent VTE, with no statically significant difference in the rate of bleeding (see **Table 5**).[37]

LMWH

High-quality evidence now indicates that patients with cancer-associated VTE should receive LMWH monotherapy for at least several months.[38] Rarely, chronic LMWH therapy may be necessary for patients without cancer; it might be appropriate for patients who cannot tolerate warfarin or for patients who experience recurrent thrombosis despite well-documented, therapeutic anticoagulation with warfarin. However, the NOAC agents may be a better alternative in these circumstances.[39,40]

Table 5
Summary of new oral anticoagulant agent trials for secondary prevention of venous thromboembolism

			Treatment		Outcome		Safety
							Fatal
		Mean	Group 1	Group 2	Recurrent VTE Events (Group 1/ Group 2)	Major Bleeding (Group 1/ Group 2)	Bleeding Events (Group 1/ Group 2)
Study (Patients)	Design	Treatment Duration	(No. of Patients)	(No. of Patients)			
ELATE[37] (VTE)	Randomized, double-blind trial	2.4 y	VKA standard dose with target INR: 2–3 (369)	VKA low dose with target INR: 1.5–1.9 (369)	6/16	8/9	0/0
PREVENT[36] (VTE)	Randomized, double-blind trial	2.1 y	Placebo (253)	VKA low dose with target INR: 1.5–2.0 (255)	37/14	2/5	1/0
RESONATE[42] (VTE)	Randomized, double-blind trial	6 mo	Placebo (662)	Dabigatran, 150 mg twice daily (681)	37/3	0/2	0/0
REMEDY[41] (VTE)	Randomized, double-blind trial	18 mo	Standard dose VKA with target INR (2–3) (1426)	Dabigatran, 150 mg twice daily (1430)	18/26	25/13	1/0
EINSTEIN-EXT[43] (VTE)	Randomized, double-blind trial	265 d	Placebo (594)	Rivaroxaban, 20 mg daily (602)	42/8	0/4	0/0
AMPLIFY-EXT[44] (VTE)	Randomized, double-blind trial	12 mo	Placebo (829)	Apixaban, 5 mg twice daily (813) or apixaban, 2.5 mg twice daily[a] (840)	73/14/14[a]	4/1/2[a]	0/0/0[a]
WARFASA[35] (VTE)	Randomized, double-blind trial	23.9 mo	Placebo (197)	Aspirin, 100 mg daily (205)	39/23	1/1	Not reported
ASPIRE[34] (VTE)	Randomized, double-blind trial	37.2 mo	Placebo (411)	Aspirin, 100 mg daily (411)	73/57	6/8	2/0

Abbreviations: INR, international normalized ratio; VKA, vitamin K antagonist; VTE, venous thromboembolism.
[a] In the AMPLIFY trial, three groups were included (Group 1, placebo; Group 2, apixaban 5 mg twice daily; Group 3, apixaban 2.5 mg twice daily). The outcome and safety data were reported in this table as (Group 1/Group 2/Group 3).

NOAC

The efficacy of the oral direct thrombin inhibitor dabigatran and the oral direct factor Xa inhibitors rivaroxaban and apixaban for treatment of unprovoked VTE for extended duration has been investigated (see **Table 5**). Although several phase III trials have demonstrated that all the NOAC (dabigatran, rivaroxaban, and apixaban [both 2.5 mg and 5 mg twice daily]) reduced the risk of recurrent VTE among patients requiring secondary prevention of VTE, so far, only one trial has compared NOACs with VKAs (dabigatran vs warfarin)[41]; the remaining trials have compared NOACs with placebo.[42-44] In addition, real world studies with longer follow-up periods are needed to evaluate the efficacy of these therapies when used for outpatient management and PE management, in addition to their efficacy in preventing major bleeding, particularly in the elderly and in patients using dual antiplatelet therapy.

SUMMARY

The exact required duration of VTE treatment is still unclear. The risk of recurrent VTE and major bleeding are fundamental considerations in a doctor's recommendation for secondary prevention of VTE and which agent to choose. Novel, target-specific oral anticoagulants have the potential to dramatically simplify and improve the existing paradigm of acute VTE treatment compared with parenteral heparin bridging therapy and VKA, with at least similar outcomes. Further research is necessary to see their effects in special patient populations, such as the elderly, patients with renal insufficiency, and patients with high bleeding risk or on multiple antithrombotic agents.

REFERENCES

1. Spyropoulos AC, Turpie A. Venous thromboembolism management: where do novel anticoagulants fit? Curr Med Res Opin 2013;29:783–90.
2. Kearon C. A conceptual framework for two phases of anticoagulant treatment of venous thromboembolism. J Thromb Haemost 2012;10:507–11.
3. Heit JA, Mohr DN, Silverstein MD, et al. Predictors of recurrence after deep vein thrombosis and pulmonary embolism: a population-based cohort study. Arch Intern Med 2000;160:761–8.
4. Kearon C. Natural history of venous thromboembolism. Circulation 2003;107: I-22–30.
5. Kearon C, Kahn SR, Agnelli G, et al. Antithrombotic therapy for venous thromboembolic disease. ACCP Evidence-Based Clinical Practice Guidelines (8th Edition). Chest 2008;133:454S–545S.
6. Kearon C, Ginsberg JS, Anderson DR, et al. Comparison of 1 month with 3 months of anticoagulation for a first episode of venous thromboembolism associated with a transient risk factor. J Thromb Haemost 2004;2:743–9.
7. Pinede L, Duhaut P, Cucherat M, et al. Comparison of long versus short duration of anticoagulant therapy after a first episode of venous thromboembolism: a meta-analysis of randomized, controlled trials. J Intern Med 2000;247:553–62.
8. Kearon C, Akl EA, Comerota AJ, et al. Antithrombotic therapy for VTE disease: antithrombotic therapy and prevention of thrombosis, 9th ed: ACCP Evidence-Based Clinical Practice Guidelines. Chest 2012;141(Suppl 2):e419S–94S.
9. Hansson PO, Sörbo J, Eriksson H. Recurrent venous thromboembolism after deep vein thrombosis: incidence and risk factors. Arch Intern Med 2000;160: 769–74.
10. Pinede L, Ninet J, Duhaut P, et al. Investigators of the (DOTAVK) Study. Comparison of 3 and 6 months of oral anticoagulant therapy after a first episode of

proximal deep vein thrombosis or pulmonary embolism and comparison of 6 and 12 weeks of therapy after isolated calf deep vein thrombosis. Circulation 2001;103:2453–60.

11. Schulman S, Rhedin AS, Lindmarker P, et al. Duration of Anticoagulation Trial Study Group. A comparison of six weeks with six months of oral anticoagulant therapy after a first episode of venous thromboembolism. N Engl J Med 1995;332: 1661–5.

12. Boutitie F, Pinede L, Schulman S, et al. Influence of preceding duration of anticoagulant treatment and initial presentation of venous thromboembolism on risk of recurrence after stopping therapy: analysis of individual participants' data from seven trials. BMJ 2011;342:d3036.

13. Lee AY, Levine MN, Baker RI, et al. Randomized comparison of low-molecular-weight heparin versus oral anticoagulant therapy for the prevention of recurrent venous thromboembolism in patients with cancer. N Engl J Med 2003;349:146–53.

14. Schulman S, Wahlander K, Lundström T, et al. THRIVE III Investigators. Secondary prevention of venous thromboembolism with the oral direct thrombin inhibitor ximelagatran. N Engl J Med 2003;349:1713–21.

15. Merli G. Anticoagulants in the treatment of deep vein thrombosis. Am J Med 2005;118(Suppl 8A):13S–20S.

16. Groce JB. Initial management of deep venous thrombosis in the outpatient setting. Am J Health Syst Pharm 2008;65:866–74.

17. Spyropoulos A, Kardos J, Wigal P. Outcomes analyses of the outpatient treatment of venous thromboembolic disease using the low-molecular weight heparin enoxaparin in a managed care organization. J Manag Care Pharm 2000;6:298–306.

18. Aujesky D, Obrosky DS, Stone RA, et al. Derivation and validation of a prognostic model for pulmonary embolism. Am J Respir Crit Care Med 2005;172: 1041–6.

19. Jimenez D, Aujesky D, Moores L, et al. Simplification of the pulmonary embolism severity index for prognostication in patients with acute symptomatic pulmonary embolism. Arch Intern Med 2010;170:1383–9.

20. Wicki J, Perrier A, Perneger TV. Predicting adverse outcome in patients with acute pulmonary embolism: a risk score. Thromb Haemost 2000;84:548–52.

21. Torbicki A, Perrier A, Konstantinides S, et al. The task force for the diagnosis and management of acute pulmonary embolism of the European Society of Cardiology (ESC). Guidelines on the diagnosis and management of acute pulmonary embolism. Eur Heart J 2008;29:2276–315.

22. Vanni S, Nazerian P, Pepe G, et al. Comparison of two prognostic models for acute pulmonary embolism: clinical vs. right ventricular dysfunction-guided approach. J Thromb Haemost 2011;9:1916–23.

23. Lankeit M, Gomez V, Wagner C, et al. A strategy combining imaging and laboratory biomarkers in comparison with a simplified clinical score for risk stratification of patients with acute pulmonary embolism. Chest 2012;141:916–22.

24. Agterof MJ, Schutgens RE, Snijder RJ, et al. Out of hospital treatment of acute pulmonary embolism in patients with a low NT-proBNP level. J Thromb Haemost 2010;8:1235–41.

25. Barra S, Paiva L, Providencia R, et al. LR-PED rule: low risk pulmonary embolism decision rule: a new decision score for low risk pulmonary embolism. Thromb Res 2012;130:327–33.

26. Aujesky D, Roy PM, Verschuren F, et al. Outpatient versus inpatient treatment for patients with acute pulmonary embolism: an international, open-label, randomized, non-inferiority trial. Lancet 2011;378:41–8.

27. Dalen JE. The uncertain role of thrombolytic therapy in the treatment of pulmonary embolism. Arch Intern Med 2002;162(22):2521.
28. Bernard J, Yi ES. Pulmonary thromboendarterectomy: a clinicopathologic study of 200 consecutive pulmonary thromboendarterectomy cases in one institution. Hum Pathol 2007;38:871-7.
29. Schulman S, Kearon C, Kakkar AK, et al. Dabigatran versus warfarin in the treatment of acute venous thromboembolism. N Engl J Med 2009;361:2342-52.
30. The Hokusai-VTE Investigators. Edoxaban versus warfarin for the treatment of symptomatic venous thromboembolism. N Engl J Med 2013;369:1406-15.
31. Agnelli G, Buller HR, AMPLIFY Investigators, et al. Oral apixaban for the treatment of acute venous thromboembolism. N Engl J Med 2013;369:799-808.
32. Bauersachs R, Berkowitz SD, Brenner B, et al. Oral rivaroxaban for symptomatic venous thromboembolism. N Engl J Med 2010;363:2499-510.
33. Prandoni P, Lensing AW, Cogo A, et al. The long-term clinical course of acute deep venous thrombosis. Ann Intern Med 1996;125:1-7.
34. Brighton AT, Eikelboom JW, Mann K, et al. Low-dose aspirin for preventing recurrent venous thromboembolism. N Engl J Med 2012;367:1979-87.
35. Becattini C, Agnelli G, Schenone A, et al. Aspirin for preventing the recurrence of venous thromboembolism. N Engl J Med 2012;366:1959-67.
36. Ridker PM, Goldhaber SZ, Danielson E, et al. Long-term, low-intensity warfarin therapy for the prevention of recurrent venous thromboembolism. N Engl J Med 2003;348:1425-34.
37. Kearon C, Ginsberg JS, Kovacs MJ, et al. Comparison of low-intensity warfarin therapy with conventional-intensity warfarin therapy for long-term prevention of recurrent venous thromboembolism. N Engl J Med 2003;349:631-9.
38. Noble SI, Shelley MD, Coles B, et al. Management of venous thromboembolism in patients with advanced cancer: a systematic review and meta-analysis. Lancet Oncol 2008;9(6):577.
39. Hull RD, Pineo GF, Brant RF, et al. Long-term low-molecular-weight heparin versus usual care in proximal-vein thrombosis patients with cancer. Am J Med 2006;119:1062-72.
40. Garcia DA, Spyropoulos AC. Update in the treatment of venous thromboembolism. Semin Respir Crit Care Med 2008;29:40-6.
41. Schulman S, Eriksson H, Goldhaber SZ, et al. Dabigatran or warfarin for extended maintenance therapy of venous thromboembolism [abstract O-TH-033]. ISTH 2011. J Thromb Haemost 2011;9(Suppl 2):731.
42. Schulman S, Baanstra D, Eriksson H, et al. Dabigatran versus placebo for extended maintenance therapy of venous thromboembolism [abstract 037]. ISTH 2011. J Thromb Haemost 2011;9(Suppl 2):731.
43. Romualdi E, Donadini MP, Ageno W. Oral rivaroxaban after symptomatic venous thromboembolism: the continued treatment study (EINSTEIN-extension study). Expert Rev Cardiovasc Ther 2011;9:841-4.
44. Agnelli G, Buller HR, Cohen A, et al. Apixaban for extended treatment of venous thromboembolism. N Engl J Med 2013;368:699-708.
45. Spyropoulos AC. Outpatient-based treatment protocols in the management of venous thromboembolic disease. Am J Manag Care 2000;6(Suppl 20): S1034-44.
46. Pradaxa (Dabigatran) [Package Insert]. Ridgefield, CT: Boehringer Ingelheim Pharmaceuticals; 2012.
47. Xarelto (Rivaroxaban) [Package Insert]. Titusville, NJ: Janssen Pharmaceuticals; 2011.

48. Eliquis (Apixaban) [Prescribing Information]. Princeton, NJ: Bristol-Myers Squibb Company; 2012.

49. Ogata K, Mendell-Harary J, Tachibana M, et al. Clinical safety, tolerability, pharmacokinetics and pharmacodynamics of the novel factor Xa inhibitor edoxaban in healthy volunteers. J Clin Pharmacol 2010;50:743–53.

50. Buller HR, Prins MH, Lensin AW, et al. Oral rivaroxaban for the treatment of symptomatic pulmonary embolism. N Engl J Med 2012;366:1287–97.

51. Schulman S, Kakkar AK, Schellong SM, et al. A randomized trial of dabigatran versus warfarin in the treatment of acute venous thromboembolism (RE-COVER II) [abstract 205]. American Society of Hematology 2011 Annual Meeting. San Diego. 2011.

Anticoagulation Strategies for the Management of Postoperative Atrial Fibrillation

Eric Anderson, MD[a], Cornelius Dyke, MD[a,b],*, Jerrold H. Levy, MD, FAHA, FCCM[c]

KEYWORDS

- Postoperative atrial fibrillation • Anticoagulation • Antiplatelet therapy • Rate control
- Risk factors

KEY POINTS

- Risk factors for postoperative atrial fibrillation (POAF) include increasing age, male gender, European ancestry, hypertension, prior myocardial infarction, heart failure, increasing grade of diastolic dysfunction, left atrial enlargement, general thoracic and cardiac procedures.
- POAF usually occurs within 5 days of surgery, with a peak onset on postoperative day 2, and is usually self-limited.
- POAF is associated with a 2- fold to 3-fold increased risk of postoperative stroke, higher 30-day mortalities, longer intensive care unit and hospital stays, higher costs, and higher complication rates compared with non-POAF patients.
- POAF is associated with an 8-fold increased risk of developing late atrial fibrillation (AF), a 2-fold increased risk of cardiovascular mortality, and is an independent risk factor for late stroke and mortality after isolated coronary artery bypass grafting.
- Rhythm control is not superior to rate control and is associated with higher adverse drug reactions and rehospitalization rates.
- Patients with persistent or paroxysmal POAF for greater than 48 hours should be anticoagulated owing to the increased risk of postoperative stroke and should be anticoagulated for at least 4 weeks after restoration of normal sinus rhythm.
- Oral anticoagulation with warfarin has been the standard of care for patients requiring anticoagulation for AF after cardiac surgery, including POAF. Newer oral factor II and factor X antagonists are indicated and available for the management of nonvalvular AF, although there is limited evidence regarding their use in the postoperative setting. Head-to-head trials between these new oral anticoagulants in a perioperative setting are needed.

Conflict of Interest Statements: None (E. Anderson, MD); Consultant: The Medicines Company, Grifols S.A; Speaker's Bureau: Pfizer, Bristol-Myers Squibb (C. Dyke, MD); Prof. J.H. Levy serves on steering committees for Boehringer Ingelheim, CSL Behring AG, Grifols, Janssen Pharmaceuticals, and The Medicines Company.

[a] Department of Surgery, University of North Dakota School of Medicine and Health Sciences, Grand Forks, 501 North Columbia Road Stop 9037, ND 58103, USA; [b] Department of Cardiothoracic Surgery, Sanford Health Fargo, 801 Broadway North, Fargo, ND 58122, USA; [c] Duke University School of Medicine, Divisions of Cardiothoracic Anesthesiology and Critical Care, Duke University Hospital, 2301 Erwin Road, Durham, NC 27710, USA
* Corresponding author. Sanford Health Fargo, 801 Broadway North, Fargo, ND 58122.
E-mail address: Cornelius.Dyke@sanfordhealth.org

Clin Lab Med 34 (2014) 537–561
http://dx.doi.org/10.1016/j.cll.2014.06.012
0272-2712/14/$ – see front matter © 2014 Elsevier Inc. All rights reserved.

INTRODUCTION
Incidence of Atrial Fibrillation

In the general population, chronic atrial fibrillation (AF) is a disease that most often occurs in the elderly. The prevalence of AF is approximately 1% to 3% in the adult population, with a doubling in the incidence of AF for each decade of life after age 50.[1–4] Risk factors for developing chronic AF include advancing age, male gender, European ancestry, diabetes mellitus, hypertension, heart failure, valvular heart disease, and history of myocardial infarction (MI).[3–5] With an aging population in the United States and around the world, the prevalence of AF is expected to increase rapidly over the next several decades. In the United States, the number of patients living with AF is expected to increase from approximately 6 million people currently to more than 10 million by 2025.[5]

Postoperative atrial fibrillation (POAF) is defined as the development of new-onset AF in the immediate postoperative period. POAF may occur in any surgical population, but is more common in patients undergoing cardiac or thoracic surgical procedures. In cardiac surgical or thoracic surgical patients, POAF usually occurs within the first 5 postoperative days, with a peak onset on postoperative day 2.[6–10] The incidence of POAF following general thoracic surgery procedures ranges from 10% to 20% of patients, compared with 20% to 40% in patients undergoing cardiac surgery.[11–25] In a study evaluating 13,696 noncardiac, nonthoracic surgical patients, the incidence of POAF was only 0.37%.[26] Similarly, in a large database analysis of more than 370,000 noncardiac surgical patients undergoing surgery (including thoracic procedures), the rate of POAF was 1%.[27] In this study, patients undergoing thoracic, intracranial, or intra-abdominal procedures were at increased risk of developing POAF when compared with patients undergoing orthopedic, spine, genitourinary, vascular, and otolaryngologic procedures. Patients who developed POAF were generally older (median age 74), had at least one cardiac risk factor, and had a positive fluid balance.[26,27]

Patients undergoing cardiac procedures have the highest incidence of POAF. Procedures associated with the highest risk (in increasing order) include isolated coronary artery bypass graft (CABG), isolated valvular procedures, combined CABG and valve procedures, and combined valve procedures. Isolated CABG surgery using traditional sternotomy and on-pump techniques is associated with a POAF rate of approximately 20% to 30%, whereas isolated valve procedures carry a higher risk of 30% to 40%; the rate is even higher in patients undergoing combined CABG and valve procedures, with a rate of 40% to 55%.[8,9,16,17,20,23] Rates of POAF as high as 80% have been reported in patients undergoing combined valvular procedures.[20]

Risk Factors for the Development of POAF

Elderly patients undergoing noncardiac surgery have been reported to have postoperative atrial arrhythmia rates as high as 6.1%.[28] Age greater than 70, history of congestive heart failure, significant valvular disease, and premature atrial contractions on preoperative electrocardiography were patient characteristics found to be independent predictors of developing POAF, with adjusted odds ratios ranging from 1.3 to 2.1. Certain noncardiac procedures have also been associated with an independent risk of developing POAF, including thoracic aortic aneurysm procedures, abdominal aortic aneurysm procedures, abdominal procedures, and vascular procedures.[28]

In thoracic, noncardiac surgical patients, increasing age (each decade after age 50), male gender, European ancestry, and history of heart failure are independently associated with the development of POAF.[6,7,11–13] Furthermore, the rate of POAF increases with increasing levels of lung resection. Wedge resection or segmental lung resection carries the lowest risk, with rates of POAF as low as 1% in this population, whereas pneumonectomy carries a risk of 20% to 25%, nearing the rates of POAF seen in patients undergoing isolated CABG.[13–15] When compared with wedge resection, the relative risk (RR) of POAF is 3.89 for patients undergoing lobectomy, 7.19 for patients undergoing bilobectomy, and 8.91 for patients undergoing pneumonectomy.[11] Esophagectomy also carries an independent increased risk of POAF, but at a rate less than that of major lung resection.[11] POAF in most general thoracic surgery patients is of short duration, with 80% of patients returning to normal sinus rhythm within 3 days of onset, and less than 3% of patients being discharged with POAF.[7,15]

Risk factors for POAF in the cardiac surgical population are well defined. European ancestry is an independent predictor of increased risk of POAF when compared with African American ancestry.[16–18] Increasing age, increasing grade of diastolic dysfunction, and combined CABG with valve procedures are the strongest independent predictors of POAF in cardiac surgery patients, whereas male gender, heart failure, hypertension, left atrial enlargement, valve procedures, and prior MI are also independent predictors of increased risk.[8,17,18,20,21] As discussed previously, the type of cardiac procedure affects the risk of developing POAF, with isolated CABG carrying the lowest risk and combined valve procedures carrying the highest risk. The surgical approach in cardiac surgical patients has also been shown to have an effect on POAF rates. Minimally invasive approaches to valve repair do appear to reduce the risk of POAF, with the use of minithoracotomy for valve replacement carrying a reduced risk when compared with traditional sternotomy or ministernotomy in similar patient populations.[19,29,30] The rates of POAF may also be reduced by almost 50% in high-risk patients undergoing transcatheter aortic valve implantation (transfemoral or transapical) when compared with a standard open approach.[31] Although the rates of POAF after any cardiac surgical procedure are high, it is usually transient, with only 5% to 8% of patients being discharged with persistent AF.[8–10]

CONSEQUENCES OF DEVELOPING POAF

AF in the general population is associated with a 3-fold to 5-fold increased stroke rate when compared with patients without AF.[2,4] The attributable risk of stroke from diabetes mellitus, heart failure, hypertension, and coronary artery disease tends to decrease with advancing age, whereas AF has an increasing rate of attributable risk as age increases, with a 1.5% to 2.6% attributable risk of stroke in patients 50 to 59 years of age, increasing to 20% to 25% in patients 80 to 89 years of age.[1,2,4] Risk factors for the development of stroke in AF patients have been well studied, with the $CHADS_2$ and CHA_2DS_2-VASc scores being commonly used for the assessment of stroke risk in AF patients (see assessment of stroke risk in later discussion). The risk of stroke or systemic thromboembolism (SSTE) is independent of the type of AF: paroxysmal versus persistent/permanent.[32–35] POAF in general thoracic surgery patients is associated with higher intensive care unit (ICU) admission rates, longer hospital stays, higher costs, higher postoperative complication rates, and higher in-hospital and 30-day mortality rates.[11–14] Even when POAF is the only postoperative complication, hospital costs are still higher.[6,11] POAF in the acute setting has not been shown to be an independent predictor of death. In cardiac surgery, POAF is associated with several adverse short-term outcomes. Large institutional studies and meta-analyses of up to 40,000 patients found that patients with POAF have an increased risk of postoperative stroke (2–3 times that of non-POAF patients), higher 30-day postoperative mortality, longer ICU stays, longer hospital stays, higher rates of postoperative acute renal failure, and higher rates of postoperative complications overall.[36–41] When studies were designed to evaluate POAF as an independent predictor of outcomes after isolated CABG, POAF was still an independent predictor of increased risk of postoperative stroke (adjusted odds ratio ~1.80), but was not an independent predictor of 30-day postoperative mortality.[24,42] When looking at isolated aortic valve replacements, POAF was not an independent predictor of either stroke or 30-day postoperative mortality.[25]

POAF is an independent predictor for the development of persistent AF after discharge.[43–45] Although rates of late AF are relatively low after cardiac surgery, POAF is associated with an 8-fold increased risk of developing late AF, at a rate of 5% per year.[43,44] POAF is also an independent risk factor for stroke and late mortality after isolated CABG, but not after valve surgery, suggesting that differences in anticoagulation in these 2 populations may play a role in long-term outcomes.[23–25,37,46] The effect of POAF on stroke and long-term mortality in patients undergoing combined procedures is less clear.[23,47]

PREVENTING POAF

Significant research has been dedicated to the prevention of POAF in the cardiothoracic surgical patient. The most commonly studied prophylactic medications including β-blockers, amiodarone, HMG-CoA reductase inhibitors (statins), magnesium, angiotensin-converting-enzyme inhibitors (ACE-Is)/angiotensin II-receptor-blockers (ARBs), and polyunsaturated fatty acids (PUFAs). There are convincing data to support the use of β-blocker prophylaxis in the prevention of POAF. At least 10 randomized controlled trials (RCTs) have evaluated the effects of β-blockers on POAF after CABG. Seven of the 10 trials found that β-blocker prophylaxis significantly reduced the risk of POAF, and a meta-analysis of these studies found a statistically significant 50% reduction in POAF.[48] Of note, 8 of the 10 trials evaluated the use of postoperative β-blockers on POAF, whereas only 2 trials evaluated the effects of preoperative β-blockers on POAF. The findings of this meta-analysis are consistent with American College of Cardiology/American Heart Association (ACC/AHA) guidelines, which have a class I recommendation for the use of oral β-blockers after cardiac surgery to prevent POAF.[49]

The prophylactic benefits of amiodarone have been well studied in both cardiac and general thoracic surgery patients. At least 23 RCTs have evaluated the effects of amiodarone on POAF, and a meta-analysis of these studies found that both oral-only and combined oral/intravenous (IV) regimens of amiodarone reduced the risk of POAF by 41% to 43%, irrespective of preoperative or postoperative administration strategies.[50] Furthermore, a meta-analysis comparing amiodarone versus β-blockers for the prevention of POAF after cardiac surgery found no statistically significant difference in preventative effects or in adverse events after surgery.[51] The beneficial effects of amiodarone are also well documented in RCTs in pulmonary resection patients, with absolute risk reductions of 18% to 23% and a relative risk reduction (RRR) greater than 50%.[52,53]

RCTs evaluating the effects of preoperative statin use in cardiac surgery patients have largely been small in size with mixed results. Two meta-analyses evaluating RCTs published in 2010 and 2012, including 8 and 11 studies, respectively, have helped clarify their benefits. Both meta-analyses found that preoperative statin use significantly reduced the risk of POAF after cardiac surgery, with an RR of 0.57 (risk difference −0.14) or an odds ratio of 0.40.[54,55]

The Use of Magnesium, PUFAs, or ACE-Is/ARB

The use of magnesium, PUFAs, or ACE-Is/ARBs is less well validated, and controversial. Early studies and smaller RCTs evaluating magnesium, and meta-analyses including these studies found prophylactic magnesium to be of benefit in reducing the risk of POAF. More recent RCTs and meta-analyses, that focused on eliminating poorly designed trials to reduce the heterogeneity among studies and evaluated the effects of prophylactic magnesium on POAF, have shown that magnesium does not provide a significant reduction in POAF.[56,57] The effects of PUFAs are even more controversial, with varying results obtained in RCTs. In addition, in various meta-analyses using the same clinical trials, differing conclusions have been reached depending on the statistical methods used.[58,59] ACE-Is and ARBs have largely been proven to be of no benefit for the prevention of POAF in cardiac surgery patients and may in fact increase the risk of POAF and other negative outcomes after cardiac surgery.[60,61]

MANAGEMENT STRATEGIES IN POAF: RATE VERSUS RHYTHM CONTROL

Several RCTs published in the early 2000s (RACE, AFFIRM, PIAF, STAF, and HOT CAFÉ) evaluated various strategies of rate control versus rhythm control in patients with AF.[62–66] Rate control strategies primarily consisted of treatment with β-blockers, calcium channel blockers, digoxin, or a combination of these drugs. Rhythm control strategies consisted of recurrent direct current cardioversion (DCC) as required, alongside the use of a large variety of antiarrhythmic agents (amiodarone, disopyramide, flecainide, moricizine, procainamide, propafenone, quinidine, sotalol, or a combination of these medications), to maintain normal sinus rhythm, allowing for adjustments in medication regimens after cardioversion for recurrent episodes. Primary outcomes evaluated in these studies included various composite outcomes focusing on death, SSTE, bleeding, and adverse cardiac outcomes. Other outcomes included rates of stroke, rehospitalization, adverse drug events, improvement of symptoms, and exercise tolerance.

None of the 5 studies found rhythm control to be superior to rate control of AF for their primary outcome, and there was no difference in stroke or SSTE rates.[62–66] Rhythm control was associated with higher rates of rehospitalization and higher rates of adverse drug reactions when compared with rate control, but was also associated with higher exercise tolerance.[63–66] In the AFFIRM study, rate control was associated with a nonsignificant, but lower 5-year mortality compared with rhythm control.[63] The most common reasons for crossover from rhythm control to rate control were inability to maintain sinus rhythm and drug intolerance, whereas uncontrolled symptoms due to AF and congestive heart failure were the most common reasons for crossover from rate control to rhythm control.[63] The lack of superiority of rhythm control over rate control for AF has been further substantiated in patients with POAF; no significant difference was observed in AF rates in short-term outpatient follow-up, ranging from 6 to 8 weeks, although patients treated with rhythm control strategies did have shorter hospital stays.[67,68]

Rate control regimens using β-blockers (with or without digoxin) are the most effective, with overall rate control (at rest and with activity) achieved in 70% of patients, whereas rate control is achieved in 54% of patients with calcium channel blocker regimens (with or without digoxin), and in 58% of patients with digoxin alone.[69] These findings are consistent with ACC/AHA guidelines, which recommend rate control strategies using β-blockers or calcium channel blockers (with or without digoxin) in patients with normal cardiac function, whereas patients with left ventricular dysfunction, heart failure, or a sedentary lifestyle should consider rate control strategies using digoxin.[49] In the acute setting, IV β-blockers (esmolol, metoprolol, propranolol) or calcium channel blockers (verapamil, diltiazem) are recommended as first-line treatment, with IV digoxin or amiodarone used in patients with hypotension or heart failure.[49]

Pharmacologic Cardioversion and/or Synchronized DCC

Rhythm control strategies with pharmacologic cardioversion and/or synchronized DCC should be undertaken in patients who have uncontrolled symptoms due to AF, developing congestive heart failure, hemodynamic instability, or a preference for rhythm control strategy. If pharmacologic cardioversion is to be undertaken, flecainide, dofetilide, propafenone, or ibutilide are recommended as first-line agents, while amiodarone is considered a reasonable alternative, and quinidine or procainamide may be considered, but fewer data exist to support these medications.[49] Synchronized DCC should be performed in patients with AF in rapid ventricular response that does not respond to pharmacologic measures, in association with active acute coronary syndrome (ACS), symptomatic hypotension, or heart failure. Antiarrhythmic agents (ACC/AHA recommend amiodarone, flecainide, ibutilide, propafenone, or sotalol) may be used in conjunction with synchronized DCC to increase the success rate of cardioversion to normal sinus rhythm or for the maintenance of normal sinus rhythm after synchronized DCC.[70–72]

Current national guidelines recommend anticoagulation (international normalized ratio [INR] 2.0–3.0) for at least 3 weeks before and 4 weeks after cardioversion (pharmacologic or synchronized DCC) in patients with AF of unknown duration or of 48 hours or more.[49] These recommendations are largely made based on the known benefits of anticoagulation on risk reduction of stroke in patients with AF, and on results from small retrospective studies that have found that although rates of SSTE in AF patients undergoing cardioversion are low (1.33%), all of the patients who had an episode of SSTE either were not on anticoagulation or had been anticoagulated for less than 1 week.[73] Patients with AF for 48 hours or more with hemodynamic instability should be treated with a heparin bolus and heparin drip until the partial thromboplastin time is 1.5 to 2.0 times the upper limit of normal or factor Xa levels are therapeutic, and undergo synchronized DCC followed by 4 weeks of postcardioversion anticoagulation (target INR 2.0–3.0).[49] Patients with AF for less than 48 hours with hemodynamic instability should undergo synchronized DCC without waiting for initiation of anticoagulation, whereas a patient-by-patient assessment of SSTE should be undertaken in stable patients with AF for less than 48 hours to determine if anticoagulation is needed before or after cardioversion.[49]

PREVENTION OF THROMBOEMBOLISM
Assessment/Risk Stratification of Stroke and Thromboembolism

Prior stroke/transient ischemic attacks/systemic thromboembolism, age 75 or more, and valvular heart disease are all considered strong predictors of stroke. Non-major risk factors for stroke are heart failure/left ventricular dysfunction, hypertension, diabetes mellitus, female gender, age 65 to 75, and vascular disease (prior MI, complex aortic plaque, and peripheral arterial disease), with the latter 3 factors considered to be less well validated.[49,74] These risk factors have been used to create risk-predicting models of stroke, with $CHAD_2$ and CHA_2DS_2-VASc being the most commonly used. The $CHADS_2$ score system was developed to unify stroke risk factors identified by the Atrial Fibrillation Investigators and the Stroke Prevention and Atrial Fibrillation (SPAF) investigators. The $CHADS_2$ score system has been well validated, with stroke rate increasing with increasing scores (**Tables 1 and 2**).[75]

Although the $CHADS_2$ scoring system provided a sensitive and easy way to predict the risk of stroke in AF patients, the system placed a large number of patients in the low (score 0) and intermediate (score 1) categories. The CHA_2DS_2-VASc scoring system was published in 2010 and includes 3 additional stroke risk factors (vascular

Table 1
CHADS$_2$ point-based scoring system

Risk Factor	Points
CHF	1
Hypertension	1
Age ≥75 y	1
Diabetes mellitus	1
Stroke/TIA (previously)	2
Total score	0–6

Table of the CHADS$_2$ scoring system used for the assessment of stroke risk in patients with AF. Patients receive 1 point for each risk factor and 2 points for the risk factor of previous stroke or TIA. Total scores range from 0 to 6.
Abbreviations: CHF, chronic heart failure; TIA, transient ischemic attack.

disease [prior MI, peripheral arterial disease, or aortic plaque], age 65–74, gender category [female]) not previously identified in the CHADS$_2$ scoring system.[76] The CHA$_2$DS$_2$-VASc scoring system was able to decrease the number of patients in the low-risk and intermediate-risk groups, more accurately predicting who was at low (score 0) and intermediate (score 1) risk of stroke and further identifying patients who were truly at high risk (score 2–9) (**Tables 3** and **4**).[76,77]

Assessment of Bleeding Risk

In the management of POAF and chronic AF, the risk of stroke must be balanced against the risk of bleeding when considering anticoagulation strategies. In an effort to reduce the impact of bleeding in patients with AF, multiple predictive models for bleeding have been developed. These systems include the ATRIA hemorrhage risk score, HEMORR$_2$HAGES, and HAS-BLED scoring systems, which are used to predict the risk of major hemorrhage (**Tables 5–8**). All of these systems have been validated with moderate ability to predict the risk of bleeding.[78–81]

Table 2
Rate of stroke and SSTE risk based on CHADS$_2$ score

CHADS$_2$ Score	Annual Stroke Rate, % (95% CI)	Annual SSTE Rate, % (95% CI)
0	1.9 (1.2, 3.0)	1.24 (1.16, 1.33)
1	2.8 (2.0, 3.8)	3.56 (3.42, 3.70)
2	4.0 (3.1, 5.1)	5.40 (5.18, 5.63)
3	5.9 (4.6, 7.3)	9.89 (9.50, 10.31)
4	8.5 (6.3, 11.1)	13.70 (12.95, 14.48)
5	12.5 (8.2, 17.5)	12.57 (11.18, 14.14)
6	18.2 (10.5, 27.4)	17.17 (12.33, 23.92)
Low risk (0)		1.24 (1.16, 1.33)
Intermediate risk (1)		3.56 (3.42, 3.70)
High risk (2–6)		7.97 (7.77, 8.17)

Table shows the annual rates of stroke or SSTE in patients with AF who are not on anticoagulation, based on their composite CHADS$_2$ score. The data in the table are based on published literature of validation studies of the CHADS$_2$ scoring system.

Table 3
CHA$_2$DS$_2$-VASc point-based scoring system

Risk Factor	Points
CHF/LV dysfunction	1
Hypertension	1
Age ≥75 y	2
Diabetes mellitus	1
SSTE/TIA (previously)	2
Vascular disease	1
Age 65–74 y	1
Sex category (female)	1
Total score	0–9

Table of the CHA$_2$DS$_2$-VASc scoring system used for the assessment of stroke risk in patients with AF. Patients receive 1 point for each risk factor and 2 points for the risk factors of previous SSTE/TIA and age ≥75. Total scores range from 0 to 9.

Abbreviations: CHF, chronic heart failure; LV, left ventricular; TIA, transient ischemic attack.

ANTITHROMBOTIC THERAPY FOR THE MANAGEMENT OF AF AND POAF
Evidence for Aspirin

Several studies have evaluated aspirin (acetylsalicylic acid; ASA) alone versus placebo or no treatment in patients with nonvalvular AF for primary and secondary prevention of stroke (**Table 9**). A meta-analysis of patients with non-valvular AF, including data from 7 studies and evaluating ASA versus placebo or no treatment (n = 3990), found that ASA had a nonsignificant reduction in stroke (RRR 19%; 95% CI: −1, 35), with an absolute risk reduction of 0.8% per year.[88] The benefits of ASA in the risk reduction of stroke in patients with AF are heavily influenced by the SPAF-I study, which found a

Table 4
Rate of SSTE based on CHA$_2$DS$_2$-VASc score

CHA$_2$DS$_2$-VASc Score	Annual SSTE Rate, % (95% CI)
0	0.66 (0.57, 0.76)
1	1.45 (1.32, 1.58)
2	2.92 (2.76, 3.09)
3	4.28 (4.10, 4.47)
4	6.46 (6.20, 6.74)
5	9.97 (9.53, 10.43)
6	12.52 (11.78, 13.31)
7	13.96 (12.57, 15.51)
8	14.10 (10.90, 18.23)
9	15.89 (7.95, 31.78)
Low risk (0)	0.66 (0.57, 0.76)
Intermediate risk (1)	1.45 (1.32, 1.58)
High risk (2–9)	5.72 (5.60, 5.84)

Table shows the annual rates of SSTE in patients with AF who are not on anticoagulation, based on their composite CHA$_2$DS$_2$-VASc Score. The data in the table are based on published literature of validation studies of the CHA$_2$DS$_2$-VASc scoring system.

Table 5	
HEMORR$_2$HAGES scoring system	
Risk Factor	**Score**
Hepatic or renal disease	1
Ethanol abuse	1
Malignancy	1
Older (age >75 y)	1
Reduced platelet count or function	1
Rebleeding risk	2
Hypertension (uncontrolled)	1
Anemia	1
Genetic factors	1
Excessive fall risk	1
Stroke	1
Total score	0–12

Table of the HEMORR$_2$HAGES scoring system for the assessment of bleeding risk in patient with AF. Patients receive 1 point for each risk factor, with 2 points awarded for rebleeding risk. Scores range from 0 to 12.

Table 6	
Major bleeding rates based on HEMORR$_2$HAGES score	
HEMORR$_2$HAGES Score	**Annual Major Bleeding Risk, % (95% CI)**
0	1.9 (0.6, 4.4)
1	2.5 (1.3, 4.3)
2	5.3 (3.4, 8.1)
3	8.4 (4.9, 13.6)
4	10.4 (5.1, 18.9)
$\geq$5	12.3 (5.8, 23.1)

Table of the annual risk of bleeding in AF patients based on their composite HEMORR$_2$HAGES score. Numbers are based on published literature for the validation of the scoring system.

Table 7	
HAS-BLED point-based scoring system	
Risk Factor	**Points**
Hypertension	1
Abnormal renal and liver function (1 point each)	1 or 2
Stroke	1
Bleeding history	1
Labile INRs	1
Elderly (Age >65 y)	1
Drugs or alcohol excess (1 point each)	1 or 2
Total score	0–9
Hypertension: systolic BP >160 Elderly: age >65 Drugs: antiplatelet agents, NSAIDs	

Table of the HAS-BLED scoring system for the assessment of bleeding risk in patient with AF. Patients receive 1 point for each risk factor. Scores range from 0 to 9.
   Abbreviations: BP, blood pressure; NSAIDs, nonsteroidal anti-inflammatory drugs.

Table 8
Major bleeding rates based on HAS-BLED score

HAS-BLED Score	Annual Major Bleeding Risk, % (95% CI)
0	1.13
1	1.02
2	1.88
3	3.74
4	8.7
≥5	12.5
Low risk	Total score 0
Moderate risk	Total score 1–2
High risk	Total score ≥3

Table of the annual risk of bleeding in AF patients based on their composite HAS-BLED score. Numbers are based on published literature for the validation of the HAS-BLED scoring system.

49% RRR in AF patients on ASA compared with placebo.[83] The study further found a 94% RRR in stroke in ASA patients who were warfarin ineligible compared with 8% in ASA patients who were warfarin eligible. In the JAST study, in which patients with lone AF were treated with ASA or received no treatment, there was no difference in primary outcomes, and ASA treatment resulted in a nonsignificant increase in major bleeding.[87]

Evidence for Vitamin K Antagonists/Warfarin

Adjusted-dose warfarin is an effective means of preventing stroke in patients with non-valvular AF, including POAF (**Table 10**). A meta-analysis including data from 5 primary prevention trials and one secondary prevention trial found that warfarin reduced the RR of stroke by 64% with an absolute risk reduction of 2.7% per year, resulting in a number needed to treat of 37 patients to prevent one stroke per year.[88] The results were similar for primary and secondary prevention. Other studies have found that most strokes in the anticoagulation arm occur in patients who are taken off anticoagulation or when the patients are subtherapeutic (INR <2). The risk of major bleeding in the 5 primary RCTs found an annual major bleeding rate of 1.2%. Warfarin is thought to double the risk of intracranial hemorrhage (ICH), but the absolute rate of ICH is quite low, ranging from 0.2% to 0.8% in RCTs and 0.1% to 0.6% in a large cohort study.[92]

Evidence for Vitamin K Antagonists/Warfarin Versus ASA

At least 8 randomized trials have evaluated vitamin K antagonists (at least 5 evaluating adjusted-dose warfarin) versus ASA in patients with nonvalvular AF, and the number of studies increases when trials using antiplatelet drugs other than ASA are included (**Table 11**). A meta-analysis of randomized trials found that adjusted-dose warfarin, when compared with ASA, reduced the RR of stroke by 38% (95% CI: 22%, 52%) with an absolute risk reduction of 0.7% per year; when compared with all antiplatelet agents, warfarin reduced the RR of stroke by 37% with an absolute risk reduction of 0.9% per year, and a 52% RRR in ischemic stroke.[88] Although patients on warfarin had higher rates of intracranial and major bleeding when compared with ASA, the absolute increased risk per year was low, at 0.2%.[88] In addition, the BAFTA trial found that well-controlled adjusted-dose warfarin treatment was not associated with an increased risk of major bleeding complications when compared with ASA.[96]

Table 9
AF ASA trials: outcomes (mortality, stroke, STE, major hemorrhage, ICH)

Study	Year	Source	Treatment	Control	Mortality Annual Rate (95% CI)	Stroke Annual Rate (95% CI)	STE Annual Rate (95% CI)	Major Hemorrhage Annual Rate (95% CI)	ICH Annual Rate (95% CI)
AFASAK-I	1989	82	ASA (75 mg/d)	Placebo	N/A	3.9% RR: 0.82 (0.42, 1.59)	0.5% RR: 0.97 (0.14, 6.91)	0.2% RR: N/A	0% RR: N/A
SPAF I	1991	83	ASA (325 mg/d)	Placebo	5.4% RR: 0.79 (0.52, 1.20)	3.2% RR: 0.56 (0.33, 0.92)	0.4% RR: 0.76 (0.17, 3.40)	1.4% RR: 0.73 (0.32, 1.63)	0.3% RR: 1.02 (0.14, 7.21)
EAFT	1993	84	ASA (300 mg/d)	Placebo	12.2% RR: 0.88 (0.67, 1.16)	10.5% RR: 0.83 (0.62, 1.12)	0.7% RR: 0.57 (0.20, 1.60)	0.7% RR: 1.28 (0.36, 4.54)	0.2% RR: 1.71 (0.15, 18.82)
ESPS II	1996	85	ASA (50 mg/d)	Placebo	N/A	13.8% RR: 0.67 (0.36, 1.25)	N/A	N/A	N/A
LASAF	1999	86	ASA (125 mg/d)	Placebo	4.8% RR: 0.72 (0.27, 1.93)	2.8% RR: 1.24 (0.28, 5.52)	N/A	N/A	N/A
LASAF	1999	86	ASA (125 mg/QOD)	Placebo	2.0% RR: 0.30 (0.08, 1.12)	0.7% RR: 0.30 (0.03, 2.92)	N/A	N/A	N/A
JAST	2006	87	ASA (150–200 mg/d)	No treatment	1.1% RR: 1.16 (0.47, 2.86)	1.9% RR: 0.99 (0.51, 1.91)	0% RR: N/A	0.8% RR: 3.66 (0.76, 17.60)	0.4% RR: 2.09 (0.38, 11.41)

Table of RCTs that evaluated the effects of ASA versus placebo/no treatment in patients with AF. Outcomes included are annual rates of mortality, stroke, systemic thromboembolism, major hemorrhage, and intracranial hemorrhage. Table includes RR calculations with their 95% CIs.
Abbreviations: CI, confidence interval; N/A, not available; QOD, every other day; STE, systemic thromboembolism.

Table 10
AF warfarin trials: outcomes (mortality, stroke, STE, major hemorrhage, ICH)

Study	Year	Source	Treatment	Control	Mortality Annual Rate (95% CI)	Stroke Annual Rate (95% CI)	STE Annual Rate (95% CI)	Major Hemorrhage Annual Rate (95% CI)	ICH Annual Rate (95% CI)
AFASAK-I	1989	82	Warfarin (INR: 2.8–4.2)	Placebo	N/A	2.7% RR: 0.56 (0.27, 1.17)	0% RR: 0	0.5% RR: N/A	0.2% RR: N/A
BAATAF	1990	89	Warfarin (INR: 1.5–2.7)	No treatment	2.3% RR: 0.38 (0.19, 0.76)	0.4% RR: 0.14 (0.03, 0.61)	0% RR: N/A	0.4% RR: 1.79 (0.16, 19.70)	0.2% RR: N/A
SPAF I	1991	83	Warfarin (INR: 2.0–4.5)	Placebo	2.3% RR: 0.70 (0.24, 2.03)	2.3% RR: 0.33 (0.13, 0.84)	0% RR: 0	1.5% RR: 0.94 (0.23, 3.75)	0.8% RR: 0.94 (0.13, 6.66)
CAFA	1991	90	Warfarin (INR: 2.0–3.0)	Placebo	5.1% RR: 1.53 (0.62, 3.73)	2.5% RR: 0.68 (0.24, 1.90)	0.4% RR: 0.51 (0.05, 5.61)	2.1% RR: 2.54 (0.49, 13.10)	0.4% RR: N/A
SPINAF	1992	91	Warfarin (INR: 1.4–2.8)	Placebo	3.5% RR: 0.67 (0.35, 1.27)	0.9% RR: 0.20 (0.07, 0.60)	0.4% RR: 1.93 (0.17, 21.26)	1.5% RR: 1.69 (0.49, 5.76)	0.2% RR: N/A

Table of RCTs that evaluated the effects of warfarin versus placebo/no treatment in patients with AF. Outcomes included are annual rates of mortality, stroke, STE, major hemorrhage, and ICH. Table includes RR calculations with their 95% CIs.
Abbreviations: CI, confidence interval; N/A, not available; STE, systemic thromboembolism.

Table 11
AF warfarin (WARF) versus ASA trials: outcomes (mortality, stroke, STE, major hemorrhage, ICH)

Study	Year	Source	Treatment: Warfarin	Treatment: ASA	Mortality Annual Rate: WARF vs ASA (95% CI)	Stroke Annual Rate: WARF vs ASA (95% CI)	STE Annual Rate: WARF vs ASA (95% CI)	Major Hemorrhage Annual Rate: WARF vs ASA (95% CI)	ICH Annual Rate: WARF vs ASA (95% CI)
AFASAK-I	1989	82	INR: 2.8–4.2	75 mg/d	N/A	2.7% vs 3.9% RR: 0.68 (0.32, 1.47)	0% vs 0.5% RR: 0	0.5% vs 0.2% RR: 1.98 (0.18, 21.84)	0.2% vs 0% RR: N/A
SPAF II (Age ≤75)	1994	93	INR: 2.0–4.5	325 mg/d	3.3% vs 3.8% RR: 0.87 (0.55, 1.35)	1.2% vs 1.8% RR: 0.67 (0.33, 1.37)	0.1% vs 0.2%: RR: 0.49 (0.04, 5.43)	1.7% vs 0.9% RR: 1.89 (not reported)	0.5% vs 0.2% RR: 2.96 (0.60, 14.65)
SPAF II (Age >75)	1994	93	INR: 2.0–4.5	325 mg/d	6.6% vs 6.4% RR: 1.04 (0.60, 1.81)	3.3% vs 4.8% RR: 0.69 (0.34, 1.41)	0.3% vs 0% RR: N/A	4.2% vs 1.6% RR: 2.63 (not reported)	1.8% vs 0.8% RR: 2.23 (0.58, 8.63)
AFASAK II	1998	94	INR: 2.0–3.0	325 mg/d	4.8% vs 3.8% RR: 1.25 (0.62, 2.53)	2.8% vs 2.5% RR: 1.14 (0.46, 2.81)	0.6% vs 0.3% RR: 2.06 (0.19, 22.68)	1.1% vs 1.4% RR: 0.82 (0.22, 3.06)	0.6% vs 0.3% RR: 2.06 (0.19, 22.68)
Hu et al	2006	95	INR: 2.0–3.0	150–160 mg/d	1.0% vs 3.2% RR: 0.45 (0.14, 1.51)	1.0% vs 3.2% RR: 0.32 (0.13, 0.81)	2.2% vs 4.1% RR: 0.54 (0.27, 1.06)	0.9% vs 0% RR: N/A	0.5% vs 0% RR: N/A
BAFTA	2007	96	INR: 2.0–3.0	75 mg/d	N/A	1.6% vs 3.4% RR: 0.47 (0.28, 0.80)	0.1% vs 0.2% RR: 0.33 (0.03, 3.19)	1.9% vs 1.9% RR: 0.99 (0.57, 1.73)	0.6% vs 0.5% RR: 1.33 (0.46, 3.82)

Table of RCTs that evaluated the effects of warfarin *versus* ASA in patients with AF. Outcomes included are annual rates of: mortality, stroke, STE, major hemorrhage, and ICH. Table includes RR calculations with their 95% CIs.
Abbreviations: CI, confidence interval; N/A, not available; STE, systemic thromboembolism.

Evidence for Warfarin Versus Dual Antiplatelet Therapy

Dual antiplatelet therapy (DAPT) has been evaluated in patients with chronic AF. In the ACTIVE W study, 6706 patients with AF and at least one risk factor for stroke were randomized to warfarin alone or ASA plus clopidogrel, with the primary composite outcome of SSTE or MI or vascular death.[97] The study was stopped early owing to the superiority of warfarin. The primary outcome occurred at a rate of 3.93% per year in the warfarin group, compared with 5.60% per year in the ASA plus clopidogrel group. Patients in the ASA plus clopidogrel group had statistically significant higher rates of stroke (RR 1.72), ischemic stroke (RR 2.17), minor bleeding (RR 1.21), and of the composite score of the primary outcome plus major bleeding (RR 1.41). There were no statistical differences in rates of hemorrhagic stroke, major bleeding, severe bleeding, or fatal bleeding between the 2 groups. The benefits of warfarin over antiplatelet therapy are independent of the type of AF. Subanalysis of the ACTIVE W study found that warfarin was superior to ASA plus clopidogrel for the prevention of SSTE in both paroxysmal and sustained AF.[33] Although DAPT has not been studied in POAF, DAPT is inferior to warfarin for the prevention of SSTE in patients with AF, and by extension should not be used for the treatment of POAF when warfarin is an option.

Evidence for Patients with AF and ACS with Stenting (Warfarin Plus Single Antiplatelet Versus Warfarin Plus DAPT)

There has been great debate about the best antithrombotic regimen in patients with AF who have had a recent MI and undergone cardiac stenting. DAPT is the standard of care for patients after cardiac stenting with drug-eluting stents and previous studies have shown that the addition of DAPT to adjusted-dose warfarin ("triple" therapy) increases the risk of bleeding. The WOEST study investigators randomized patients to warfarin plus DAPT (ASA plus clopidogrel) versus warfarin plus clodipogrel and found that patients on warfarin plus clopidogrel had a significant 64% RRR in bleeding (due to a decreased risk of minor bleeding), no difference in major bleeding rates, low rates of multiple bleeding episodes (2.2% vs 12.0%) with lower rates of blood transfusions (3.5% vs 9.5%), and a significantly lower mortality (2.5% vs 6.3%).[98] They also found a nonsignificant lower stent thrombosis rate (1.4% vs 3.2%). These findings were supported by results from a study of 12,165 Danish patients with AF who had an MI with or without cardiac stenting.[99] In the study, compared with triple therapy, patients treated with an oral anticoagulant (OAC) plus clopidogrel or OAC plus ASA had no increased risk of recurrent coronary events; a nonsignificant reduction in bleeding was observed in the OAC plus clopidogrel group, and a significant reduction in bleeding was observed in the OAC plus ASA group. Patients in the OAC plus ASA group did have a significantly increased risk of all-cause mortality. The effects of DAPT alone were also investigated and, when compared with triple therapy, DAPT was associated with higher rates of ischemic stroke and all-cause mortality, but lower rates of bleeding. In both studies, triple therapy (OAC plus ASA plus clopidogrel) was associated with unacceptable rates of bleeding with no clear benefit.

Evidence for New Oral Anticoagulants Versus Warfarin

In the United States, 3 new oral anticoagulants (NOACs) have been approved by the Food and Drug Administration (FDA) for the treatment of nonvalvular AF (**Table 12**). Dabigatran is a competitive, direct thrombin inhibitor (DTI) that is primarily excreted through the urine and has a 12- to 17-hour half-life.[103] Apixaban and rivaroxaban are competitive factor Xa inhibitors and are metabolized in the blood; apixaban has a 12-hour half-life, whereas the half-life of rivaroxaban varies with age, with an

Table 12
NOACs versus warfarin trials: outcomes (stroke, STE, major hemorrhage, ICH)

Study	Year	Source	Treatment: NOAC	Treatment: Warfarin	Mortality Annual Rate: NOAC vs Warfarin (95% CI)	Stroke/STE Annual Rate: NOAC vs Warfarin (95% CI)	Major Hemorrhage Annual Rate: NOAC vs Warfarin (95% CI)	ICH Annual Rate: NOAC vs Warfarin (95% CI)
RE-LY (110 mg)	2009	100	Dabigatran 110 mg BID	INR: 2.0–3.0	3.75% vs 4.13% RR: 0.91 (0.80, 1.03)	1.53% vs 1.69% RR: 0.91 (0.74, 1.11)	2.71% vs 3.36% RR: 0.80 (0.69, 0.93)	0.23% vs 0.74% RR: 0.31 (0.20, 0.47)
RE-LY (150 mg)	2009	100	Dabigatran 150 mg BID	INR: 2.0–3.0	3.64% vs 4.13% RR: 0.88 (0.77, 1.00)	1.11% vs 1.69% RR: 0.66 (0.53, 0.82)	3.11% vs 3.36% RR: 0.93 (0.81, 1.07)	0.30% vs 0.74% RR: 0.40 (0.27, 0.60)
ROCKET AF	2011	101	Rivaroxaban 20 mg once daily	INR: 2.0–3.0	1.9% vs 2.2% HR: 0.85 (0.70, 1.02)	2.1% vs 2.4% HR: 0.88 (0.74, 1.03)	3.6% vs 3.4% HR: 1.04 (0.90, 1.20)	0.5% vs 0.7% HR: 0.67 (0.47, 0.93)
ARISTOTLE	2011	102	Apixaban 5 mg BID	INR: 2.0–3.0	3.52% vs 3.94% HR: 0.89 (0.80, 1.0)	1.27% vs 1.60% HR: 0.79 (0.66, 0.95)	2.13% vs 3.09% HR: 0.69 (0.60, 0.80)	0.33% vs 0.80% HR: 0.42 (0.30, 0.58)

Table of RCTs that evaluated the effects of the NOACs versus warfarin in the management of patients with nonvalvular AF. Outcomes included are annual rates of: mortality, stroke, STE, major hemorrhage, and ICH. Table includes RR and HR calculations with their 95% CIs.

Abbreviations: BID, twice a day; CI, confidence interval; HR, hazard ratio; STE, systemic thromboembolism.

11- to 13-hour half-life in the elderly population.[104–106] Apixaban is dosed twice daily, whereas rivaroxaban is dosed once a day.

Dabigatran was studied against adjusted-dose warfarin for the treatment of non-valvular AF at 150 mg twice daily and 110 mg twice daily in the RE-LY trial.[100] Dabigatran 150 mg is available in the United States for SSTE prophylaxis in nonvalvular AF and was found to be superior to warfarin in preventing SSTE, with similar rates of major bleeding. Both doses of dabigatran were associated with significantly lower rates of life-threatening bleeding and intracranial bleeding, but higher rates of gastrointestinal (GI) bleeding were observed with dabigatran 150 mg. Similar findings were found in the ROCKET AF trial evaluating rivaroxaban 20 mg once daily. Rivaroxaban was found to be noninferior to warfarin for the prevention of SSTE, but had similar major and nonmajor bleeding rates, lower rates of ICH and fatal bleeding, and higher rates of major GI bleeding.[101]

In contrast to dabigatran 150 mg twice daily and rivaroxaban 20 mg once daily, apixaban 5 mg twice daily (2.5 mg twice daily in selected patients), when compared with adjusted-dose warfarin in the ARISTOTLE trial, was found to be superior (as opposed to noninferior) to warfarin for the prevention of SSTE.[102] Apixaban treatment was also associated with significantly lower rates of major bleeding, hemorrhagic stroke, and death from any cause. Based on findings from the AVERROES study, which evaluated apixaban versus ASA in the treatment of nonvalvular AF, administration of apixaban resulted in similar bleeding rates to those obtained with ASA.[107] In this study, treatment with apixaban was also reported to be associated with a similar rate of GI bleeding to ASA; GI bleeding rates were not reported in the ARISTOTLE trial. No direct comparative trials of the NOACs have been conducted.

All of the major RCTs evaluating the currently available NOACs for the treatment of nonvalvular AF excluded patients that had reversible causes of AF (including POAF), or who had plans to undergo surgery at the time of enrollment in the study.[100–102] For this reason, it is hard to directly apply the results of these studies to patients with POAF. Despite the exclusion criteria at admission, nearly a quarter of the patients in the RE-LY study underwent a surgical procedure during the 2-year study period. There was no difference in rates of periprocedural major, minor, or fatal bleeding between patients on dabigatran and those on warfarin, and dabigatran treatment was associated with significantly lower rates of bleeding in cases where dabigatran or warfarin was stopped within 48 hours of surgery.[108] The rates of bleeding were also not affected by minor or major procedures, or urgent or elective procures. In addition, postmarketing information and one RCT of dabigatran (RE-ALIGN study) has demonstrated that NOACs are not appropriate for patients with valvular heart disease who have undergone valve replacement, as NOAC treatment in this patient population is associated with increased rates of thromboembolic and bleeding complications, as compared with warfarin.[109]

Management of bleeding for any of the 3 NOACs approved for the treatment of nonvalvular AF is covered in other articles in this publication. However, management of acute bleeding in this patient population is based on case studies or correction of anticoagulation in volunteers, and no human studies evaluating different treatment regimens and their effectiveness for the control of bleeding have been published to date. Recommendations for the management of uncontrolled bleeding in patients on DTIs or factor Xa inhibitors include cessation of the OAC, localized control of bleeding if possible, fluid resuscitation, and blood products as needed. In instances of severe or life-threatening bleeding, activated and nonactivated 4-factor prothrombin complex concentrates, now FDA-approved in the United States, are potential therapeutic approaches and are covered more extensively in other sections.[110–113]

Hemodialysis may also be considered in severe or life-threatening bleeding in patients on dabigatran because it has an 80% renal excretion and is dialyzable.[114] Additional research efforts into the development of an antidote for factor Xa and thrombin inhibitors are currently in phase II proof-of-concept trials for the purpose of reversal of anticoagulation in bleeding patients on factor Xa inhibitors and dabigatran.[115]

Evidence of Anticoagulation in POAF Patients

Studies evaluating the benefits and risks of oral anticoagulation for the treatment of POAF are limited, largely retrospective, and lack the power to detect small differences in stroke rates between various treatments. The results of these studies are also conflicting. One study by Makhija and colleagues[116] at the Mayo Clinic reviewed 759 general thoracic surgery patients who developed POAF: 228 patients were anticoagulated and 531 patients were not anticoagulated. Patients were followed for a median of 27.6 months. Patients who were anticoagulated had higher rates of pulmonary hypertension, heart failure, and peripheral vascular disease. There was no statistical difference in stroke rates between the 2 groups, but patients who received anticoagulation had a significantly higher rate of bleeding complications when compared with those who received no anticoagulation (9.6% vs 5.1%, respectively). No direct correlation between increasing $CHADS_2$ scores and the incidence of stroke was noted, but the difference in $CHADS_2$ scores in patients experiencing strokes versus those not experiencing strokes was not statistically significant.

Further literature questioning the benefits of anticoagulation in the postoperative period were published by Kollar and colleagues,[117] who reviewed 2960 CABG patients and identified 32 patients who had a postoperative stroke (1.1%). Of the 32 patients that had a stroke, 12 (37.5%) woke up with an immediate stroke noted on extubation, 11 (34.4%) had postoperative strokes but no episodes of AF or atrial flutter (AFL), and 4 (12.5%) had strokes before their first episode of AF or AFL. Of the remaining 5 patients (15.6%) who had POAF or AFL before their stroke, 2 had strokes related to atrial septal defects or patent foramen ovale with pulmonary embolism, one had a massive stroke due to carotid artery occlusion, one had bilateral axional brain injury secondary to respiratory arrest, and only one patient had AF/AFL-related stroke, which occurred on the same day as the onset of the arrhythmia. The average time to stroke onset after surgery was 21 hours. Based on these findings, the authors concluded that the attributable risk of POAF to postoperative stroke was low and that starting anticoagulation at 48 hours, as recommended in the AHA/ACC guidelines, would not have prevented most of the strokes. Support for the use of anticoagulation has been published by El-Chami and colleagues,[36] who evaluated the effects of POAF on long-term outcomes. Patients were followed for an average of 6 years, and POAF was found to be an independent risk factor for late mortality. Patients with POAF who were discharged on warfarin had an independent 22% relative decrease in mortality compared with patients who were not discharged on warfarin. In addition, a small study performed in Japan evaluated the risk of stroke in status post-CABG in 151 paroxysmal POAF patients who were either treated with 2 antiplatelet drugs (ASA plus ticlopidine) or warfarin plus ASA.[118] The warfarin plus ASA group had a significantly higher mean $CHADS_2$ score but had a lower rate of postoperative stroke and, on multivariate analysis, the absence of warfarin was an independent risk factor for postoperative stroke in patients with paroxysmal POAF.

National consensus guidelines for the treatment POAF do exist. The ACC/AHA, European Society of Cardiology (ESC), and American College of Chest Physicians (ACCP) guidelines for the management of POAF recommend systemic anticoagulation with warfarin with or without heparin bridging when POAF persists for more than

48 hours to prevent thromboembolic events and stroke.[49,74,119,120] Guidelines also recommend continuing anticoagulation for 30 days after restoration of sinus rhythm. In the postoperative period, after 30 days of stable sinus rhythm, OACs may be discontinued. For patients with persistent or intermittent AF that persists after surgery, treatment is similar to that for patients with chronic AF who have not undergone an operation.

Patients who have undergone valve surgery are not candidates for NOACs, and warfarin is indicated for the management of POAF in these patients. For patients with nonvalvular POAF (eg, after lung resection or coronary bypass surgery), NOACs have an attractive pharmacologic profile that may support their utility in this population, similar to their use in patients with chronic AF, with the ability to rapidly establish anticoagulation levels, no need for routine monitoring, and the ability to avoid heparin in patient populations at great risk for heparin-induced thrombocytopenia. Whether there are differences between the NOACs (apixaban, rivaroxaban, dabigatran) in this setting remains speculative, but NOACs provide an important therapeutic option for anticoagulation that requires additional investigation.

REFERENCES

1. Björck S, Palaszewski B, Friberg L, et al. Atrial fibrillation, stroke risk, and warfarin therapy revisited: a population-based study. Stroke 2013;44(11): 3103–8.
2. Naccarelli GV, Varker H, Lin J, et al. Increasing prevalence of atrial fibrillation and flutter in the United States. Am J Cardiol 2009;104(11):1534–9.
3. Go AS, Hylek EM, Phillips KA, et al. Prevalence of diagnosed atrial fibrillation in adults: national implications for rhythm management and stroke prevention: the AnTicoagulation and Risk Factors in Atrial Fibrillation (ATRIA) Study. JAMA 2001;285(18):2370–5.
4. Kannel WB, Wolf PA, Benjamin EJ, et al. Prevalence, incidence, prognosis, and predisposing conditions for atrial fibrillation: population-based estimates. Am J Cardiol 1998;82(8A):2N–9N.
5. Miyasaka Y, Barnes ME, Gersh BJ, et al. Secular trends in incidence of atrial fibrillation in Olmsted County, Minnesota, 1980 to 2000, and implications on the projections for future prevalence. Circulation 2006;114(2):119–25.
6. Roselli EE, Murthy SC, Rice TW, et al. Atrial fibrillation complicating lung cancer resection. J Thorac Cardiovasc Surg 2005;130(2):438–44.
7. Rena O, Papalia E, Oliaro A, et al. Supraventricular arrhythmias after resection surgery of the lung. Eur J Cardiothorac Surg 2001;20(4):688–93.
8. Rostagno C, La Meir M, Gelsomino S, et al. Atrial fibrillation after cardiac surgery: incidence, risk factors, and economic burden. J Cardiothorac Vasc Anesth 2010;24(6):952–8.
9. Piccini JP, Zhao Y, Steinberg BA, et al. Comparative effectiveness of pharmacotherapies for prevention of atrial fibrillation following coronary artery bypass surgery. Am J Cardiol 2013;112(7):954–60.
10. Al-Khatib SM, Hafley G, Harrington RA, et al. Patterns of management of atrial fibrillation complicating coronary artery bypass grafting: results from the PRoject of Ex-vivo Vein graft ENgineering via Transfection IV (PREVENT-IV) Trial. Am Heart J 2009;158(5):792–8.
11. Vaporciyan AA, Correa AM, Rice DC, et al. Risk factors associated with atrial fibrillation after noncardiac thoracic surgery: analysis of 2588 patients. J Thorac Cardiovasc Surg 2004;127(3):779–86.

12. Passman RS, Gingold DS, Amar D, et al. Prediction rule for atrial fibrillation after major noncardiac thoracic surgery. Ann Thorac Surg 2005;79(5):1698–703.
13. Onaitis M, D'Amico T, Zhao Y, et al. Risk factors for atrial fibrillation after lung cancer surgery: analysis of the Society of Thoracic Surgeons general thoracic surgery database. Ann Thorac Surg 2010;90(2):368–74.
14. Harpole DH, Liptay MJ, DeCamp MM Jr, et al. Prospective analysis of pneumonectomy: risk factors for major morbidity and cardiac dysrhythmias. Ann Thorac Surg 1996;61(3):977–82.
15. Dyszkiewicz W, Skrzypczak M. Atrial fibrillation after surgery of the lung: clinical analysis of risk factors. Eur J Cardiothorac Surg 1998;13(6):625–8.
16. Lahiri MK, Fang K, Lamerato L, et al. Effect of race on the frequency of postoperative atrial fibrillation following coronary artery bypass grafting. Am J Cardiol 2011;107(3):383–6.
17. Sun X, Hill PC, Lowery R, et al. Comparison of frequency of atrial fibrillation after coronary artery bypass grafting in African Americans versus European Americans. Am J Cardiol 2011;108(5):669–72.
18. Rader F, Van Wagoner DR, Ellinor PT, et al. Influence of race on atrial fibrillation after cardiac surgery. Circ Arrhythm Electrophysiol 2011;4(5):644–52.
19. Gilmanov D, Bevilacqua S, Murzi M, et al. Minimally invasive and conventional aortic valve replacement: a propensity score analysis. Ann Thorac Surg 2013; 96(3):837–43.
20. Melduni RM, Suri RM, Seward JB, et al. Diastolic dysfunction in patients undergoing cardiac surgery: a pathophysiological mechanism underlying the initiation of new-onset post-operative atrial fibrillation. J Am Coll Cardiol 2011;58(9): 953–61.
21. Thorén E, Hellgren L, Jidéus L, et al. Prediction of postoperative atrial fibrillation in a large coronary artery bypass grafting cohort. Interact Cardiovasc Thorac Surg 2012;14(5):588–93.
22. Almassi GH, Pecsi SA, Collins JF, et al. Predictors and impact of postoperative atrial fibrillation on patients' outcomes: a report from the randomized on versus off bypass trial. J Thorac Cardiovasc Surg 2012;143(1):93–102.
23. Mariscalco G, Engström KG. Postoperative atrial fibrillation is associated with late mortality after coronary surgery, but not after valvular surgery. Ann Thorac Surg 2009;88(6):1871–6.
24. Saxena A, Dinh DT, Smith JA, et al. Usefulness of postoperative atrial fibrillation as an independent predictor for worse early and late outcomes after isolated coronary artery bypass grafting (multicenter Australian study of 19,497 patients). Am J Cardiol 2012;109(2):219–25.
25. Saxena A, Shi WY, Bappayya S, et al. Postoperative atrial fibrillation after isolated aortic valve replacement: a cause for concern? Ann Thorac Surg 2013; 95(1):133–40.
26. Christians KK, Wu B, Quebbeman EJ, et al. Postoperative atrial fibrillation in noncardiothoracic surgical patients. Am J Surg 2001;182(6):713–5.
27. Bhave PD, Goldman LE, Vittinghoff E, et al. Incidence, predictors, and outcomes associated with postoperative atrial fibrillation after major noncardiac surgery. Am Heart J 2012;164(6):918–24.
28. Polanczyk CA, Goldman L, Marcantonio ER, et al. Supraventricular arrhythmia in patients having noncardiac surgery: clinical correlates and effect on length of stay. Ann Intern Med 1998;129(4):279–85.
29. Miceli A, Murzi M, Gilmanov D, et al. Minimally invasive aortic valve replacement using right minithoracotomy is associated with better outcomes than ministernotomy.

J Thorac Cardiovasc Surg 2014;148(1):133–7. http://dx.doi.org/10.1016/j.jtcvs. 2013.07.060.

30. Mihos CG, Santana O, Lamas GA, et al. Incidence of postoperative atrial in patients undergoing minimally invasive versus median sternotomy valve surgery. J Thorac Cardiovasc Surg 2013;146(6):1436–41.

31. Smith CR, Leon MB, Mack MJ, et al, PARTNER Trial Investigators. Transcatheter versus surgical aortic-valve replacement in high-risk patients. N Engl J Med 2011;364(23):2187–98.

32. Hart RG, Pearce LA, Rothbart RM, et al. Stroke with intermittent atrial fibrillation: incidence and predictors during aspirin therapy. Stroke prevention in Atrial Fibrillation Investigators. J Am Coll Cardiol 2000;35(1):183–7.

33. Hohnloser SH, Pajitnev D, Pogue J, et al, ACTIVE W Investigators. Incidence of stroke in paroxysmal versus sustained atrial fibrillation in patients taking oral anticoagulation or combined antiplatelet therapy: an ACTIVE W Substudy. J Am Coll Cardiol 2007;50(22):2156–61.

34. Friberg L, Hammar N, Rosenqvist M. Stroke in paroxysmal atrial fibrillation: report from the stockholm cohort of atrial fibrillation. Eur Heart J 2010;31(8): 967–75.

35. Nieuwlaat R, Dinh T, Olsson SB, et al, Euro Heart Survey Investigators. Should we abandon the common practice of withholding oral anticoagulation in paroxysmal atrial fibrillation? Eur Heart J 2008;29(7):915–22.

36. El-Chami MF, Kilgo P, Thourani V, et al. New-onset atrial fibrillation predicts long-term mortality after coronary artery bypass graft. J Am Coll Cardiol 2010;55(13): 1370–6.

37. Horwich P, Buth KJ, Légaré JF. New onset postoperative atrial fibrillation is associated with a long-term risk for stroke and death following cardiac surgery. J Card Surg 2013;28(1):8–13.

38. Bramer S, van Straten AH, Soliman Hamad MA, et al. The impact of new-onset postoperative atrial fibrillation on mortality after coronary artery bypass grafting. Ann Thorac Surg 2010;90(2):443–9.

39. Villareal RP, Hariharan R, Liu BC, et al. Postoperative atrial fibrillation and mortality after coronary artery bypass surgery. J Am Coll Cardiol 2004;43(5):742–8.

40. Efird JT, Davies SW, O'Neal WT, et al. The impact of race and postoperative atrial fibrillation on operative mortality after elective coronary artery bypass grafting. Eur J Cardiothorac Surg 2014;45(2):e20–5.

41. Lahtinen J, Biancari F, Salmela E, et al. Postoperative atrial fibrillation is a major cause of stroke after on-pump coronary artery bypass surgery. Ann Thorac Surg 2004;77(4):1241–4.

42. Likosky DS, Leavitt BJ, Marrin CA, et al, Northern New England Cardiovascular Disease Study Group. Intra- and postoperative predictors of stroke after coronary artery bypass grafting. Ann Thorac Surg 2003;76(2):428–34.

43. Ahlsson A, Fengsrud E, Bodin L, et al. Postoperative atrial fibrillation in patients undergoing aortocoronary bypass surgery carries an eightfold risk of future atrial fibrillation and a doubled cardiovascular mortality. Eur J Cardiothorac Surg 2010;37(6):1353–9.

44. Antonelli D, Peres D, Freedberg NA, et al. Incidence of postdischarge symptomatic paroxysmal atrial fibrillation in patients who underwent coronary artery bypass graft: long-term follow-up. Pacing Clin Electrophysiol 2004;27(3): 365–7.

45. Ambrosetti M, Tramarin R, Griffo R, et al, ISYDE and ICAROS Investigators of the Italian Society for Cardiovascular Prevention, Rehabilitation and Epidemiology

(IACPR-GICR). Late postoperative atrial fibrillation after cardiac surgery: a national survey within the cardiac rehabilitation setting. J Cardiovasc Med 2011; 12(6):390–5.

46. Hedberg M, Boivie P, Engström KG. Early and delayed stroke after coronary surgery - an analysis of risk factors and the impact on short- and long-term survival. Eur J Cardiothorac Surg 2011;40(2):379–87.

47. Filardo G, Hamilton C, Hamman B, et al. New-onset postoperative atrial fibrillation and long-term survival after aortic valve replacement surgery. Ann Thorac Surg 2010;90(2):474–9.

48. Khan MF, Wendel CS, Movahed MR. Prevention of post-coronary artery bypass grafting (CABG) atrial fibrillation: efficacy of prophylactic beta-blockers in the modern era: a meta-analysis of latest randomized controlled trials. Ann Noninvasive Electrocardiol 2013;18(1):58–68.

49. Fuster V, Rydén LE, Cannom DS, et al, American College of Cardiology Foundation/American Heart Association Task Force. 2011 ACCF/AHA/HRS focused updates incorporated into the ACC/AHA/ESC 2006 guidelines for the management of patients with atrial fibrillation: a report of the American College of Cardiology Foundation/American Heart Association Task Force on practice guidelines. Circulation 2011;123(10):e269–367.

50. Chatterjee S, Sardar P, Mukherjee D, et al. Timing and route of amiodarone for prevention of postoperative atrial fibrillation after cardiac surgery: a network regression meta-analysis. Pacing Clin Electrophysiol 2013;36(8):1017–23.

51. Zhu J, Wang C, Gao D, et al. Meta-analysis of amiodarone versus β-blocker as a prophylactic therapy against atrial fibrillation following cardiac surgery. Intern Med J 2012;42(10):1078–87.

52. Riber LP, Christensen TD, Jensen HK, et al. Amiodarone significantly decreases atrial fibrillation in patients undergoing surgery for lung cancer. Ann Thorac Surg 2012;94(2):339–44.

53. Tisdale JE, Wroblewski HA, Wall DS, et al. A randomized trial evaluating amiodarone for prevention of atrial fibrillation after pulmonary resection. Ann Thorac Surg 2009;88(3):886–93 [discussion: 894–5].

54. Chen WT, Krishnan GM, Sood N, et al. Effect of statins on atrial fibrillation after cardiac surgery: a duration- and dose-response meta-analysis. J Thorac Cardiovasc Surg 2010;140(2):364–72.

55. Liakopoulos OJ, Kuhn EW, Slottosch I, et al. Preoperative statin therapy for patients undergoing cardiac surgery. Cochrane Database Syst Rev 2012;(4):CD008493.

56. De Oliveira GS Jr, Knautz JS, Sherwani S, et al. Systemic magnesium to reduce postoperative arrhythmias after coronary artery bypass graft surgery: a meta-analysis of randomized controlled trials. J Cardiothorac Vasc Anesth 2012; 26(4):643–50.

57. Cook RC, Yamashita MH, Kearns M, et al. Prophylactic magnesium does not prevent atrial fibrillation after cardiac surgery: a meta-analysis. Ann Thorac Surg 2013;95(2):533–41.

58. Mariani J, Doval HC, Nul D, et al. N-3 polyunsaturated fatty acids to prevent atrial fibrillation: updated systematic review and meta-analysis of randomized controlled trials. J Am Heart Assoc 2013;2(1):e005033.

59. Costanzo S, di Niro V, Di Castelnuovo A, et al. Prevention of postoperative atrial fibrillation in open heart surgery patients by preoperative supplementation of n-3 polyunsaturated fatty acids: an updated meta-analysis. J Thorac Cardiovasc Surg 2013;146(4):906–11.

60. Bandeali SJ, Kayani WT, Lee VV, et al. Outcomes of preoperative angiotensin-converting enzyme inhibitor therapy in patients undergoing isolated coronary artery bypass grafting. Am J Cardiol 2012;110(7):919–23.

61. Chin JH, Lee EH, Son HJ, et al. Preoperative treatment with an angiotensin-converting enzyme inhibitor or an angiotensin receptor blocker has no beneficial effect on the development of new-onset atrial fibrillation after off-pump coronary artery bypass graft surgery. Clin Cardiol 2012;35(1):37–42.

62. Van Gelder IC, Hagens VE, Bosker HA, et al, Rate Control versus Electrical Cardioversion for Persistent Atrial Fibrillation Study Group. A comparison of rate control and rhythm control in patients with recurrent persistent atrial fibrillation. N Engl J Med 2002;347(23):1834–40.

63. Wyse DG, Waldo AL, DiMarco JP, et al, Atrial Fibrillation Follow-up Investigation of Rhythm Management (AFFIRM) Investigators. A comparison of rate control and rhythm control in patients with atrial fibrillation. N Engl J Med 2002; 347(23):1825–33.

64. Hohnloser SH, Kuck KH, Lilienthal J. Rhythm or rate control in atrial fibrillation–Pharmacological Intervention in Atrial Fibrillation (PIAF): a randomised trial. Lancet 2000;356(9244):1789–94.

65. Carlsson J, Miketic S, Windeler J, et al, STAF Investigators. Randomized trial of rate-control versus rhythm-control in persistent atrial fibrillation: the Strategies of Treatment of Atrial Fibrillation (STAF) Study. J Am Coll Cardiol 2003;41(10):1690–6.

66. Opolski G, Torbicki A, Kosior D, et al. Rhythm control versus rate control in patients with persistent atrial fibrillation. Results of the HOT CAFE Polish Study. Kardiol Pol 2003;59(7):1–16.

67. Lee JK, Klein GJ, Krahn AD, et al. Rate-control versus conversion strategy in postoperative atrial fibrillation: a prospective, randomized pilot study. Am Heart J 2000;140(6):871–7.

68. Kowey PR, Stebbins D, Igidbashian L, et al. Clinical outcome of patients who develop PAF after CABG surgery. Pacing Clin Electrophysiol 2001;24(2):191–3.

69. Olshansky B, Rosenfeld LE, Warner AL, et al, AFFIRM Investigators. The Atrial Fibrillation Follow-up Investigation of Rhythm Management (AFFIRM) Study: approaches to control rate in atrial fibrillation. J Am Coll Cardiol 2004;43(7):1201–8.

70. Manios EG, Mavrakis HE, Kanoupakis EM, et al. Effects of amiodarone and diltiazem on persistent atrial fibrillation conversion and recurrence rates: a randomized controlled study. Cardiovasc Drugs Ther 2003;17(1):31–9.

71. Bianconi L, Mennuni M, Lukic V, et al. Effects of oral propafenone administration before electrical cardioversion of chronic atrial fibrillation: a placebo-controlled study. J Am Coll Cardiol 1996;28:700–6.

72. Oral H, Souza JJ, Michaud GF, et al. Facilitating transthoracic cardioversion of atrial fibrillation with ibutilide pretreatment. N Engl J Med 1999;340:1849–54.

73. Arnold AZ, Mick MJ, Mazurek RP, et al. Role of prophylactic anticoagulation for direct current cardioversion in patients with atrial fibrillation or atrial flutter. J Am Coll Cardiol 1992;19:851–5.

74. European Heart Rhythm Association, European Association for Cardio-Thoracic Surgery, Camm AJ, Kirchhof P, Lip GY, et al. Guidelines for the management of atrial fibrillation: the Task Force for the Management of Atrial Fibrillation of the European Society of Cardiology (ESC). Eur Heart J 2010;31(19):2369–429.

75. Gage BF, Waterman AD, Shannon W, et al. Validation of clinical classification schemes for predicting stroke: results from the National Registry of Atrial Fibrillation. JAMA 2001;285(22):2864–70.

76. Lip GY, Nieuwlaat R, Pisters R, et al. Refining clinical risk stratification for predicting stroke and thromboembolism in atrial fibrillation using a novel risk factor-based approach: the Euro Heart Survey on atrial fibrillation. Chest 2010;137(2): 263–72.
77. Olesen JB, Lip GY, Hansen ML, et al. Validation of risk stratification schemes for predicting stroke and thromboembolism in patients with atrial fibrillation: nationwide cohort study. BMJ 2011;342:d124.
78. Pisters R, Lane DA, Nieuwlaat R, et al. A novel user-friendly score (HAS-BLED) to assess 1-year risk of major bleeding in patients with atrial fibrillation: the Euro Heart Survey. Chest 2010;138(5):1093–100.
79. Lip GY, Frison L, Halperin JL, et al. Comparative validation of a novel risk score for predicting bleeding risk in anticoagulated patients with atrial fibrillation: the HAS-BLED (Hypertension, Abnormal Renal/Liver Function, Stroke, Bleeding History or Predisposition, Labile INR, Elderly, Drugs/Alcohol Concomitantly) score. J Am Coll Cardiol 2011;57(2):173–80.
80. Fang MC, Go AS, Chang Y, et al. A new risk scheme to predict warfarin-associated hemorrhage: the ATRIA (Anticoagulation and Risk Factors in Atrial Fibrillation) Study. J Am Coll Cardiol 2011;58(4):395–401.
81. Clinical Gage BF, Yan Y, Milligan PE, et al. Classification schemes for predicting hemorrhage: results from the National Registry of Atrial Fibrillation (NRAF). Am Heart J 2006;151(3):713–9.
82. Petersen P, Boysen G, Godtfredsen J, et al. Placebo-controlled, randomised trial of warfarin and aspirin for prevention of thromboembolic complications in chronic atrial fibrillation. The Copenhagen AFASAK Study. Lancet 1989;1(8631): 175–9.
83. Stroke prevention in Atrial Fibrillation Study. Final results. Circulation 1991;84(2): 527–39.
84. Secondary prevention in non-rheumatic atrial fibrillation after transient ischaemic attack or minor stroke. EAFT (European Atrial Fibrillation Trial) Study Group. Lancet 1993;342(8882):1255–62.
85. Diener HC, Cunha L, Forbes C, et al. European Stroke Prevention Study. 2. Dipyridamole and acetylsalicylic acid in the secondary prevention of stroke. J Neurol Sci 1996;143(1–2):1–13.
86. Posada IS, Barriales V. Alternate-day dosing of aspirin in atrial fibrillation. LASAF Pilot Study Group. Am Heart J 1999;138(1 Pt 1):137–43.
87. Sato H, Ishikawa K, Kitabatake A, et al, Japan Atrial Fibrillation Stroke Trial Group. Low-dose aspirin for prevention of stroke in low-risk patients with atrial fibrillation: Japan Atrial Fibrillation Stroke Trial. Stroke 2006;37(2):447–51.
88. Hart RG, Pearce LA, Aguilar MI. Meta-analysis: antithrombotic therapy to prevent stroke in patients who have nonvalvular atrial fibrillation. Ann Intern Med 2007;146(12):857–67.
89. The effect of low-dose warfarin on the risk of stroke in patients with nonrheumatic atrial fibrillation. The Boston Area Anticoagulation Trial for Atrial Fibrillation Investigators. N Engl J Med 1990;323(22):1505–11.
90. Connolly SJ, Laupacis A, Gent M, et al. Canadian Atrial Fibrillation Anticoagulation (CAFA) Study. J Am Coll Cardiol 1991;18(2):349–55.
91. Ezekowitz MD, Bridgers SL, James KE, et al. Warfarin in the prevention of stroke associated with nonrheumatic atrial fibrillation. Veterans Affairs Stroke Prevention in Nonrheumatic Atrial Fibrillation Investigators. N Engl J Med 1992; 327(20):1406–12.

92. Go AS, Hylek EM, Chang Y, et al. Anticoagulation therapy for stroke prevention in atrial fibrillation: how well do randomized trials translate into clinical practice? JAMA 2003;290:2685–92.

93. Halperin JL, Hart RG, Kronmal RA, et al. Warfarin versus aspirin for prevention of thromboembolism in atrial fibrillation: Stroke Prevention in Atrial Fibrillation II Study. Lancet 1994;343(8899):687–91.

94. Gulløv AL, Koefoed BG, Petersen P, et al. Fixed minidose warfarin and aspirin alone and in combination vs adjusted-dose warfarin for stroke prevention in atrial fibrillation: Second Copenhagen Atrial Fibrillation, Aspirin, and Anticoagulation Study. Arch Intern Med 1998;158(14):1513–21.

95. Hu DY, Zhang HP, Sun YH, et al, Antithrombotic Therapy in Atrial Fibrillation Study Group. The randomized study of efficiency and safety of antithrombotic therapy in nonvalvular atrial fibrillation: warfarin compared with aspirin. Zhonghua Xin Xue Guan Bing Za Zhi 2006;34(4):295–8 [in Chinese].

96. Mant J, Hobbs FD, Fletcher K, et al. Warfarin versus aspirin for stroke prevention in an elderly community population with atrial fibrillation (the Birmingham Atrial Fibrillation Treatment of the Aged Study, BAFTA): a randomised controlled trial. Lancet 2007;370:493–503.

97. ACTIVE Writing Group of the ACTIVE Investigators, Connolly S, Pogue J, et al. Clopidogrel plus aspirin versus oral anticoagulation for atrial fibrillation in the Atrial fibrillation Clopidogrel Trial with Irbesartan for prevention of Vascular Events (ACTIVE W): a randomised controlled trial. Lancet 2006;367(9526):1903–12.

98. Dewilde WJ, Oirbans T, Verheugt FW, et al, WOEST Study Investigators. Use of clopidogrel with or without aspirin in patients taking oral anticoagulant therapy and undergoing percutaneous coronary intervention: an open-label, randomised, controlled trial. Lancet 2013;381(9872):1107–15.

99. Lamberts M, Gislason GH, Olesen JB, et al. Oral anticoagulation and antiplatelets in atrial fibrillation patients after myocardial infarction and coronary intervention. J Am Coll Cardiol 2013;62(11):981–9.

100. Connolly SJ, Ezekowitz MD, Yusuf S, et al, RE-LY Steering Committee and Investigators. Dabigatran versus warfarin in patients with atrial fibrillation. N Engl J Med 2009;361(12):1139–51.

101. Patel MR, Mahaffey KW, Garg J, et al, ROCKET AF Investigators. Rivaroxaban versus warfarin in nonvalvular atrial fibrillation. N Engl J Med 2011;365(10):883–91.

102. Granger CB, Alexander JH, McMurray JJ, et al, ARISTOTLE Committees and Investigators. Apixaban versus warfarin in patients with atrial fibrillation. N Engl J Med 2011;365(11):981–92.

103. Stangier J, Clemens A. Pharmacology, pharmacokinetics, and pharmacodynamics of dabigatran etexilate, an oral direct thrombin inhibitor. Clin Appl Thromb Hemost 2009;15(Suppl 1):9S–16S.

104. Raghavan N, Frost CE, Yu Z, et al. Apixaban metabolism and pharmacokinetics after oral administration to humans. Drug Metab Dispos 2009;37(1):74–81.

105. Kubitza D, Becka M, Wensing G, et al. Safety, pharmacodynamics, and pharmacokinetics of BAY 59-7939–an oral, direct Factor Xa inhibitor–after multiple dosing in healthy male subjects. Eur J Clin Pharmacol 2005;61(12):873–80.

106. Kubitza D, Becka M, Roth A, et al. Dose-escalation study of the pharmacokinetics and pharmacodynamics of rivaroxaban in healthy elderly subjects. Curr Med Res Opin 2008;24(10):2757–65.

107. Connolly SJ, Eikelboom J, Joyner C, et al, AVERROES Steering Committee and Investigators. Apixaban in patients with atrial fibrillation. N Engl J Med 2011; 364(9):806–17.

108. Healey JS, Eikelboom J, Douketis J, et al, RE-LY Investigators. Periprocedural bleeding and thromboembolic events with dabigatran compared with warfarin: results from the Randomized Evaluation of Long-Term Anticoagulation Therapy (RE-LY) randomized trial. Circulation 2012;126(3):343–8.

109. Eikelboom JW, Connolly SJ, Brueckmann M, et al, RE-ALIGN Investigators. Dabigatran versus warfarin in patients with mechanical heart valves. N Engl J Med 2013;369(13):1206–14.

110. Marlu R, Hodaj E, Paris A, et al. Effect of non-specific reversal agents on anticoagulant activity of dabigatran and rivaroxaban: a randomised crossover ex vivo study in healthy volunteers. Thromb Haemost 2012;108(2):217–24.

111. Eerenberg ES, Kamphuisen PW, Sijpkens MK, et al. Reversal of rivaroxaban and dabigatran by prothrombin complex concentrate: a randomized, placebo-controlled, crossover study in healthy subjects. Circulation 2011;124(14):1573–9.

112. Escolar G, Fernandez-Gallego V, Arellano-Rodrigo E, et al. Reversal of apixaban induced alterations in hemostasis by different coagulation factor concentrates: significance of studies in vitro with circulating human blood. PLoS One 2013; 8(11):e78696.

113. Körber MK, Langer E, Ziemer S, et al. Measurement and reversal of prophylactic and therapeutic peak levels of rivaroxaban: an In Vitro Study. Clin Appl Thromb Hemost 2013. http://dx.doi.org/10.1177/1076029613494468.

114. Warkentin TE, Margetts P, Connolly SJ, et al. Recombinant factor VIIa (rFVIIa) and hemodialysis to manage massive dabigatran-associated postcardiac surgery bleeding. Blood 2012;119(9):2172–4.

115. Lu G, DeGuzman FR, Hollenbach SJ, et al. A specific antidote for reversal of anticoagulation by direct and indirect inhibitors of coagulation factor Xa. Nat Med 2013;19(4):446–51.

116. Makhija Z, Allen MS, Wigle DA, et al. Routine anticoagulation is not indicated for postoperative general thoracic surgical patients with new-onset atrial fibrillation. Ann Thorac Surg 2011;92(2):421–6.

117. Kollar A, Lick SD, Vasquez KN, et al. Relationship of atrial fibrillation and stroke after coronary artery bypass graft surgery: when is anticoagulation indicated? Ann Thorac Surg 2006;82(2):515–23.

118. Hata M, Akiyama K, Wakui S, et al. Does warfarin help prevent ischemic stroke in patients presenting with post coronary bypass paroxysmal atrial fibrillation? Ann Thorac Cardiovasc Surg 2013;19(3):207–11.

119. Epstein AE, Alexander JC, Gutterman DD, et al, American College of Chest Physicians. Anticoagulation: American College of Chest Physicians guidelines for the prevention and management of postoperative atrial fibrillation after cardiac surgery. Chest 2005;128(2 Suppl):24S–7S.

120. You JJ, Singer DE, Howard PA, et al, American College of Chest Physicians. Antithrombotic therapy for atrial fibrillation: antithrombotic therapy and prevention of thrombosis, 9th ed: American College of Chest Physicians Evidence-Based Clinical Practice Guidelines. Chest 2012;141(2 Suppl):e531S–75S.

Management of Anticoagulation Agents in Trauma Patients

C. Cameron McCoy, MD[a],*, Jeffrey H. Lawson, MD, PhD[b],
Mark L. Shapiro, MD[c]

KEYWORDS

- Trauma • Anticoagulation • Thromboelastography • Hemorrhage • Hemostasis

KEY POINTS

- Early identification of anticoagulation status is key to injury management in the trauma patient.
- Whereas some anticoagulant effects are detected on standard assays, such as prothrombin time and activated partial thromboplastin time, the effect of other, newer agents is only evident on specialized assays or thromboelastography.
- Knowledge of specific reversal strategies for individual agents such as direct thrombin and factor Xa inhibitors is essential in managing acute, traumatic hemorrhage.
- Direct antidotes are not available for many newer anticoagulants; the management of hemorrhage is complicated by these drugs, and is currently focused on resuscitation and factor replacement.

INTRODUCTION

Anticoagulation adds additional complexity to the assessment and management of the trauma patient.[1,2] Trauma clinicians must act quickly to determine the patient's medications, complexity of injury, coagulation status, and the most appropriate reversal strategy. The broad range of anticoagulants encountered includes antiplatelet agents, low molecular weight heparin (LMWH), vitamin K antagonists (VKAs), and newer, direct inhibitors of factors in the coagulation cascade. The use of particular agents may suggest concurrent medical comorbidities that should be taken into

The authors have no disclosures or conflicts of interest to declare.
[a] Department of Surgery, Duke University Medical Center, Duke University, Box 3443, Room 3581, White Zone, Duke South, Durham, NC 27710, USA; [b] Division of Vascular Surgery, Department of Surgery, Duke University Medical Center, Duke University, Box 2622, Room 481 MSRB 1 Research Drive, Durham, NC 27710, USA; [c] Division of Trauma & Critical Care, Department of Surgery, Duke University Medical Center, Duke University, 1557 F Duke South, Blue Zone Box 2837, Durham, NC 27710, USA
* Corresponding author.
E-mail address: Christopher.mccoy@dm.duke.edu

Clin Lab Med 34 (2014) 563–574
http://dx.doi.org/10.1016/j.cll.2014.06.013   labmed.theclinics.com
0272-2712/14/$ – see front matter © 2014 Elsevier Inc. All rights reserved.

consideration during the initial phase of trauma assessment and care. Once anticoagulant medications are identified, the patient's assessment should include laboratory assessment of their coagulation state. Traditional studies such as activated partial thromboplastin time (aPTT) and international normalized ratio (INR) may be augmented by functional assays of coagulation such as thromboelastography (TEG). Simultaneously, the patient's complexity of injury should be assessed for any indications to administer reversal. In addition to an accurate physical examination, radiographic studies should be used to determine the presence of occult hemorrhage in the setting of anticoagulation. Once the clinician has determined the patient's anticoagulation status and complexity of injury, reversal of anticoagulation can be targeted to specific agents and injuries. Failure to rapidly assess these factors can result in delays in restoring hemostasis, and increased morbidity and mortality from injury.

INITIAL ASSESSMENT OF THE ANTICOAGULATED TRAUMA PATIENT

The identification of injuries and determination of the extent of anticoagulation are essential steps in the initial assessment of any trauma patient. The coagulation status should be identified early during ascertainment of the medical history. Injuries exacerbated by therapeutic coagulation will also be identified on examination and will guide further diagnostics. Laboratory studies should also be drawn to ensure their availability at the earliest opportunity to guide possible reversal. Based on the patient's history and results from the primary survey and physical examination, radiographic studies should be performed to identify occult injuries that could also be complicated by the patient's anticoagulation status.

Patient's History and Physical Examination

It is essential to identify patients on therapeutic anticoagulation during the secondary trauma survey. Special attention should be paid to current home medications to identify agents affecting coagulation. This information may be available from the patient, the patient's family, or prehospital care providers. Other clues to medical conditions requiring anticoagulation treatment include previous surgical scars for procedures such as valve replacement and medical alert badges. Suspicion of anticoagulation based on clinical presentation and medical comorbidities may also be sufficient to warrant further investigation of a patient's coagulation status. Failure to obtain a complete history, including medication, may result in serious complications from uncontrolled hemorrhage.

Laboratory Analysis

Laboratory analysis to determine the extent of anticoagulation in the trauma patient is a crucial early assessment step. The initial laboratory analysis for most trauma patients, regardless of known coagulation status, often includes prothrombin time (PT), aPTT, and platelet count as the sole indicators of coagulation status.[3] For some anticoagulants, such as VKAs, these data may be sufficient to determine the level of anticoagulation and guide reversal. With other agents, such as direct thrombin and factor Xa inhibitors, these assays provide unreliable means of identifying the level of anticoagulation and drug activity. Details regarding the laboratory assessment of specific anticoagulant medications during trauma are described in a subsequent section.

Functional assays of coagulation such as TEG are also becoming more readily available and can guide care for patients on anticoagulants. TEG (TEG 5000; Haemonetics,

Braintree, MA, USA) and rotational thromboelastometry (ROTEM; TEM Systems Inc, Durham, NC, USA) are increasingly used to provide a more complete assessment of coagulation status for trauma patients.[4–6] These newer assays provide results more rapidly (15–20 minutes) than traditional assays such as aPTT or platelet count (45–60 minutes).[4,7] Originally described in 1948, TEG and ROTEM provide information on clot formation, propagation, stabilization, and dissolution.[6] Various therapeutic anticoagulants produce distinct effects on these assays (**Fig. 1**). Thromboelastographic changes specific to individual agents are discussed in a subsequent section.

Radiographic Studies

Following the initial assessment, and often run concurrently with laboratory assays, radiographic studies are used to detect occult injuries and internal hemorrhage in the anticoagulated trauma patient. Computed tomography (CT) is the most widely used diagnostic method for this purpose.[8,9] In particular, anticoagulated patients suspected of traumatic brain injury should undergo a head CT scan to assess for occult intracranial hemorrhage (ICH). Although the UK National Institute for Health and Care Excellence guidelines suggest that routine head CT scanning is not necessary for all patients on therapeutic anticoagulation with head trauma,[10] multiple studies have demonstrated missed ICH and current practice in many institutions is to obtain a head CT scan on presentation for these patients.[11,12] Demonstration of ICH by the initial head CT scan of the anticoagulated trauma patient indicates the need for urgent anticoagulation reversal, unless the risk is prohibitive owing to the likelihood of thromboembolic complications for an individual patient.

MANAGEMENT OF THE ANTICOAGULATED TRAUMA PATIENT
Vitamin K Antagonists

Some of the most commonly used therapeutic anticoagulants are VKAs such as warfarin. Indications for warfarin use are some forms of atrial fibrillation, the presence of a metallic valve or ventricular assist device, deep vein thrombosis, and pulmonary embolism.[13] Approximately 3% of patients presenting to Level 1 trauma centers in one study were anticoagulated with this agent. In these patients, warfarin treatment was associated with a 3-fold increase in mortality compared with those not taking warfarin or antiplatelet agents.[14] Based on this evidence, trauma patients on warfarin should receive urgent reversal if an indication exists.

Warfarin's anticoagulation effect is monitored via the INR. Some guidelines recommend a target INR of 1.6 for anticoagulation reversal, with stepwise administration of

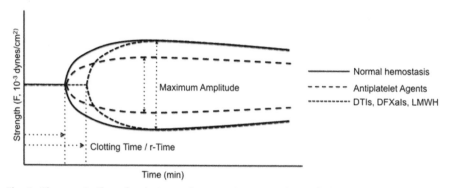

Fig. 1. Changes in thromboelastography secondary to anticoagulation. DFXaI, direct factor Xa inhibitor; DTI, direct thrombin inhibitor; LMWH, low molecular weight heparin.

a reversal agent followed by repeat INR measurement before additional administration.[15] Indications for the reversal of warfarin in trauma patients include ICH and uncontrolled hemorrhage elsewhere in the body. The Eastern Association for the Surgery of Trauma guidelines state that patients with posttraumatic ICH should begin therapy to correct their INR to less than 1.6 within 2 hours of arrival, and reach an INR of less than 1.6 within 4 hours.[15] Early reversal has been demonstrated to reduce hemorrhage progression and mortality.[16] Anticoagulated patients with head trauma but without radiographic evidence of ICH should not receive preventive reversal. Patients presenting with a hemorrhage in other locations aside from the brain should have reversal considered on a patient-by-patient basis, taking into account the extent of injury and the potential risks associated with anticoagulation reversal.

Fresh frozen plasma (FFP) has been the traditional reversal agent for warfarin in trauma patients.[17] FFP, as a blood product, requires frozen storage and associated thawing time in addition to ABO compatibility testing, and carries a risk of transfusion-related complications.[18,19] Thawing time and ABO compatibility testing may not pose a delay at centers capable of maintaining thawed FFP stores of type AB, but availability in large volumes or at smaller centers is not guaranteed.[16] In addition, multiple doses of FFP are often required to reduce the INR to levels necessary for normal hemostasis. Administration of large volumes of FFP poses a risk for patients with medical comorbidities such as congestive heart failure who do not require volume resuscitation. Because of these issues, prothrombin complex concentrate (PCC) has gained favor as the agent of choice for emergent warfarin reversal.

PCCs are available as 3-factor (factors II, IX, X) or 4-factor (factors II, VII, IX, X) concentrates. These agents have a low risk of infection because of viral inactivation, do not require cross-matching, and are administered in low volumes; moreover, therapeutic doses can be infused within 15 to 30 minutes.[20,21] The current American College of Chest Physicians guidelines recommend the use of PCC over FFP for reversal of warfarin in patients with serious hemorrhage.[22] Kcentra (CSL Behring, King of Prussia, PA, USA), a 4-factor PCC, has recently been licensed for urgent warfarin reversal in the United States.[23] The lack of cross-matching and speed of correction make PCCs the ideal agents for correction of warfarin anticoagulation in trauma patients (**Table 1**).

Limited evidence exists regarding the use of recombinant activated factor VII (rFVIIa) for reversal of VKA-related hemorrhage.[17] Use of rFVIIa in VKA-anticoagulated patients presenting with a traumatic hemorrhage should be reserved for cases when first-line agents are not available.[24] rFVIIa carries a significant risk of thrombosis. By comparison, PCCs contain minimal levels of activated clotting factors in addition to some level of Protein C and S. As a result, PCCs carry a theoretically lower risk of thrombosis than rFVIIa.

Direct Thrombin Inhibitors

Direct thrombin inhibitors (DTIs) are reversible, competitive inhibitors that block the active site of thrombin, and do not require a cofactor to exert their effect on the coagulation cascade. As DTIs are relatively new oral anticoagulants, fewer data exist regarding the management of posttraumatic hemorrhage in patients taking these agents. One such agent, dabigatran etexilate, is approved in several countries for the prevention of venous thromboembolism in patients undergoing total hip or knee replacement and the prevention of stroke or embolism in patients with nonvalvular atrial fibrillation.[25–27] Dabigatran is mainly eliminated by renal clearance, and blood levels can be decreased through diuresis and dialysis.[28]

Table 1
Anticoagulants and urgent reversal strategies

Anticoagulant	Mechanism	Urgent Reversal Strategy
VKA (eg, warfarin)	Epoxide reductase inhibition	First line: PCC Second line: FFP
Oral DTI (eg, dabigatran)	Competitive, reversible direct inhibition of thrombin	First line: PCC including FEIBA, rFVIIa Second line: hemodialysis *Pending: direct inhibitors (eg, anti-Dabi Fab)*
Direct factor Xa inhibitor (eg, rivaroxaban)	Competitive, reversible direct inhibition of factor Xa	First line: PCC *Poorly removed by hemodialysis*
LMWH (eg, enoxaparin)	Potentiation of antithrombin III	First line: protamine (temporary, partial), rFVIIa
Aspirin	Cyclooxygenase-1 inhibition	First line: platelet transfusion Second line: desmopressin
Clopidogrel	Irreversible inhibition of platelet P2Y$_{12}$ ADP receptor	First line: platelet transfusion Second line: desmopressin

Abbreviations: ADP, adenosine diphosphate; DTI, direct thrombin inhibitor; FEIBA, factor VIII inhibitor bypassing activity; FFP, fresh frozen plasma; LMWH, low molecular weight heparin; PCC, prothrombin complex concentrate; rFVIIa, recombinant activated factor VII; VKA, vitamin K antagonist.

DTIs affect multiple coagulation studies, including thrombin clotting time (TCT), PT, aPTT and ecarin clotting time (ECT).[29,30] The aPTT does not provide a linear representation of plasma DTI levels. The aPTT underestimates DTI activity at high plasma concentrations, whereas TCT may overestimate DTI levels; its use should be reserved to ruling out the presence of any residual DTI activity, as a normal TCT ensures that no DTI anticoagulation effect is present. The preferred assay for quantitative assessment of DTI activity is ECT, which was originally developed to monitor hirudin-type DTI activity. ECT is the only dose-responsive assay for DTIs. Unfortunately, it is uncommon and its availability in smaller institutions may be limited. DTIs such as dabigatran and argatroban produce dose-dependent increases in clotting time on InTEM (ellagic acid–activated intrinsic pathway thromboelastometry) (see **Fig. 1**).[31] These changes in clotting time are based on direct inhibition of thrombin by the drug.

Initial management of uncontrolled bleeding complicated by DTIs should focus on volume and blood product resuscitation. Although the manufacturer recommends FFP to assist with restoring circulating coagulation factors, it is unlikely to reverse the drug effect based on its mechanism.[32,33] Animal models and case study reports suggest that rFVIIa significantly reduces bleeding time and may be useful in treating hemorrhage in subjects receiving a DTI, but this effect is agent-dependent and dose-dependent.[34–38]

Both activated and nonactivated PCCs have also been evaluated as agents for emergency reversal of dabigatran (see **Table 1**). Animal models suggest that these agents significantly reduce dabigatran-induced prolongation of bleeding time. However, clinical data regarding their use in hemorrhaging patients are limited to case reports.[39,40] Further details on results from these case reports are available in the article by Levy and Levi elsewhere in this issue. Looking forward, a true antidote (anti-Dabi Fab), which complexes with dabigatran in a similar manner to that of thrombin and functions as a high-affinity competitive inhibitor, is under development for emergency reversal of dabigatran anticoagulation.[41] At present, PCCs are the agent of choice to treat posttraumatic hemorrhage in patients on DTIs.

Direct Factor Xa Inhibitors

Another class of new oral anticoagulants, direct factor Xa inhibitors, are associated with many of the same difficulties in controlling posttraumatic hemorrhage as DTIs. Direct factor Xa inhibitors, like DTIs with thrombin, are capable of accessing not only free factor Xa but also factor Xa associated with the prothrombinase complex and established clot.[42,43] One direct factor Xa inhibitor, rivaroxaban, is currently approved in the United States for the prevention of venous thromboembolism in patients undergoing total hip or knee replacement surgery.[44,45] In clinical practice, rivaroxaban is replacing LMWH as the agent of choice in this role.

Treatment with direct factor Xa inhibitors results in prolongation of the PT and aPTT. Platelet aggregation does not seem to be affected.[46] Direct factor Xa inhibitor treatment also produces dose-dependent increases in clotting time on InTEM (see **Fig. 1**). These changes in clotting time also mirror dose-dependent changes in PT and are similar to changes seen with DTIs.[47,48]

FFP is unlikely to provide direct factor Xa reversal, but will help to maintain coagulation factor levels during an ongoing hemorrhage. High-dose PCC (50 IU/kg) and activated PCC (50 IU/kg) administration have demonstrated efficacy in normalizing bleeding time in an animal model (see **Table 1**).[49] This dose is approximately twice the amount of PCC administered to reverse hemorrhage secondary to VKAs in patients with a pretreatment INR of 2 to 4 (25 IU/kg).[23] High-affinity competitive inhibitors, such as those for DTIs, are also under development and are being tested in animal models, with promising results showing complete PT normalization. Similarly to DTI reversal, PCCs are currently the best available agents for reversal of direct factor Xa inhibitors.

Low Molecular Weight Heparin

Enoxaparin is the most widely used LMWH for outpatient anticoagulation, and the heparinoid most likely to be encountered in the setting of acute trauma.[50] Owing to their lighter weight compared with unfractionated heparin, LMWHs exhibit anti-thrombin III–dependent coagulation factor inactivation but also significant anti–factor Xa activity.

LMWH activity may be assessed using an anti–factor Xa assay, available in many hospital clinical laboratories.[51] Unfortunately, this assay takes a minimum of 1 to 2 hours to complete and does not provide timely data in acute trauma care. Patients taking heparinoid anticoagulation demonstrate prolonged clotting time on the InTEM assay of ROTEM and prolonged reaction time on TEG (see **Fig. 1**). These changes represent inhibition of thrombin burst formation by the circulating anticoagulant.[52] This finding can be confirmed in ROTEM by performing the HEPTEM (heparinase-modified thromboelastometry) test.

There is no US Food and Drug Administration (FDA)-approved antidote for LMWHs, but protamine sulfate exhibits partial, temporary reversal of anti–factor IIa activity (see **Table 1**).[20,53] Anticoagulant activity may return as soon as 3 hours following reversal, so ongoing administration is vital. Case reports, small series, and in vitro studies have documented successful outcomes and laboratory assay normalization using rFVIIa.[54] However, the risk of thrombosis must be balanced with the possibility of ongoing hemorrhage when using this agent for the reversal of LMWHs.

Antiplatelet Agents

Antiplatelet agents such as aspirin and clopidogrel are used individually and in combination for the treatment of cardiovascular disease.[55,56] Patients who have undergone percutaneous coronary intervention are often temporarily or permanently dependent on these medications to maintain stent patency. As a result, caution must be used during attempted reversal of traumatic hemorrhage, owing to the risk of stent thrombosis and subsequent myocardial infarction. Numerous studies have demonstrated a greater degree of progression of ICH and worse outcomes in trauma patients taking antiplatelet agents.[57,58]

Aspirin irreversibly acetylates a specific serine moiety of platelet cyclooxygenase (COX)-1, thereby reducing the synthesis of thromboxane A_2.[59] Thromboxane A_2 acts as a potent platelet aggregator and vasoconstrictor. Aspirin's effect is clinically evident in arachidonic acid (AA)-based or collagen-based aggregation assays, but bleeding time is rarely prolonged.[60] The platelet function assay using collagen-based and adenosine diphosphate (ADP)-based activation also demonstrates aspirin inactivation, but results are not available in the acute setting owing to the test duration. Newer assays, such as VerifyNow (Accumetrics, San Diego, CA, USA), aim to provide faster results that reflect the true bleeding potential of patients taking antiplatelet agents.[61]

Clopidogrel irreversibly blocks the binding of ADP to platelet $P2Y_{12}$ receptors and thereby inhibits further release of ADP from platelets.[59] ADP is a potent platelet activator, and clopidogrel interrupts the self-feedback activation loop normally established by ADP release from platelet dense bodies.[62] Unlike aspirin, clopidogrel demonstrates both inhibition of platelet aggregation assays and a prolongation in bleeding time.[59] Early TEG poorly detected changes in platelet activation secondary to antiplatelet agents such as aspirin and clopidogrel. Modern TEG for platelet function uses platelet-specific activators. TEG Platelet Mapping (Haemonetics) using AA-based or ADP-based assays of blood from patients taking as little as 75 mg of aspirin daily for 1 week demonstrates significant time-dependent reductions in maximum amplitude and curve area (see **Fig. 1**).[63,64] Similar reductions are seen in patients on clopidogrel using the ADP-based assay, but not the AA-based assay.

Owing to their irreversible mechanisms of action, aspirin and clopidogrel do not have direct antidotes. When traumatic hemorrhage is present, the traditional belief is that platelet function may be reestablished by the transfusion of nonacetylated platelets. Some studies have demonstrated restoration of platelet activity with transfusion for patients on a low-dose (75–81 mg/d) aspirin regimen, whereas others have demonstrated failure of transfusion to halt ICH progression in patients on a high-dose (325 mg/d) aspirin regimen.[61,65] In the event of clinically significant bleeding, such as traumatic ICH, older literature recommends the urgent transfusion of multiple units of platelets for patients on clopidogrel.[20]

Numerous subsequent studies and reviews have now demonstrated that platelet transfusion is not effective in reducing mortality or altering outcomes from traumatic ICH complicated by some antiplatelet agents.[65,66] Because many of these studies were based at institutions without specific protocols for platelet transfusion, recent studies have hypothesized that the extent and duration of platelet transfusion were insufficient to affect outcomes.[57] As a result a new protocol was developed, recommending 5 platelet concentrate units for patients with small ICH on aspirin and 10 platelet concentrate units for patients with small ICH on clopidogrel. In more severe cases of ICH, this protocol recommends the addition of desmopressin and serial platelet transfusions every 12 hours for 48 hours (see **Table 1**). Additional platelet transfusion for up to 5 days may be necessary in patients on clopidogrel, owing to the persistence of the drug's active metabolite.

SUMMARY

Therapeutic anticoagulation presents unique challenges during the care of trauma patients. Failure of normal hemostatic measures secondary to pharmacologic blockade may turn clinically insignificant hemorrhage into an organ-threatening or life-threatening situation. The spectrum of agents encountered by trauma clinicians requires familiarity with coagulation physiology, drug mechanisms, and appropriate reversal strategies. The advent of new anticoagulation agents poses additional challenges because of the lack of adequate reversal agents. To provide optimal trauma care for the anticoagulated patient, research and clinician education must continue to match pace with drug development and transition to these newer agents.

REFERENCES

1. Coimbra R, Hoyt DB, Anjaria DJ, et al. Reversal of anticoagulation in trauma: a North-American survey on clinical practices among trauma surgeons. J Trauma 2005;59(2):375–82.
2. Fortuna GR, Mueller EW, James LE, et al. The impact of preinjury antiplatelet and anticoagulant pharmacotherapy on outcomes in elderly patients with hemorrhagic brain injury. Surgery 2008;144(4):598–603 [discussion: 603–5].
3. Kutcher ME, Ferguson AR, Cohen MJ. A principal component analysis of coagulation after trauma. J Trauma Acute Care Surg 2013;74(5):1223–9 [discussion: 1229–30].
4. Romlin BS, Wahlander H, Synnergren M, et al. Earlier detection of coagulopathy with thromboelastometry during pediatric cardiac surgery: a prospective observational study. Paediatr Anaesth 2013;23(3):222–7.
5. McCully SP, Fabricant LJ, Kunio NR, et al. The International Normalized Ratio overestimates coagulopathy in stable trauma and surgical patients. J Trauma Acute Care Surg 2013;75(6):947–53.
6. Whiting D, Dinardo JA. TEG and ROTEM: technology and clinical applications. Am J Hematol 2014;89(2):228–32.
7. Solomon C, Sorensen B, Hochleitner G, et al. Comparison of whole blood fibrin-based clot tests in thrombelastography and thromboelastometry. Anesth Analg 2012;114(4):721–30.
8. Ahmed N, Kassavin D, Kuo YH, et al. Sensitivity and specificity of CT scan and angiogram for ongoing internal bleeding following torso trauma. Emerg Med J 2013;30(3):e14.
9. Roudsari B, Psoter KJ, Fine GC, et al. Falls, older adults, and the trend in utilization of CT in a level I trauma center. AJR Am J Roentgenol 2012;198(5):985–91.
10. Prowse SJ, Sloan J. NICE guidelines for the investigation of head injuries–an anticoagulant loop hole? Emerg Med J 2010;27(4):277–8.
11. National Institute for Health and Care Excellence. Head injury clinical guidelines (CG56): triage, assessment, investigation and early management of head injury in infants, children and adults. 2007. Available at: http://www.nice.org.uk/guidance/index.jsp?action=byID&o=11836. Accessed February 10, 2014.
12. Cohen DB, Rinker C, Wilberger JE. Traumatic brain injury in anticoagulated patients. J Trauma 2006;60(3):553–7.

13. Hirsh J, Dalen J, Anderson DR, et al. Oral anticoagulants: mechanism of action, clinical effectiveness, and optimal therapeutic range. Chest 2001;119(1 Suppl): 8S–21S.

14. Bonville DJ, Ata A, Jahraus CB, et al. Impact of preinjury warfarin and antiplatelet agents on outcomes of trauma patients. Surgery 2011;150(4):861–8.

15. Calland JF, Ingraham AM, Martin N, et al. Evaluation and management of geriatric trauma: an Eastern Association for the Surgery of Trauma practice management guideline. J Trauma Acute Care Surg 2012;73(5 Suppl 4):S345–50.

16. Ivascu FA, Howells GA, Junn FS, et al. Rapid warfarin reversal in anticoagulated patients with traumatic intracranial hemorrhage reduces hemorrhage progression and mortality. J Trauma 2005;59(5):1131–7 [discussion: 1137–9].

17. Ageno W, Garcia D, Aguilar MI, et al. Prevention and treatment of bleeding complications in patients receiving vitamin K antagonists, part 2: treatment. Am J Hematol 2009;84(9):584–8.

18. Contreras M, Ala FA, Greaves M, et al. Guidelines for the use of fresh frozen plasma. British Committee for Standards in Haematology, Working Party of the Blood Transfusion Task Force. Transfus Med 1992;2(1):57–63.

19. Popovsky MA. Transfusion-related acute lung injury: incidence, pathogenesis and the role of multicomponent apheresis in its prevention. Transfus Med Hemother 2008;35(2):76–9.

20. Beshay JE, Morgan H, Madden C, et al. Emergency reversal of anticoagulation and antiplatelet therapies in neurosurgical patients. J Neurosurg 2010;112(2): 307–18.

21. Sarode R, Matevosyan K, Bhagat R, et al. Rapid warfarin reversal: a 3-factor prothrombin complex concentrate and recombinant factor VIIa cocktail for intracerebral hemorrhage. J Neurosurg 2012;116(3):491–7.

22. Ageno W, Gallus AS, Wittkowsky A, et al. Oral anticoagulant therapy: antithrombotic therapy and prevention of thrombosis, 9th ed: American College of Chest Physicians evidence-based clinical practice guidelines. Chest 2012;141(2 Suppl):e44S–88S.

23. CSL Behring GmbH. Kcentra prescribing information. 2013. Available at: http://www.kcentra.com/prescribing-information.aspx. Accessed February 27, 2014.

24. Rosovsky RP, Crowther MA. What is the evidence for the off-label use of recombinant factor VIIa (rFVIIa) in the acute reversal of warfarin? ASH evidence-based review 2008. Hematology Am Soc Hematol Educ Program 2008;36–8. http://dx.doi.org/10.1182/asheducation-2008.1.36.

25. Lazo-Langner A, Rodger MA, Wells PS. Lessons from ximelagatran: issues for future studies evaluating new oral direct thrombin inhibitors for venous thromboembolism prophylaxis in orthopedic surgery. Clin Appl Thromb Hemost 2009; 15(3):316–26.

26. Boudes PF. The challenges of new drugs benefits and risks analysis: lessons from the ximelagatran FDA Cardiovascular Advisory Committee. Contemp Clin Trials 2006;27(5):432–40.

27. Nutescu EA, Shapiro NL, Chevalier A. New anticoagulant agents: direct thrombin inhibitors. Cardiol Clin 2008;26(2):169–87, v–vi.

28. Blech S, Ebner T, Ludwig-Schwellinger E, et al. The metabolism and disposition of the oral direct thrombin inhibitor, dabigatran, in humans. Drug Metab Dispos 2008;36(2):386–99.

29. Wienen W, Stassen JM, Priepke H, et al. In-vitro profile and ex-vivo anticoagulant activity of the direct thrombin inhibitor dabigatran and its orally active prodrug, dabigatran etexilate. Thromb Haemost 2007;98(1):155–62.

30. Lange U, Nowak G, Bucha E. Ecarin chromogenic assay–a new method for quantitative determination of direct thrombin inhibitors like hirudin. Pathophysiol Haemost Thromb 2003;33(4):184–91.

31. Engstrom M, Rundgren M, Schott U. An evaluation of monitoring possibilities of argatroban using rotational thromboelastometry and activated partial thromboplastin time. Acta Anaesthesiol Scand 2010;54(1):86–91.

32. van Ryn J, Stangier J, Haertter S, et al. Dabigatran etexilate–a novel, reversible, oral direct thrombin inhibitor: interpretation of coagulation assays and reversal of anticoagulant activity. Thromb Haemost 2010;103(6):1116–27.

33. Boehringer Ingelheim Pharmaceuticals. Pradaxa prescribing information. 2013. Available at: http://bidocs.boehringer-ingelheim.com/BIWebAccess/ViewServlet.ser?docBase=renetnt&folderPath=/Prescribing%20Information/PIs/Pradaxa/Pradaxa.pdf. Accessed February 27, 2014.

34. Crowther MA, Warkentin TE. Managing bleeding in anticoagulated patients with a focus on novel therapeutic agents. J Thromb Haemost 2009;7(Suppl 1):107–10.

35. Garber ST, Sivakumar W, Schmidt RH. Neurosurgical complications of direct thrombin inhibitors–catastrophic hemorrhage after mild traumatic brain injury in a patient receiving dabigatran. J Neurosurg 2012;116(5):1093–6.

36. Gruber A, Carlsson S, Kotze HF, et al. Hemostatic effect of activated factor VII without promotion of thrombus growth in melagatran-anticoagulated primates. Thromb Res 2007;119(1):121–7.

37. Oh JJ, Akers WS, Lewis D, et al. Recombinant factor VIIa for refractory bleeding after cardiac surgery secondary to anticoagulation with the direct thrombin inhibitor lepirudin. Pharmacotherapy 2006;26(4):569–77.

38. Wolzt M, Levi M, Sarich TC, et al. Effect of recombinant factor VIIa on melagatran-induced inhibition of thrombin generation and platelet activation in healthy volunteers. Thromb Haemost 2004;91(6):1090–6.

39. Faust AC, Peterson EJ. Management of dabigatran-associated intracerebral and intraventricular hemorrhage: a case report. J Emerg Med 2014;46(4):525–9. http://dx.doi.org/10.1016/j.jemermed.2013.11.097.

40. Dumkow LE, Voss JR, Peters M, et al. Reversal of dabigatran-induced bleeding with a prothrombin complex concentrate and fresh frozen plasma. Am J Health Syst Pharm 2012;69(19):1646–50.

41. Schiele F, van Ryn J, Canada K, et al. A specific antidote for dabigatran: functional and structural characterization. Blood 2013;121(18):3554–62.

42. Perzborn E, Roehrig S, Straub A, et al. Rivaroxaban: a new oral factor Xa inhibitor. Arterioscler Thromb Vasc Biol 2010;30(3):376–81.

43. Gerotziafas GT, Elalamy I, Depasse F, et al. In vitro inhibition of thrombin generation, after tissue factor pathway activation, by the oral, direct factor Xa inhibitor rivaroxaban. J Thromb Haemost 2007;5(4):886–8.

44. Kakkar AK, Brenner B, Dahl OE, et al. Extended duration rivaroxaban versus short-term enoxaparin for the prevention of venous thromboembolism after total hip arthroplasty: a double-blind, randomised controlled trial. Lancet 2008;372(9632):31–9.

45. Eriksson BI, Borris LC, Friedman RJ, et al. Rivaroxaban versus enoxaparin for thromboprophylaxis after hip arthroplasty. N Engl J Med 2008;358(26):2765–75.

46. Samama MM, Martinoli JL, LeFlem L, et al. Assessment of laboratory assays to measure rivaroxaban–an oral, direct factor Xa inhibitor. Thromb Haemost 2010;103(4):815–25.

47. Martin AC, Le Bonniec B, Fischer AM, et al. Evaluation of recombinant activated factor VII, prothrombin complex concentrate, and fibrinogen concentrate to

reverse apixaban in a rabbit model of bleeding and thrombosis. Int J Cardiol 2013;168(4):4228–33.

48. Escolar G, Fernandez-Gallego V, Arellano-Rodrigo E, et al. Reversal of apixaban induced alterations in hemostasis by different coagulation factor concentrates: significance of studies in vitro with circulating human blood. PLoS One 2013; 8(11):e78696.

49. Perzborn E, Gruber A, Tinel H, et al. Reversal of rivaroxaban anticoagulation by haemostatic agents in rats and primates. Thromb Haemost 2013;110(1):162–72.

50. Garcia DA, Baglin TP, Weitz JI, et al. Parenteral anticoagulants: antithrombotic therapy and prevention of thrombosis, 9th ed: American College of Chest Physicians evidence-based clinical practice guidelines. Chest 2012;141(2 Suppl): e24S–43S.

51. Abbate R, Gori AM, Farsi A, et al. Monitoring of low-molecular-weight heparins in cardiovascular disease. Am J Cardiol 1998;82(5B):33L–6L.

52. Mittermayr M, Velik-Salchner C, Stalzer B, et al. Detection of protamine and heparin after termination of cardiopulmonary bypass by thrombelastometry (RO-TEM): results of a pilot study. Anesth Analg 2009;108(3):743–50.

53. Pai M, Crowther MA. Neutralization of heparin activity. Handb Exp Pharmacol 2012;(207):265–77.

54. Young G, Yonekawa KE, Nakagawa PA, et al. Recombinant activated factor VII effectively reverses the anticoagulant effects of heparin, enoxaparin, fondaparinux, argatroban, and bivalirudin ex vivo as measured using thromboelastography. Blood Coagul Fibrinolysis 2007;18(6):547–53.

55. Doyal L, Wilsher D. Towards guidelines for withholding and withdrawal of life prolonging treatment in neonatal medicine. Arch Dis Child Fetal Neonatal Ed 1994;70(1):F66–70.

56. Yusuf S, Zhao F, Mehta SR, et al. Effects of clopidogrel in addition to aspirin in patients with acute coronary syndromes without ST-segment elevation. N Engl J Med 2001;345(7):494–502.

57. Campbell PG, Sen A, Yadla S, et al. Emergency reversal of antiplatelet agents in patients presenting with an intracranial hemorrhage: a clinical review. World Neurosurg 2010;74(2–3):279–85.

58. Ohm C, Mina A, Howells G, et al. Effects of antiplatelet agents on outcomes for elderly patients with traumatic intracranial hemorrhage. J Trauma 2005;58(3): 518–22.

59. Harder S, Klinkhardt U, Alvarez JM. Avoidance of bleeding during surgery in patients receiving anticoagulant and/or antiplatelet therapy: pharmacokinetic and pharmacodynamic considerations. Clin Pharmacokinet 2004;43(14):963–81.

60. Grove EL, Hvas AM, Johnsen HL, et al. A comparison of platelet function tests and thromboxane metabolites to evaluate aspirin response in healthy individuals and patients with coronary artery disease. Thromb Haemost 2010;103(6):1245–53.

61. Joseph B, Pandit V, Sadoun M, et al. A prospective evaluation of platelet function in patients on antiplatelet therapy with traumatic intracranial hemorrhage. J Trauma Acute Care Surg 2013;75(6):990–4.

62. Murugappa S, Kunapuli SP. The role of ADP receptors in platelet function. Front Biosci 2006;11:1977–86.

63. Swallow RA, Agarwala RA, Dawkins KD, et al. Thromboelastography: potential bedside tool to assess the effects of antiplatelet therapy? Platelets 2006; 17(6):385–92.

64. Collyer TC, Gray DJ, Sandhu R, et al. Assessment of platelet inhibition secondary to clopidogrel and aspirin therapy in preoperative acute surgical patients

measured by thrombelastography platelet mapping. Br J Anaesth 2009;102(4): 492–8.

65. Taylor G, Osinski D, Thevenin A, et al. Is platelet transfusion efficient to restore platelet reactivity in patients who are responders to aspirin and/or clopidogrel before emergency surgery? J Trauma Acute Care Surg 2013;74(5):1367–9.

66. Nishijima DK, Zehtabchi S, Berrong J, et al. Utility of platelet transfusion in adult patients with traumatic intracranial hemorrhage and preinjury antiplatelet use: a systematic review. J Trauma Acute Care Surg 2012;72(6):1658–63.

New Oral Anticoagulant–Induced Bleeding

Clinical Presentation and Management

Jerrold H. Levy, MD, FAHA, FCCM[a],*, Marcel Levi, MD, PhD, FRCP[b]

KEYWORDS

- Anticoagulation • New oral anticoagulants • Reversal • Safety • Bleeding
- Hemorrhage

KEY POINTS

- Bleeding is a significant complication of anticoagulant therapy, and the ever-increasing use of anticoagulants means that even small risks of major or fatal bleeding cannot be ignored.
- With the emergence of new oral anticoagulants (NOACs; ie, direct factor IIa or Xa inhibitors), this risk is further compounded by the lack of validated reversal strategies for these agents.
- Recent post-marketing data on NOAC-associated bleeding risk are consistent with those observed in head-to-head clinical trials of NOACs vs traditional anticoagulants.
- Despite the lack of clinical evidence in bleeding patients, several guidelines have recommended the use of hemostatic agents, such as prothrombin complex concentrates and recombinant activated factor VII, for NOAC reversal in patients with life-threatening bleeding.
- Ultimately, adequately powered studies will be crucial in assessing fully the effectiveness and safety of any proposed reversal strategies.

Conflict of Interest Statements: Prof. J.H. Levy serves on steering committees for Boehringer Ingelheim, CSL Behring AG, Grifols, Janssen Pharmaceuticals, and The Medicines Company. Prof. M. Levi has received research grants from Sanquin and CSL Behring, and has been on advisory boards of Bayer, LFB, and Johnson & Johnson.
Editorial assistance was provided by Chrystelle Rasamison at Fishawack Communications Ltd, UK, with a grant from CSL Behring, Marburg, Germany.
[a] Duke University School of Medicine, Divisions of Cardiothoracic Anesthesiology and Critical Care, Duke University Hospital, 2301 Erwin Road, Durham, NC 27710, USA; [b] Faculty of Medicine, Academic Medical Center, University of Amsterdam, Meibergdreef 9, Amsterdam 1105AZ, The Netherlands
* Corresponding author.
E-mail address: jerrold.levy@duke.edu

Clin Lab Med 34 (2014) 575–586
http://dx.doi.org/10.1016/j.cll.2014.06.004
labmed.theclinics.com
0272-2712/14/$ – see front matter © 2014 Elsevier Inc. All rights reserved.

INTRODUCTION

There is a substantial and ever-increasing need for anticoagulation treatment for the prevention of thromboembolic events in patients at risk. The prevalence of atrial fibrillation (AF) in the United States is projected to increase to 7.56 million by 2050[1] while it is estimated that greater than 900,000 fatal and nonfatal symptomatic venous thromboembolism (VTE) events occur in the United States every year.[2] Although warfarin, a vitamin K antagonist (VKA), has been a mainstay of oral anticoagulation therapy for many years, its use is associated with significant limitations, such as a slow onset and offset of action, food and drug interactions, and a need for frequent monitoring.[3] New oral anticoagulants (NOACs; ie, direct factor [F] IIa and FXa inhibitors) have been developed to alleviate these issues, and have recently emerged as effective alternatives to traditional anticoagulants such as warfarin and low molecular weight heparins (LMWHs; eg, enoxaparin). However, these older agents are still commonly prescribed.

Clinical trials of NOACs have demonstrated equivalence or superiority to VKAs and LMWHs for the prevention of stroke or systemic embolism in patients with AF,[4–6] and the prevention of VTE in patients with deep vein thrombosis or pulmonary embolism.[7,8] However, their original appeal (ie, owing to ease of use there is no requirement for laboratory monitoring, and less food and drug interaction than with traditional agents) is partially offset by concerns over the reported incidence of bleeding events in clinical practice, particularly considering the lack of validated reversal agents.[9–11]

Several agents currently used for VKA reversal, such as activated and nonactivated prothrombin complex concentrates (PCCs) and recombinant activated FVII (rFVIIa), have been evaluated for the reversal of NOAC-induced anticoagulation. Overall, the results obtained have provided valuable evidence for the use of these agents for NOAC reversal, although data are mostly limited to preclinical models of anticoagulation and NOAC-related bleeding.[12]

There is still a need for clinical data and clear strategies for the management of patients receiving these new agents, particularly in bleeding patients, and this holds especially true for NOAC reversal in the emergency setting. This article aims to provide some clarity with regard to the following questions: what is the prevalence and severity of bleeding events with both traditional anticoagulants and NOACs, what is the current available clinical evidence for anticoagulation reversal, and what do guidelines recommend?

PREVALENCE AND SEVERITY OF BLEEDING EVENTS WITH TRADITIONAL AND NEW ORAL ANTICOAGULANTS

Traditional Anticoagulants and Bleeding Risk

Bleeding is a major complication of anticoagulant therapy,[13] and the use of traditional anticoagulants during hospitalization, or after discharge, has been associated with an increased risk of major bleeding.[14] Annually, more than 4 million patients are prescribed warfarin in the United States for the treatment and prevention of thromboembolic events,[15] and warfarin treatment is the principal cause of adverse drug events that require emergency department treatment in people 65 years or older in the United States.[16] In particular, warfarin use is associated with an increased risk of bleeding: from 2007 to 2009, warfarin-related hemorrhages accounted for 63.3% of all warfarin-related hospitalizations in patients 65 years and older in the United States.[17]

Warfarin-induced bleeding events are associated with significant morbidity and mortality. A study of adverse events recorded between 1993 and 2006 by the Food and Drug Administration (FDA) Adverse Events Reporting System found that 86% of warfarin-related bleeding cases resulted in a serious outcome (including death, hospitalization, and disability), with 10% of cases resulting in a fatal outcome.[18] Of particular concern is the increased risk for intracranial bleeding, because the use of traditional anticoagulants has been associated with increased intracranial hematoma volumes in comparison with nonanticoagulated patients,[19,20] in turn leading to worse patient outcomes.[21] This finding is consistent with studies showing that warfarin treatment was an independent predictor of mortality in patients with intracranial hemorrhage (ICH).[22,23]

A population-based cohort study of 116,288 patients with AF conducted in the United Kingdom evaluated the association between antithrombotic therapy and the risk of bleeding.[24] This study reported an incidence rate of 4.5 per 100 person-years for any bleeding event. ICH and gastrointestinal (GI) bleeding events occurred with an incidence of 0.25 and 1.2 per 100 person-years, respectively. In this patient population, warfarin monotherapy was associated with a greater than 2-fold increase in the risk of any bleeding event compared with nonuse, while dual antithrombotic therapy with warfarin and 1 of 2 antiplatelet agents (aspirin, clopidogrel) increased the risk of bleeding by nearly 3-fold. Of interest, in this study only dual and triple therapy with warfarin and antiplatelet agents was found to be associated with an increased risk for ICH, whereas warfarin monotherapy was not. By contrast, all warfarin therapy combinations were associated with an increased risk for GI bleeds.

The association between anticoagulant treatment and risk of hemorrhage was also evaluated in a 5-year population-based cohort study, conducted in Canada, of 125,195 patients with AF who had recently been prescribed warfarin.[25] Warfarin treatment was associated with an overall risk of major hemorrhage of 3.8% per person-year; the risk of major hemorrhage was highest (11.8% per person-year) in the first month of therapy. Of note, 18.1% of hemorrhagic patients who were hospitalized died in hospital or within 7 days of discharge. As expected, patients presenting with ICH had a higher mortality risk than patients with an upper or lower GI bleed (41.7% vs 14.4% and 15.0%, respectively).

NOACs and Bleeding Risk

The severity and incidence of bleeding events in NOAC-treated patients has been evaluated in several clinical studies, which demonstrated similar or lower rates of major bleeding with NOACs when compared with traditional anticoagulants.[4–6,8] An overview of the safety results obtained with NOACs in clinical trials is available in the article by Levy elsewhere in this issue. Of note, NOAC treatment was associated with a reduced ICH incidence compared with warfarin therapy, whereas some analyses showed an increased risk for GI bleeds.[26–28] These results are consistent with recent post-marketing data on NOAC-associated bleeding risk.

The safety and efficacy of dabigatran versus warfarin was evaluated in a meta-analysis of 14 prospective and retrospective studies in patients with AF undergoing catheter ablation (4782 patients in total).[29] Overall, no significant difference was observed in terms of thromboembolic events or major bleeding events between the warfarin and dabigatran treatment arms, although minor bleeding events occurred significantly less frequently with dabigatran than with warfarin. The 2 approved dabigatran doses (110 mg or 150 mg, twice daily) were also compared in this meta-analysis, and no differences were reported in the incidence of thromboembolic events or major bleeding events, although minor bleeding occurred significantly more frequently in the 110-mg group.

Berger and colleagues[11] have also reported on their experience with bleeding complications in patients treated with dabigatran in comparison with patients on warfarin. This prospective chart review of 15 emergency department patients treated with dabigatran and 123 patients treated with warfarin showed that patients on dabigatran had a shorter length of stay, fewer major bleeding events, and fewer life-threatening complications compared with patients on warfarin. In addition, dabigatran use was more frequently associated with GI bleeds and less frequently associated with ICH when compared with warfarin in this patient population. This finding is in contrast to results from an analysis of insurance claim and administrative data from the FDA Mini-Sentinel database, which showed that dabigatran was associated with reduced incidences of GI bleeds in comparison with warfarin.[9]

The Australian Therapeutic Goods Administration has been monitoring the safety profile of dabigatran, and reported 361 serious bleeding events with this agent between January 2011 and February 2013.[30] The most commonly reported bleeding site was the GI tract, and a smaller proportion of ICHs were reported for dabigatran versus warfarin.[30] Following reports of fatal cases of dabigatran-related bleeding in Japan, the European Medicines Agency commissioned an in-depth assessment of the latest available data to determine whether the risk associated with dabigatran use was higher than perceived at the time of authorization.[31] This report concluded that the incidence of fatal bleeding events with dabigatran was lower than had been observed in clinical trials, but should continue to be closely monitored.

Of note, Boehringer Ingelheim recently announced that they were entering a multi-year partnership with Brigham and Women's Hospital, Boston, to conduct a long-term study of the comparative effectiveness, safety, and prescribing patterns of oral anticoagulants.[32]

CURRENTLY AVAILABLE OPTIONS FOR ANTICOAGULATION REVERSAL AND BLEEDING MANAGEMENT
Warfarin Reversal

The current recommendations for warfarin reversal include administration of PCCs or plasma, both concomitant with vitamin K.[33–37] Several published guidelines recommend PCCs over plasma for VKA reversal, owing to the risk of viral transmission and adverse transfusion reactions (eg, volume overload) associated with plasma use.[34–36] Of note, a recent phase IIIb trial comparing a 4F-PCC (Beriplex/Kcentra) and plasma for VKA reversal in patients with acute major bleeding demonstrated that 4F-PCC was noninferior to plasma for hemostatic efficacy, and superior for rapid reduction of international normalized ratio (INR). This study also reported an increased incidence of fluid overload events in the plasma group compared with the 4F-PCC group.[38]

NOAC Reversal

A large number of guidelines aim to provide clinicians with recommendations for the urgent reversal of NOAC-induced anticoagulation in patients presenting with major bleeding or requiring emergency surgery.[39–50] These recommendations include the use of hemostatic agents, such as rFVIIa and activated or nonactivated PCCs, in patients with life-threatening bleeding. Because the prothrombotic potential of activated PCCs and rFVIIa might be higher than that of nonactivated PCCs, nonactivated PCCs may be preferred.[43,51]

However, these recommendations are primarily based on preclinical or early clinical evidence, and no NOAC reversal strategies have yet been fully validated. Preclinical data suggest that rFVIIa and PCCs (activated and nonactivated) may be useful for the reversal of NOAC-induced anticoagulation.[52–54] A phase I study of NOAC reversal in healthy volunteers also showed that a 4F-PCC (Cofact) was able to reverse rivaroxaban-induced, but not dabigatran-induced anticoagulant effects, as measured by laboratory assays of coagulation; bleeding was not assessed in this study.[55] Similarly, another 4F-PCC (Beriplex) and a 3F-PCC (Profilnine) were also evaluated for rivaroxaban reversal in a study in healthy volunteers, and were shown to be able to correct some of the rivaroxaban-induced effects on coagulation parameters.[56]

Baumann Kreuziger and Reding recently published a survey of current NOAC reversal practices.[57] Physician members of the Hemostasis and Thrombosis Research Society and US Hemophilia Center directors provided feedback on bleeding management and perceived effectiveness of reversal strategies for patients on dabigatran and rivaroxaban therapy. Dabigatran-related bleeding was controlled in all 43 reported cases, with dialysis considered the most effective strategy in patients with renal failure. Activated PCCs and rFVIIa were considered effective in 50% to 80% of dabigatran-related bleeding episodes, while coadministration of PCC and rFVIIa was effective in the 2 cases where this strategy was used. Fewer cases of rivaroxaban-related bleeding were reported (n = 5); withholding treatment, local measures, and administration of activated PCC (1 case) were all considered effective by the treating physicians. It is interesting that most physicians (91%) reported moderate to high concern regarding their ability to manage bleeding patients on NOACs, emphasizing the need for adequately powered clinical studies to determine the best strategies for NOAC reversal.

CASE STUDIES OF NOAC REVERSAL

There are limited data on the use of NOAC reversal strategies in actively bleeding patients. As mentioned previously, most of the available data in support of the proposed reversal strategies come from studies of reversal of anticoagulation in volunteers receiving NOACs, from in vitro studies using blood samples, or from in vivo animal studies. Several case studies of NOAC-related bleeding management have been published, but it should be noted that most of these studies focus on dabigatran reversal (**Table 1**). Several of these case studies are reviewed here.

Dager and Colleagues

Dager and colleagues[58] reported on the use of the activated PCC FEIBA (Factor VIII Inhibitor Bypassing Activity) for dabigatran reversal in a 67-year-old patient with a history of symptomatic AF presenting for repeat ablation. This patient developed a major bleed after heparinization and, following volume replacement therapy and administration of blood products, reversal of dabigatran-induced coagulation was attempted. Treatment with 26 IU/kg FEIBA was able to significantly slow bleeding, with a notable effect occurring as early as 5 minutes after treatment, and bleeding had stopped by the end of the infusion; ablation was not ultimately performed. An additional infusion of 16 IU/kg FEIBA was also administered approximately 30 hours after attempted surgery, following concerns about rebleeding. Treatment with FEIBA was not associated with any evidence of thrombosis in this patient.

Diaz and Colleagues

The effectiveness of dabigatran-related bleeding management using a nonactivated 4F-PCC (Octaplex) was recently evaluated by Diaz and colleagues.[59] Five patients receiving dabigatran, 76 to 88 years of age, were administered 4F-PCC to manage dabigatran-related GI bleeding complications. Treatment with 4F-PCC was able to adequately control bleeding in 4 of 5 patients; the fifth patient died of septic shock and coagulopathy secondary to severe hemorrhage. No thromboembolic events

Table 1
Case studies of dabigatran reversal: methods and results

Authors,[Ref.] Year	Possible Dabigatran Reversal Strategies (As Discussed in Guidelines)						Total Additional Blood Product Transfusions	Results
	3F-PCC	4F-PCC	Activated PCC	rFVIIa	FFP	Dialysis		
Cano & Miyares,[63] 2012	50 IU/kg					CVVHD	PRBCs (12 U) FFP (14 U) CP (60 U) Platelets (15 U)	Reversal strategy did not control hemorrhage in this patient
Dager et al,[58] 2013			26 IU/kg				PRBCs (6 U) FFP (2 U)	Bleeding stopped by the end of the 15-min infusion of activated PCC
Diaz et al,[59] 2013		15–25 IU/kg					RBC (0–2 U)	Adequate control of bleeding in 4/5 patients.
Dumkow et al,[60] 2012	20 IU/kg				4 U		PRBCs (5 U) FFP (12 U)	Only slight reduction in INR although hemoglobin levels restored and bleeding stopped
Harinstein et al,[61] 2013				30 mg/kg		CVVHD followed by CVVHDF	PRBCs (14 U) FFP (9 U) + 24-h infusion (50 mL/h) CP (20 U) Platelets (1 U)	rFVIIa, FFP, and CVVHD were unable to correct coagulopathy and bleeding CVVHDF + blood products restored hemostasis
Warkentin et al,[64] 2012				3 × 2.4 mg then 2 × 7.2 mg		High-flux dialysis filter	PRBCs (26 U) Plasma (22 U) CP (50 U) Platelets (5 adult doses)	High-dose rFVIIa and hemodialysis controlled bleeding in this patient

Abbreviations: CP, cryoprecipitate; CVVHD, continuous venovenous hemodialysis; CVVHDF, continuous venovenous hemodiafiltration; FFP, fresh frozen plasma; INR, international normalized ratio; IU, international unit; PCC, prothrombin complex concentrate; PRBCs, packed red blood cells; rFVIIa, recombinant activated factor VII; U, unit; 3F-PCC, 3-factor prothrombin complex concentrate; 4F-PCC, 4-factor prothrombin complex concentrate.

were reported in the next 6 months of follow-up in these patients. Interestingly, the investigators also reported that, in the one patient presenting with a prolonged activated partial thromboplastin time as a result of dabigatran treatment, administration of 4F-PCC was able to partially normalize this laboratory parameter, in contrast with results previously reported in a study in healthy volunteers.[55]

Concomitant administration of a nonactivated 3F-PCC (Profilnine) and fresh frozen plasma (FFP) was evaluated as a dabigatran reversal strategy in an 85-year-old patient with AF presenting with acute GI bleeding and multiorgan failure.[60] Following unsuccessful attempts to control bleeding via administration of packed red blood cells (PRBCs), FFP, and vitamin K, dabigatran reversal was attempted as per hospital guidelines, using 20 IU/kg of 3F-PCC with concurrent FFP infusion (4 U). This strategy resulted in only a slight reduction in INR at 30 minutes after treatment, followed by an increase on the next day (FFP [4 U] was subsequently administered to restore hemodynamic stability). However, this reversal protocol did successfully stabilize hemoglobin levels and stop the GI bleed, even though the patient later died of multiorgan failure.

Harinstein and Colleagues

Harinstein and colleagues[61] reported on dabigatran reversal in an 84-year-old patient with AF presenting with rectal bleeding from cecal perforation, which was subsequently corrected by hemicolectomy. Administration of FFP or cryoprecipitate had very little impact on coagulation parameters or transfusion requirements in this patient. Indeed, despite treatment with FFP and a single dose of rFVIIa before surgery and administration of blood products after surgery (including PRBCs, FFP, and cryoprecipitate), the patient still presented with continued bleeding and persistent coagulopathy. Continuous venovenous hemodialysis (CVVHD) was also unsuccessful in controlling bleeding or improving coagulopathy, and the patient was then switched to continuous venovenous hemodiafiltration (CVVHDF). Continued CVVHDF, alongside administration of additional blood products (2 U PRBCs, 1 U platelets, and 10 U cryoprecipitate), eventually resulted in hemodynamic stability 4 days after initial surgery. These particular hemodialysis methods were chosen because of the patient's hemodynamic instability; however, it is interesting that they removed negligible amounts of dabigatran, in contrast to the successful results obtained in other studies of dabigatran removal by hemodialysis.[62] Nevertheless, the investigators hypothesized that their approach may have had a small beneficial impact on the patient's recovery time.

Cano and Miyares

CVVHD was also used by Cano and Miyares,[63] in combination with 3F-PCC (Profilnine) for dabigatran reversal in a 78-year-old patient with AF presenting with rectal bleeding. Despite aggressive concomitant transfusion of blood products, this strategy proved ineffective in reversing dabigatran-induced anticoagulation and controlling bleeding, and the patient later died after withdrawal of care. Of note, the investigators did not comment on the effectiveness of the dialysis method for dabigatran removal in this patient. However, they did hypothesize that the use of rFVIIa in combination with 3F-PCC might have proved to be effective (3F-PCC was used in this study because 4F-PCCs were not available in the United States at that time).

Warkentin and Colleagues

Warkentin and colleagues[64] reported on a case study of a 79-year-old patient enrolled in the RE-LY trial (NCT00262600) who presented with severe postoperative bleeding following cardiac surgery; dabigatran had been discontinued 2 days prior. Administration of blood products, including cryoprecipitate, plasma, PRBCs, and platelets, and treatment with three 2.4-mg doses of rFVIIa were unable to control the bleeding. Administration of 2 additional 7.2-mg doses of rFVIIa decreased bleeding to levels sufficient to initiate hemodialysis, and, in contrast to results reported by Harinstein and colleagues,[61] hemodialysis effectively decreased dabigatran levels in this patient. Overall, this life-threatening bleeding episode was successfully managed by administration of high-dose rFVIIa followed by hemodialysis.

DISCUSSION

NOACs have emerged as effective alternatives to traditional VKAs, but are still associated with a risk of major bleeding. This risk is compounded by the absence of validated NOAC reversal strategies. Recent population-based evidence on NOAC-associated bleeding risk is consistent with data observed in head-to-head clinical trials of NOACs vs traditional anticoagulants. Nevertheless, the safety profile of NOACs should continue to be closely monitored. Continued surveillance, in addition to the study recently commissioned by Boehringer Ingelheim,[32] should provide additional evidence regarding the risk of major or fatal bleeding with these agents.

Whereas VKA reversal methods are well established, the current recommendations for NOAC reversal are based on preclinical or early clinical data, and no studies in bleeding patients have yet been performed. General hemostatic agents (eg, rFVIIa, activated and nonactivated PCCs) have been recommended for urgent reversal in patients with life-threatening bleeding, and emerging case-study reports provide some evidence for the effectiveness of these proposed reversal agents. Most of the published literature seems to be focused on dabigatran reversal, whereas similar studies seem to be lacking for the other NOACs. Ultimately, adequately powered studies in bleeding patients are warranted to assess the efficacy of these agents in the clinical setting.

Specific and selective NOAC reversal agents are also being developed, and have demonstrated promising results in preclinical in vitro, ex vivo, and in vivo models of hemostasis. A dabigatran antibody fragment was demonstrated to successfully reverse dabigatran-induced anticoagulation in vitro, and dabigatran-induced bleeding in a rat in vivo model of blood loss.[65] Similarly, administration of a specific FXa inhibitor antidote (PRT064445) successfully reversed rivaroxaban-induced anticoagulation in in vitro and ex vivo models, and restored hemostasis in animal models of blood loss.[66]

Finally, clinicians need to consider when to resume NOAC treatment in this patient population, who are prone to thromboembolic events without adequate antithrombotic therapy.[67] NOAC manufacturers generally recommend postoperative resumption of treatment as soon as possible, providing adequate hemostasis has been established.[68–70] To mitigate bleeding and thromboembolic risks, restarting with a lower dose than the recommended maintenance dose has also been suggested.[71] Ultimately, the decision to resume treatment depends on the risk of bleeding. Further details on current recommendations for the resumption of treatment can be found in the article by Levy elsewhere in this issue.

REFERENCES

1. Naccarelli GV, Varker H, Lin J, et al. Increasing prevalence of atrial fibrillation and flutter in the United States. Am J Cardiol 2009;104(11):1534–9.

2. Heit JA, Cohen AT, Anderson FA. Estimated annual number of incident and recurrent, non-fatal and fatal venous thromboembolism (VTE) events in the US. Blood 2005;106:910.
3. Nutescu EA, Shapiro NL, Chevalier A, et al. A pharmacologic overview of current and emerging anticoagulants. Cleve Clin J Med 2005;72(Suppl 1):S2–6.
4. Connolly SJ, Ezekowitz MD, Yusuf S, et al. Dabigatran versus warfarin in patients with atrial fibrillation. N Engl J Med 2009;361:1139–51.
5. Granger CB, Alexander JH, McMurray JJ, et al. Apixaban versus warfarin in patients with atrial fibrillation. N Engl J Med 2011;365:981–92.
6. Patel MR, Mahaffey KW, Garg J, et al. Rivaroxaban versus warfarin in nonvalvular atrial fibrillation. N Engl J Med 2011;365:883–91.
7. Büller HR, Prins MH, Lensin AW, et al. Oral rivaroxaban for the treatment of symptomatic pulmonary embolism. N Engl J Med 2012;366:1287–97.
8. Schulman S, Kearon C, Kakkar AK, et al. Dabigatran versus warfarin in the treatment of acute venous thromboembolism. N Engl J Med 2009;361:2342–52.
9. Southworth MR, Reichman ME, Unger EF. Dabigatran and postmarketing reports of bleeding. N Engl J Med 2013;368(14):1272–4.
10. U.S. Food and Drug Administration. Pradaxa (dabigatran etexilate meslate): drug safety communication - safety review of post-market reports of serious bleeding events. 2012. Available at: http://www.fda.gov/safety/medwatch/safetyinformation/safetyalertsforhumanmedicalproducts/ucm282820.htm. Accessed August 6, 2013.
11. Berger R, Salhanick SD, Chase M, et al. Hemorrhagic complications in emergency department patients who are receiving dabigatran compared with warfarin. Ann Emerg Med 2013;61(4):475–9.
12. Dickneite G, Hoffman M. Reversing the new oral anticoagulants with prothrombin complex concentrates (PCCs): what is the evidence? Thromb Haemost 2014;111(2):189–98.
13. Levine MN, Raskob G, Beyth RJ, et al. Hemorrhagic complications of anticoagulant treatment: the Seventh ACCP Conference on Antithrombotic and Thrombolytic Therapy. Chest 2004;126(Suppl 3):287S–310S.
14. Eikelboom JW, Mehta SR, Anand SS, et al. Adverse impact of bleeding on prognosis in patients with acute coronary syndromes. Circulation 2006;114(8):774–82.
15. IMS. IMS data US National Prescription Audit; MAT (moving annual total) 2011–2012.
16. Budnitz DS, Shehab N, Kegler SR, et al. Medication use leading to emergency department visits for adverse drug events in older adults. Ann Intern Med 2007;147(11):755–65.
17. Budnitz DS, Lovegrove MC, Shehab N, et al. Emergency hospitalizations for adverse drug events in older Americans. N Engl J Med 2011;365(21):2002–12.
18. Wysowski DK, Nourjah P, Swartz L. Bleeding complications with warfarin use: a prevalent adverse effect resulting in regulatory action. Arch Intern Med 2007;167(13):1414–9.
19. Stead LG, Jain A, Bellolio MF, et al. Effect of anticoagulant and antiplatelet therapy in patients with spontaneous intra-cerebral hemorrhage: does medication use predict worse outcome? Clin Neurol Neurosurg 2010;112(4):275–81.
20. Flaherty ML, Tao H, Haverbusch M, et al. Warfarin use leads to larger intracerebral hematomas. Neurology 2008;71(14):1084–9.
21. Broderick JP, Brott TG, Duldner JE, et al. Volume of intracerebral hemorrhage. A powerful and easy-to-use predictor of 30-day mortality. Stroke 1993;24(7):987–93.

22. Huhtakangas J, Tetri S, Juvela S, et al. Effect of increased warfarin use on warfarin-related cerebral hemorrhage: a longitudinal population-based study. Stroke 2011;42(9):2431–5.
23. Rosand J, Eckman MH, Knudsen KA, et al. The effect of warfarin and intensity of anticoagulation on outcome of intracerebral hemorrhage. Arch Intern Med 2004; 164(8):880–4.
24. Azoulay L, Dell'Aniello S, Simon T, et al. The concurrent use of antithrombotic therapies and the risk of bleeding in patients with atrial fibrillation. Thromb Haemost 2013;109(3):431–9.
25. Gomes T, Mamdani MM, Holbrook AM, et al. Rates of hemorrhage during warfarin therapy for atrial fibrillation. CMAJ 2013;185(2):E121–7.
26. Desai J, Granger CB, Weitz JI, et al. Novel oral anticoagulants in gastroenterology practice. Gastrointest Endosc 2013;78(2):227–39.
27. Capodanno D, Capranzano P, Giacchi G, et al. Novel oral anticoagulants versus warfarin in non-valvular atrial fibrillation: a meta-analysis of 50,578 patients. Int J Cardiol 2013;167(4):1237–41.
28. Miller CS, Grandi SM, Shimony A, et al. Meta-analysis of efficacy and safety of new oral anticoagulants (dabigatran, rivaroxaban, apixaban) versus warfarin in patients with atrial fibrillation. Am J Cardiol 2012;110(3):453–60.
29. Providencia R, Albenque JP, Combes S, et al. Safety and efficacy of dabigatran versus warfarin in patients undergoing catheter ablation of atrial fibrillation: a systematic review and meta-analysis. Heart 2013;100(4):324–35.
30. Australian Therapeutic Goods Administration (TGA). Dabigatran (Pradaxa) and risk of bleeding: information for health professionals. 2013. Available at: http://www.tga.gov.au/safety/alerts-medicine-dabigatran-111005.htm. Accessed September 3, 2013.
31. European Medicines Agency (EMA). European Medicines Agency updates patient and prescriber information for Pradaxa. 2012. Available at: http://www.ema.europa.eu/ema/index.jsp?curl=pages/news_and_events/news/2012/05/news_detail_001518.jsp&mid=WC0b01ac058004d5c1. Accessed September 4, 2013.
32. Boehringer Ingelheim. Boehringer Ingelheim announces agreement to study real-world use of oral anticoagulants. 2013. Available at: http://us.boehringer-ingelheim.com/news_events/press_releases/press_release_archive/2013/08-15-13-boehringer-ingelheim-announces-agreement-study-real-world-use-oral-anticoagulants.html. Accessed September 9, 2013.
33. Board of the German Medical Association. Cross-sectional guidelines for therapy with blood components and blood derivatives; plasma for therapeutic use. Transfus Med Hemother 2009;26:388–97.
34. Holbrook A, Schulman S, Witt DM, et al. Evidence-based management of anticoagulant therapy: antithrombotic therapy and prevention of thrombosis, 9th ed: American College of Chest Physicians Evidence-Based Clinical Practice Guidelines. Chest 2012;141:e152S–84S.
35. Keeling D, Baglin T, Tait C, et al. Guidelines on oral anticoagulation with warfarin - fourth edition. Br J Haematol 2011;154:311–24.
36. Pernod G, Godier A, Gozalo C, et al. French clinical practice guidelines on the management of patients on vitamin K antagonists in at-risk situations (overdose, risk of bleeding, and active bleeding). Thromb Res 2010;126:e167–74.
37. Spahn DR, Bouillon B, Cerny V, et al. Management of bleeding and coagulopathy following major trauma: an updated European guideline. Crit Care 2013; 17:R76.

38. Sarode R, Milling TJ Jr, Refaai MA, et al. Efficacy and safety of a 4-factor pro-thrombin complex concentrate in patients on vitamin K antagonists presenting with major bleeding: a randomized, plasma-controlled, phase IIIb study. Circulation 2013;128(11):1234–43.

39. Heidbuchel H, Verhamme P, Alings M, et al. European Heart Rhythm Association practical guide on the use of new oral anticoagulants in patients with non-valvular atrial fibrillation. Europace 2013;15:625–51.

40. Huisman MV, Lip GY, Diener HC, et al. Dabigatran etexilate for stroke prevention in patients with atrial fibrillation: resolving uncertainties in routine practice. Thromb Haemost 2012;107:838–47.

41. Levy JH, Faraoni D, Spring JL, et al. Managing new oral anticoagulants in the perioperative and intensive care unit setting. Anesthesiology 2013;118: 1466–74.

42. Pengo V, Crippa L, Falanga A, et al. Questions and answers on the use of dabigatran and perspectives on the use of other new oral anticoagulants in patients with atrial fibrillation. A consensus document of the Italian Federation of Thrombosis Centers (FCSA). Thromb Haemost 2011;106:868–76.

43. Turpie AG, Kreutz R, Llau J, et al. Management consensus guidance for the use of rivaroxaban – an oral, direct factor Xa inhibitor. Thromb Haemost 2012;108: 876–86.

44. Pernod G, Albaladejo P, Godier A, et al. Management of major bleeding complications and emergency surgery in patients on long-term treatment with direct oral anticoagulants, thrombin or factor-Xa inhibitors: proposals of the working group on perioperative haemostasis (GIHP) - March 2013. Arch Cardiovasc Dis 2013;106(6–7):382–93.

45. Ageno W, Gallus AS, Wittkowsky A, et al. Oral anticoagulant therapy: antithrombotic therapy and prevention of thrombosis, 9th ed: American College of Chest Physicians Evidence-Based Clinical Practice Guidelines. Chest 2012;141(Suppl 2):e44S–88S.

46. Kaatz S, Kouides PA, Garcia DA, et al. Guidance on the emergent reversal of oral thrombin and factor Xa inhibitors. Am J Hematol 2012;87(Suppl 1):S141–5.

47. Fawole A, Daw HA, Crowther MA. Practical management of bleeding due to the anticoagulants dabigatran, rivaroxaban, and apixaban. Cleve Clin J Med 2013; 80(7):443–51.

48. Queensland Health. Guideline for managing patients on dabigatran (Pradaxa®). 2013. Available at: http://www.health.qld.gov.au/qhcss/mapsu/documents/dabigatran_info.pdf. Accessed September 9, 2013.

49. Peacock WF, Gearhart MM, Mills RM. Emergency management of bleeding associated with old and new oral anticoagulants. Clin Cardiol 2012;35(12): 730–7.

50. Pollack CV Jr. Managing bleeding in anticoagulated patients in the emergency care setting. J Emerg Med 2013;45(3):467–77.

51. Miesbach W, Seifried E. New direct oral anticoagulants – current therapeutic options and treatment recommendations for bleeding complications. Thromb Haemost 2012;108(4):625–32.

52. Marlu R, Hodaj E, Paris A, et al. Effect of non-specific reversal agents on anti-coagulant activity of dabigatran and rivaroxaban. A randomised crossover ex vivo study in healthy volunteers. Thromb Haemost 2012;108:217–24.

53. Perzborn E, Gruber A, Tinel H, et al. Reversal of rivaroxaban anticoagulation by haemostatic agents in rats and primates. Thromb Haemost 2013;110:162–72.

54. Zhou W, Zorn M, Nawroth P, et al. Hemostatic therapy in experimental intracerebral hemorrhage associated with rivaroxaban. Stroke 2013;44:771–8.

55. Eerenberg ES, Kamphuisen PW, Sijpkens MK, et al. Reversal of rivaroxaban and dabigatran by prothrombin complex concentrate: a randomized, placebo-controlled, crossover study in healthy subjects. Circulation 2011;124:1573–9.

56. Levi M, Moore T, Castillejos CF, et al. Effects of three-factor and four-factor prothrombin complex concentrates on the pharmacodynamics of rivaroxaban (2013 ISTH abstracts). J Thromb Haemost 2013;11(Suppl s2):167.

57. Baumann Kreuziger LM, Reding MT. Management of bleeding associated with dabigatran and rivaroxaban: a survey of current practices. Thromb Res 2013; 132(2):e161–3.

58. Dager WE, Gosselin RC, Roberts AJ. Reversing dabigatran in life-threatening bleeding occurring during cardiac ablation with factor eight inhibitor bypassing activity. Crit Care Med 2013;41(5):e42–6.

59. Diaz MQ, Borobia AM, Nunez MA, et al. Use of prothrombin complex concentrates for urgent reversal of dabigatran in the Emergency Department. Haematologica 2013;98(11):e143–4.

60. Dumkow LE, Voss JR, Peters M, et al. Reversal of dabigatran-induced bleeding with a prothrombin complex concentrate and fresh frozen plasma. Am J Health Syst Pharm 2012;69(19):1646–50.

61. Harinstein LM, Morgan JW, Russo N. Treatment of dabigatran-associated bleeding: case report and review of the literature. J Pharm Pract 2013;26(3):264–9.

62. Khadzhynov D, Wagner F, Formella S, et al. Effective elimination of dabigatran by haemodialysis. A phase I single-centre study in patients with end-stage renal disease. Thromb Haemost 2013;109(4):596–605.

63. Cano EL, Miyares MA. Clinical challenges in a patient with dabigatran-induced fatal hemorrhage. Am J Geriatr Pharmacother 2012;10(2):160–3.

64. Warkentin TE, Margetts P, Connolly SJ, et al. Recombinant factor VIIa (rFVIIa) and hemodialysis to manage massive dabigatran-associated postcardiac surgery bleeding. Blood 2012;119(9):2172–4.

65. van Ryn J, Litzenburger T, Waterman A, et al. An antibody selective to dabigatran safely neutralizes both dabigatran-induced anticoagulant and bleeding activity in in vitro and in vivo models. J Thromb Haemost 2011;9(Suppl 2):1–970.

66. Lu G, DeGuzman FR, Hollenbach SJ, et al. A specific antidote for reversal of anticoagulation by direct and indirect inhibitors of coagulation factor Xa. Nat Med 2013;19:446–51.

67. Prandoni P, Noventa F, Ghirarduzzi A, et al. The risk of recurrent venous thromboembolism after discontinuing anticoagulation in patients with acute proximal deep vein thrombosis or pulmonary embolism. A prospective cohort study in 1,626 patients. Haematologica 2007;92(2):199–205.

68. Bayer Pharma AG. Xarelto® – Summary of product characteristics. Available at: http://www.ema.europa.eu/docs/en_GB/document_library/EPAR_-_Product_Information/human/000944/WC500057108.pdf. Accessed September 10, 2013.

69. Boehringer Ingelheim. Pradaxa® – Summary of product characteristics. Available at: http://www.ema.europa.eu/docs/en_GB/document_library/Other/2012/05/WC500127777.pdf. Accessed September 10, 2013.

70. Bristol-Myers Squibb. Eliquis® – Summary of product characteristics. Available at: http://www.ema.europa.eu/docs/en_GB/document_library/EPAR_-_Product_Information/human/002148/WC500107728.pdf. Accessed September 10, 2013.

71. Schulman S, Crowther MA. How I treat with anticoagulants in 2012: new and old anticoagulants, and when and how to switch. Blood 2012;119(13):3016–23.

Treatment of Intracerebral Hemorrhage Associated with New Oral Anticoagulant Use

The Neurologist's View

Roland Veltkamp, MD, FESO[a,b,*], Solveig Horstmann, MD[b]

KEYWORDS

- Intracerebral hemorrhage • Warfarin • Oral anticoagulation
- New oral anticoagulants

KEY POINTS

- The mortality rate associated with intracerebral hemorrhage (ICH) in patients treated with oral anticoagulants (OAC-ICH) is high.
- Secondary hematoma enlargement is one of the main reasons for poor outcome in patients with OAC-ICH.
- The key therapeutic target in OAC-ICH is rapid restoration of normal coagulation.
- In ICH associated with vitamin K antagonist therapy, hemostatic factors can be used.
- Optimal management of ICH associated with new direct OAC treatment is currently unknown.

INTRODUCTION

Intracerebral hemorrhage (ICH) associated with the use of oral anticoagulants (OAC-ICH) is an increasingly frequent challenge for emergency management. This mini-review summarizes the epidemiology of and predisposing factors for OAC-ICH. Current recommendations are reviewed for the management of OAC-ICH in patients using vitamin K antagonists (VKAs) or new direct oral anticoagulants (NOACs).

Disclosure Statement: R. Veltkamp has received consulting honoraria, research support, travel grants, and speakers' honoraria from Bayer HealthCare, Boehringer Ingelheim, Bristol-Myers Squibb, Pfizer, Roche Diagnostics Corporation, CSL Behring, St. Jude Medical, and Sanofi-Aventis. S. Horstmann is supported by an Olympia Morata Fellowship of the Medical Faculty, University of Heidelberg, Germany.

[a] Department of Stroke Medicine, Charing Cross Hospital, Imperial College London, Fulham Palace Road, London W6 8RF, UK; [b] Department of Neurology, University of Heidelberg, INF 400, Heidelberg 69120, Germany

* Corresponding author. Department of Stroke Medicine, Charing Cross Hospital, Imperial College London, Fulham Palace Road, London SW, UK.
E-mail address: roland.veltkamp@imperial.nhs.uk

Abbreviations	
AF	Atrial fibrillation
aPCC	Activated PCC
APOE	Apolipoprotein E
ICH	Intracerebral hemorrhage
INR	International normalized ratio
NOAC	New direct oral anticoagulant
OAC-ICH	Intracerebral hemorrhage associated with the use of oral anticoagulants
PCC	Prothrombin complex concentrate
rFVIIa	Recombinant activated factor VII
VKA	Vitamin K antagonists

EPIDEMIOLOGY AND PROGNOSIS OF OAC-ICH

Older epidemiologic studies suggest that OAC-ICH associated with VKA treatment occurs at a rate of 2 to 9 per 100,000 population per year.[1] The incidence of OAC-ICH is 7- to 10-fold higher than the incidence of ICH in patients who do not receive OACs.[1] Furthermore, the incidence of OAC-ICH has increased considerably over the past few years, reaching 12% to 15% in the general population, and up to 24% in tertiary care centers.[2–6] This increase reflects the increasing prevalence of atrial fibrillation (AF) in aging populations,[7–10] which is the predominant reason for long-term oral anticoagulation. Currently, 1% to 2% of the general population have AF.[7] The rate of ICH in patients treated with VKAs is up to 1.8% per year.[11,12] The rate of ICH during treatment with NOACs is 40% to 70% lower compared with warfarin, based on results from 4 large trials of stroke prevention in patients with AF.[8,13,14]

Mortality rates in patients with OAC-ICH range from 52% to 67%, and are higher than those observed in patients with spontaneous ICH without OAC therapy.[15] Survivors of OAC-ICH also more frequently remain severely disabled compared with patients recovering from spontaneous ICH unrelated to OAC therapy.[3,4,11] OAC-ICH is responsible for 60% to 90% of all bleeding-associated deaths in patients receiving VKA therapy.[16,17] Based on data from the RE-LY trial, mortality seems to be as high in ICH associated with NOAC therapy as in ICH during VKA treatment.[18]

PREDISPOSING FACTORS FOR OAC-ICH

Spontaneous ICH and OAC-ICH share the same risk factors. Advanced age, hypertension, and previous ischemic stroke have the strongest association with ICH.[19] Up to 70% of ICH is attributed to hypertensive small penetrating vessel arteriopathy, whereas cerebral amyloid angiopathy is associated with 5% to 20% of ICH cases.[20] Additional risk factors for OAC-ICH are concomitant use of aspirin, smoking, alcohol consumption, and severe heart and liver disease.[21–23]

The risk of ICH during anticoagulation therapy increases markedly when the international normalized ratio (INR) exceeds 4,[24] whereas the estimated annual risk of OAC-ICH is 0.3% to 3.7% when the target INR is between 2.0 and 4.5.[1] Each increase in the INR by 0.5 increases the bleeding risk by a factor of 1.4 and, although the intensity of anticoagulation therapy is related to a greater risk of OAC-ICH,[24–26] most ICH associated with VKA treatment occurs while patients are in the therapeutic range (ie, INR 2–3).[6] Data from epidemiologic studies of ICH in patients undergoing NOAC treatment are not yet available.

One further aspect of the risk factors for ICH is the hematoma location. For example, strong evidence shows that genetic risk factors influence ICH location and, in genetic association studies, apolipoprotein E (APOE) ε2 more than APOE ε4 was associated with lobar hemorrhage.[27–29]

The individual risk of experiencing any bleeding event when using a VKA can be determined using the HAS-BLED score[30]; evidence suggests that the score also moderately correlates with ICH risk.[31] The use of cerebral microbleeds detected on magnetic resonance imaging as indicators of an increased risk of hemorrhagic complications is currently under investigation.[32]

EMERGENCY TREATMENT OF ICH ASSOCIATED WITH VKA THERAPY

Hematoma size is a major prognostic factor in ICH because early secondary hematoma growth occurs in approximately one-third of patients experiencing a spontaneous ICH without OAC and is even more frequent in patients with OAC-ICH.[3,4,11] Therefore, prevention of hematoma expansion is a major therapeutic target. Another factor determining prognosis after ICH is expansion of the hematoma into the ventricles, which is more frequent and prolonged in patients receiving OACs.[6,33]

The use of VKAs reduces the plasma level of the clotting factors II, VII, IX, and X, but also of the anticoagulant proteins C and S. The anticoagulant effect of VKAs can be measured easily by routine coagulation tests (eg, INR), and point-of-care testing is available in emergency settings, allowing for prompt initiation and monitoring of reversal with coagulation factor concentrates.[34,35] In ICH associated with VKA therapy, coagulation can be restored by substitution of hemostatic factors using prothrombin complex concentrate (PCC) or fresh frozen plasma.[36–39] Because the efficacy and safety of these treatments have not been evaluated in randomized controlled trials in patients with OAC-ICH,[40,41] the recommendation to reverse VKA-induced anticoagulation with these agents during ICH is mainly based on plausibility and expert opinion.

EMERGENCY TREATMENT OF ICH ASSOCIATED WITH NOAC THERAPY

NOACs inhibit either factor Xa (rivaroxaban, apixaban, edoxaban), which is responsible for the generation of thrombin from prothrombin, or thrombin (factor IIa; dabigatran), which converts fibrinogen to fibrin.[42,43] The mechanism of action of NOACs differs substantially from that of VKAs, as described previously and in other articles elsewhere in this issue by Samama and colleagues and van Ryn and colleagues. The onset of anticoagulation occurs within 1 to 4 hours after first dosing, and the anticoagulant effect of NOACs is much shorter than that of VKAs. NOACs have limited interaction with other drugs[44] and none with food. The anticoagulant effect does not require monitoring and, unlike VKAs, dose-adjustments are usually unnecessary. NOAC-specific antidotes are in preclinical and clinical testing, but they are not yet available in routine practice.[45,46]

It is currently unknown whether NOACs increase the risk of secondary hematoma enlargement in ICH compared with non-anticoagulated patients. In a murine collagenase injection model of OAC-ICH, high doses of dabigatran or rivaroxaban led to excess hematoma expansion,[47,48] whereas another study with lower doses of dabigatran reported no effect.[49] Despite the current uncertainty, most stroke specialists assume that ICH occurring during NOAC therapy confers an additional risk of hematoma expansion.[50–52] Consequently, prevention of hematoma expansion is considered a major therapeutic target in ICH associated with NOACs.

Comparable to the treatment of ICH during VKA treatment, reversal of the anticoagulant effect of NOACs using hemostatic factors may be an effective approach to treat ICH during NOAC treatment as well.[47,48] However, no specific antidote is currently available to reverse the activity of NOACs in major bleeding, including ICH, and coagulation tests may not be predictive of bleeding (**Table 1**). Moreover, laboratory monitoring procedures have not been established to assess the effectiveness of nonspecific hemostatic reversal agents for NOACs. Further details on this topic have been extensively addressed in the 15 articles included in this issue.

The activated partial thromboplastin time provides a qualitative assessment of dabigatran levels. However, the sensitivity of different reagents used in this assay varies widely. The anticoagulant effect of dabigatran can also be quantified by the diluted thrombin time and the ecarin clotting time, as discussed by van Ryn and colleagues elsewhere in this issue.

Anticoagulation induced by rivaroxaban and apixaban can be assessed using prothrombin time when specific reagents are used (eg, neoplastin) (see **Table 1**). However, the anticoagulant effect of these factor Xa inhibitors is best evaluated through measuring substance-specific anti–factor Xa activity (see **Table 1** and the article by Samama and colleagues in this issue).

In experimental studies of ICH associated with NOAC treatment, PCCs and, less consistently, fresh frozen plasma and recombinant activated factor VII (rFVIIa) prevented excess hematoma enlargement.[47,48] A study in healthy human volunteers reported that PCC (50 U/kg) completely normalized prolongation of the prothrombin time after pretreatment with rivaroxaban, but had no effect on coagulation tests that were altered after the intake of dabigatran.[53] Administration of activated PCC (aPCC) to healthy volunteers pretreated with rivaroxaban, apixaban, or dabigatran had a more profound effect on coagulation parameters than PCC.[54] However, whether these parameters sufficiently reflect the effects of these reversal agents on the coagulation system in patients with ICH remains to be shown.

Current Treatment Recommendations

Current treatment recommendations for the management of ICH associated with NOAC use are based on expert opinion (**Fig. 1**).[55–57] In patients presenting with ICH, NOAC treatment should be discontinued. Because of the short half-lives of

Table 1
Laboratory diagnostics

	Dabigatran	Rivaroxaban	Apixaban
aPTT	↑↑	↑(↑)	↑
PT	↑	↑ to ↑↑	↑
Quick test	↓	↓ to ↓↓	↓
INR	(↑)	↑ to ↑↑	↑
TT	↑↑↑↑	↔	(↑)
ECT	↑↑↑↑	↔	↔
Anti–factor Xa Activity	↔ to ↑	↑↑↑	↑↑↑
Peak value test	aPTT	Anti–factor Xa activity (PT, aPTT)	Anti–factor Xa activity (PT, aPTT)
Trough test	TT	Anti–factor Xa activity	Anti–factor Xa activity
Substance-specific test system	Hemoclot, dabigatran concentration	Anti–factor Xa activity (calibrated)	Anti–factor Xa activity (calibrated)

↑, Prolonged/increased; (↑), may be prolonged/increased; ↓, decreased; ↔, equal/no change.
Abbreviations: aPTT, activated partial thromboplastin time; ECT, ecarin clotting time; PT, prothrombin time; TT, thrombin time.

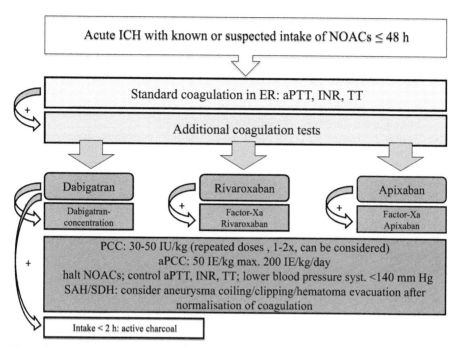

Fig. 1. Emergency management of ICH associated with NOAC therapy. aPTT, activated partial thromboplastin time; ER, emergency room; SAH/SDH, subarachnoid/subdural hemorrhage; TT, thrombin time. (*Courtesy of* Roland Veltkamp, MD, London, United Kingdom and Jan Purrucker, MD, Heidelberg, Germany.)

NOACs, time is the most important elimination factor, and the time of last intake should be identified to estimate the current coagulation status. In the case of recent (<2 hours) intake of NOACs, enteric uptake of NOACs may be reduced using activated charcoal. Coagulation factor concentrates should be administered. A single intravenous administration of PCC at a dose of 30 to 50 IU/kg is recommended.[55–57] Alternatively, aPCC at a dose of 50 IU/kg (maximum 200 IU/kg/d) can be considered.[55,56] The administration of PCC can be repeated if clinically indicated by hematoma expansion.[55,56] The use of rFVIIa for the treatment of ICH associated with NOAC therapy needs further evaluation, whereas vitamin K or protamine therapy are ineffective for the acute management of ICH in this context.[55,56] Elimination of NOACs from the blood through renal dialysis (dabigatran) or plasmapheresis (rivaroxaban, apixaban) is possible, but the practicability of this approach in acute ICH is limited.

In addition to the recommendations given earlier, the management of OAC-ICH should follow the recommendations for ICH treatment in patients not receiving anticoagulants.[1,58] In subarachnoid and subdural hemorrhages, aneurysm coiling or clipping and evacuation of the hematoma must be considered, respectively, after restoration of coagulation.[57] Structured collection of clinical experience relating to the management of ICH associated with NOACs in prospective clinical studies is needed.[59]

REFERENCES

1. Steiner T, Kaste M, Forsting M, et al. Recommendations for the management of intracranial haemorrhage - part I: spontaneous intracerebral haemorrhage. The

European Stroke Initiative Writing Committee and the Writing Committee for the EUSI Executive Committee. Cerebrovasc Dis 2006;22(4):294–316.

2. Go A, Hylek E, Phillips K, et al. Prevalence of diagnosed atrial fibrillation in adults: national implications for rhythm management and stroke prevention: the AnTicoagulation and Risk factors in Atrial Fibrillation (ATRIA) Study. JAMA 2001;285:2370–5.

3. Franke CL, de Jonge J, van Swieten JC, et al. Intracerebral hematomas during anticoagulant treatment. Stroke 1990;21(5):726–30.

4. Flibotte JJ, Hagan N, O'Donnell J, et al. Warfarin, hematoma expansion, and outcome of intracerebral hemorrhage. Neurology 2004;63(6):1059–64.

5. Sacco S, Marini C, Toni D, et al. Incidence and 10-year survival of intracerebral hemorrhage in a population-based registry. Stroke 2009;40:394–9.

6. Horstmann S, Rizos T, Lauseker M, et al. Intracerebral hemorrhage during anti-coagulation with vitamin K antagonists: a consecutive observational study. J Neurol 2013;260(8):2046–51.

7. Hohnloser SH, Crijns HJ, van Eickels M, et al. Effect of dronedarone on cardio-vascular events in atrial fibrillation. N Engl J Med 2009;360(7):668–78.

8. Connolly SJ, Ezekowitz MD, Yusuf S, et al. Dabigatran versus warfarin in pa-tients with atrial fibrillation. N Engl J Med 2009;361(12):1139–51.

9. Wolf PA, Abbott RD, Kannel WB. Atrial fibrillation: a major contributor to stroke in the elderly. The Framingham Study. Arch Intern Med 1987;147:1561–4.

10. Heeringa J, van der Kuip DA, Hofman A, et al. Prevalence, incidence and life-time risk of atrial fibrillation: the Rotterdam study. Eur Heart J 2006;27:949–53.

11. Rosand J, Eckman MH, Knudsen KA, et al. The effect of warfarin and intensity of anticoagulation on outcome of intracerebral hemorrhage. Arch Intern Med 2004; 164(8):880–4.

12. Hart RG, Boop BS, Anderson DC. Oral anticoagulants and intracranial hemor-rhage. Facts and hypotheses. Stroke 1995;26(8):1471–7.

13. Granger CB, Alexander JH, McMurray JJ, et al. Apixaban versus warfarin in patients with atrial fibrillation. N Engl J Med 2011;365(11):981–92.

14. Patel MR, Mahaffey KW, Garg J, et al. Rivaroxaban versus warfarin in nonvalv-ular atrial fibrillation. N Engl J Med 2011;365(10):883–91.

15. Veltkamp R, Rizos T, Horstmann S. Intracerebral bleeding in patients on antith-rombotic agents. Semin Thromb Hemost 2013;39(8):963–71.

16. Levine MN, Raskob G, Beyth RJ, et al. Hemorrhagic complications of anticoag-ulant treatment: the Seventh ACCP Conference on Antithrombotic and Thrombo-lytic Therapy. Chest 2004;126(3 Suppl):287S–310S.

17. Steiner T, Rosand J, Diringer M. Intracerebral hemorrhage associated with oral anticoagulant therapy: current practices and unresolved questions. Stroke 2006;37(1):256–62.

18. Hart RG, Diener HC, Yang S, et al. Intracranial hemorrhage in atrial fibrillation patients during anticoagulation with warfarin or dabigatran: the RE-LY trial. Stroke 2012;43(6):1511–7.

19. Hart RG, Tonarelli SB, Pearce LA. Avoiding central nervous system bleeding during antithrombotic therapy: recent data and ideas. Stroke 2005;36(7): 1588–93.

20. Revesz T, Holton JL, Lashley T, et al. Sporadic and familial cerebral amyloid an-giopathies. Brain Pathol 2002;12(3):343–57.

21. O'Donnell MJ, Xavier D, Liu L, et al. Risk factors for ischaemic and intracerebral haemorrhagic stroke in 22 countries (the INTERSTROKE study): a case-control study. Lancet 2010;376(9735):112–23.

22. Ariesen MJ, Claus SP, Rinkel GJ, et al. Risk factors for intracerebral hemorrhage in the general population: a systematic review. Stroke 2003;34(8):2060–5.
23. Schulman S, Beyth RJ, Kearon C, et al. Hemorrhagic complications of anticoagulant and thrombolytic treatment: American College of Chest Physicians Evidence-Based Clinical Practice Guidelines (8th edition). Chest 2008;133(6 Suppl): 257S–98S.
24. Hylek EM, Go AS, Chang Y, et al. Effect of intensity of oral anticoagulation on stroke severity and mortality in atrial fibrillation. N Engl J Med 2003;349: 1019–26.
25. Smith EE, Rosand J, Knudsen KA, et al. Leukoaraiosis is associated with warfarin-related hemorrhage following ischemic stroke. Neurology 2002;59: 193–7.
26. Lee GH, Kwon SU, Kang DW. Warfarin-induced intracerebral hemorrhage associated with microbleeds. J Clin Neurol 2008;4(3):131–3.
27. Rosand J, Hylek EM, O'Donnell HC, et al. Warfarin-associated hemorrhage and cerebral amyloid angiopathy: a genetic and pathologic study. Neurology 2000; 55(7):947–51.
28. Biffi A, Sonni A, Anderson CD, et al. Variants at APOE influence risk of deep and lobar intracerebral hemorrhage. Ann Neurol 2010;68(6):934–43.
29. Woo D, Sauerbeck LR, Kissela BM, et al. Genetic and environmental risk factors for intracerebral hemorrhage: preliminary results of a population-based study. Stroke 2002;33(5):1190–5.
30. Pisters R, Lane DA, Nieuwlaat R, et al. A novel user-friendly score (HAS-BLED) to assess 1-year risk of major bleeding in patients with atrial fibrillation: the Euro Heart Survey. Chest 2010;138(5):1093–100.
31. Friberg L, Rosenqvist M, Lip GY. Evaluation of risk stratification schemes for ischaemic stroke and bleeding in 182 678 patients with atrial fibrillation: the Swedish Atrial Fibrillation cohort study. Eur Heart J 2012;33(12):1500–10.
32. Charidimou A, Shakeshaft C, Werring DJ. Cerebral microbleeds on magnetic resonance imaging and anticoagulant-associated intracerebral hemorrhage risk. Front Neurol 2012;3:133.
33. Biffi A, Battey TW, Ayres AM, et al. Warfarin-related intraventricular hemorrhage: imaging and outcome. Neurology 2011;77(20):1840–6.
34. Rizos T, Jenetzky E, Herweh C, et al. Point-of-care reversal treatment in phenprocoumon-related intracerebral hemorrhage. Ann Neurol 2010;67(6): 788–93.
35. Rizos T, Jenetzky E, Herweh C, et al. Fast point-of-care coagulometer guided reversal of oral anticoagulation at the bedside hastens management of acute subdural hemorrhage. Neurocrit Care 2010;13(3):321–5.
36. Freeman WD, Brott TG, Barrett KM, et al. Recombinant factor VIIa for rapid reversal of warfarin anticoagulation in acute intracranial hemorrhage. Mayo Clin Proc 2004;79:1495–500.
37. Butler AC, Tait RC. Management of oral anticoagulant-induced intracranial haemorrhage. Blood Rev 1998;12:35–44.
38. Ansell J, Hirsh J, Hylek E, et al. Pharmacology and management of the vitamin K antagonists: American College of Chest Physicians Evidence-Based Clinical Practice Guidelines (8th edition). Chest 2008;133:160S–98S.
39. Baglin TP, Keeling DM, Watson HG. Guidelines on oral anticoagulation (warfarin): third edition – 2005 update. Br J Haematol 2006;132:277–85.
40. Freeman WD, Aguilar MI. Management of warfarin-related intracerebral hemorrhage. Expert Rev Neurother 2008;8:271–90.

41. Kessler CM. Urgent reversal of warfarin with prothrombin complex concentrate: where are the evidence-based data? J Thromb Haemost 2006;4:963–6.
42. Eisert WG, Hauel N, Stangier J, et al. Dabigatran: an oral novel potent reversible nonpeptide inhibitor of thrombin. Arterioscler Thromb Vasc Biol 2010;30(10): 1885–9.
43. Weitz JI. New oral anticoagulants in development. Thromb Haemost 2010;103: 62–70.
44. Weitz JI. Factor Xa and thrombin as targets for new oral anticoagulants. Thromb Res 2011;127(Suppl 2):S5–12.
45. Schiele F, van Ryn J, Canada K, et al. A specific antidote for dabigatran: functional and structural characterization. Blood 2013;121(18):3554–62.
46. Dolgin E. Antidotes edge closer to reversing effects of new blood thinners. Nat Med 2013;19(3):251.
47. Zhou W, Schwarting S, Illanes S, et al. Hemostatic therapy in experimental intracerebral hemorrhage associated with the direct thrombin inhibitor dabigatran. Stroke 2011;42:3594–9.
48. Zhou W, Zorn M, Nawroth P, et al. Hemostatic therapy in experimental intracerebral hemorrhage associated with rivaroxaban. Stroke 2013;44(3):771–8.
49. Lauer A, Cianchetti FA, Van Cott EM, et al. Anticoagulation with the oral direct thrombin inhibitor dabigatran does not enlarge hematoma volume in experimental intracerebral hemorrhage. Circulation 2011;124:1654–62.
50. Steiner T, Bosel J. Options to restrict hematoma expansion after spontaneous intracerebral hemorrhage. Stroke 2010;41(2):402–9.
51. Qureshi AI, Tuhrim S, Broderick JP, et al. Spontaneous intracerebral hemorrhage. N Engl J Med 2001;344(19):1450–60.
52. Alberts MJ, Eikelboom JW, Hankey GJ. Antithrombotic therapy for stroke prevention in non-valvular atrial fibrillation. Lancet Neurol 2012;11(12):1066–81.
53. Eerenberg ES, Kamphuisen PW, Sijpkens MK, et al. Reversal of rivaroxaban and dabigatran by prothrombin complex concentrate: a randomized, placebo-controlled, crossover study in healthy subjects. Circulation 2011;124:1573–9.
54. Marlu R, Hodaj E, Paris A, et al. Effect of non-specific reversal agents on anticoagulant activity of dabigatran and rivaroxaban: a randomised crossover ex vivo study in healthy volunteers. Thromb Haemost 2012;108(2):217–24.
55. Heidbuchel H, Verhamme P, Alings M, et al. EHRA practical guide on the use of new oral anticoagulants in patients with non-valvular atrial fibrillation: executive summary. Eur Heart J 2013;34(27):2094–106.
56. Heidbuchel H, Verhamme P, Alings M, et al. European Heart Rhythm Association Practical Guide on the use of new oral anticoagulants in patients with non-valvular atrial fibrillation. Europace 2013;15(5):625–51.
57. Steiner T, Bohm M, Dichgans M, et al. Recommendations for the emergency management of complications associated with the new direct oral anticoagulants (DOACs), apixaban, dabigatran and rivaroxaban. Clin Res Cardiol 2013; 102(6):399–412.
58. Morgenstern LB, Hemphill JC 3rd, Anderson C, et al. Guidelines for the management of spontaneous intracerebral hemorrhage: a guideline for healthcare professionals from the American Heart Association/American Stroke Association. Stroke 2010;41(9):2108–29.
59. Veltkamp R, Juttler E, Pfefferkorn T, et al. Current registry studies of acute ischemic stroke. Nervenarzt 2012;83(10):1270–4 [in German].

Periprocedural Management of Patients on Anticoagulants

Lance A. Williams III, MD[a],*, James M. Hunter Jr, MD[b],
Marisa B. Marques, MD[c], Thomas R. Vetter, MD, MPH[d]

KEYWORDS

- Anticoagulant • Antiplatelet • Periprocedural • Atrial fibrillation • CHA$_2$DS$_2$-VASc

KEY POINTS

- The risk of recurrent thrombosis and of significant surgical bleeding must be considered when deciding on the periprocedural management of anticoagulation.
- Caution must be used when interpreting laboratory values in patients taking older and newer anticoagulants owing to variability in in vivo and in vitro assay results.
- Minor surgeries often require no adjustment of anticoagulant therapy, whereas major surgeries may require complex management, including bridging therapy with heparin.
- The CHA$_2$DS$_2$-VASc (congestive heart failure, hypertension, age ≥75 years, diabetes mellitus, stroke, vascular disease, age 65–74 years, sex category) and HAS-BLED (hypertension, abnormal renal/liver function, stroke, bleeding history or predisposition, labile International Normalized Ratio, elderly, drugs/alcohol concomitantly) scores are useful in evaluating patient risk for thromboembolism and surgical bleeding, respectively.
- Although novel oral anticoagulants may simplify periprocedural anticoagulation in the future, the management of novel oral anticoagulant–induced anticoagulation is currently difficult owing to the lack of validated reversal strategies and of laboratory tests that can accurately determine dose responses.

INTRODUCTION

Over the past decade, the periprocedural management of patients on anticoagulants has become increasingly complex, especially with the advent of novel agents with

The authors have no relevant financial disclosures.
[a] Department of Pathology, University of Alabama at Birmingham, 619 19th Street South, WPP230F, Birmingham, AL 35249-7331, USA; [b] Department of Anesthesiology, University of Alabama at Birmingham, 1720 2nd Avenue South, JT926C, Birmingham, AL 35249-6810, USA; [c] Department of Pathology, University of Alabama at Birmingham, 619 19th Street South, WPP230G, Birmingham, AL 35249-7331, USA; [d] Department of Anesthesiology, University of Alabama at Birmingham, 619 19th Street South, JT865, Birmingham, AL 35249, USA
* Corresponding author.
E-mail address: law3@uab.edu

varying mechanisms of action and half-lives. Some of the most common indications for anticoagulant treatment include deep vein thrombosis (DVT), venous thromboembolism (VTE), atrial fibrillation (AF), and mechanical heart valves.

VTE affects approximately 1 to 2 per 1000 adults in the United States[1] and the annual prevalence increases greatly in patients 65 years of age and older (1382 vs 231 per 100,000 patients ≥65 and <65 years old, respectively, in 2006).[2] Long-term anticoagulation is used to prevent recurrences, which affect approximately 30% of patients.[3] As documented by the Anticoagulation and Risk Factors in Atrial Fibrillation (ATRIA) study, the prevalence of AF varies widely with age, ranging from 0.1% in individuals less than or equal to 55 years old to approximately 9% in those 80 years of age and older.[4] In addition, as safety and efficacy improve, the use of mechanical heart valves is becoming more common, exposing patients to an annual risk of valve-associated thrombosis that varies depending on the interval since placement. During the first year following implantation of heart valves, the risk of thrombosis is approximately 24%, decreasing to 15% by the fourth year.[5]

Although a multitude of studies and evidence exists regarding the general management of patients on anticoagulants, periprocedural risk stratification and decision making remain difficult owing to a lack of controlled trials. Achieving the delicate balance between preventing thrombosis and minimizing surgical bleeding is challenging in the preprocedural, intraprocedural, and postprocedural periods. In addition, as external pressures to reduce discharge times mount, the need for efficient but safe periprocedural management protocols is paramount.

Recognizing the importance of this issue, this article reviews the current evidence and recommendations for how best to manage anticoagulated patients requiring a nonemergent surgical procedure. Although some controversy still exists regarding the appropriate measures to implement, this article presents guidelines/algorithms to assist clinicians in the management of these challenging situations.

ORAL ANTICOAGULANTS AND LABORATORY TESTS

The practice of prescribing outpatient oral anticoagulants is less than 60 years old, and until a few years ago was almost exclusively limited to the use of warfarin, a vitamin K antagonist. Exceptions exist, such as in pregnant women, who cannot receive warfarin and thus require a safer alternative such as subcutaneous low-molecular-weight heparin (LMWH). Because this practice is typically handled by maternal health specialists, periprocedural management of these patients is not discussed in this article.

Warfarin, the most commonly prescribed oral anticoagulant, has an unpredictable anticoagulant effect and must be monitored using the prothrombin time (PT) and the International Normalized Ratio (INR), derived from the PT. Although an INR between 2.0 and 3.0 (2.5–3.5 for patients with mechanical mitral or mitral and aortic heart valves) is desirable in order to avoid thrombosis and minimize the risk of serious bleeding,[6] the higher the INR, the greater the likelihood of hemorrhage. Health care providers are familiar with this concept and monitor the INR of patients on warfarin monthly (or less frequently as appropriate) on an ongoing basis.

If a nonemergent procedure is planned, patient management will depend on various factors, such as the indication for anticoagulation and the type of procedure. Because warfarin causes deficiencies of the vitamin K–dependent factors, administration of vitamin K and replenishment of these factors are effective measures for reversal of its anticoagulant effects, if required.

Laboratory Testing in Patient Management

The role of laboratory testing in patient management has changed greatly with the introduction of new oral anticoagulants, which include dabigatran (a direct thrombin inhibitor) and rivaroxaban and apixaban (direct factor Xa inhibitors). First, these agents have a more predictable dose response compared with traditional anticoagulants and thus do not require routine monitoring. Second, there is a misconception among clinicians that because laboratory testing is not indicated, these drugs have no effect on coagulation parameters such as PT and partial thromboplastin time (PTT). On the contrary, as coagulation inhibitors, they prolong various clotting assay parameters, although these values are not used for dose adjustment, unlike the practice with warfarin. Third, the effects of new oral anticoagulants on PT and PTT vary among laboratories, depending on the method used to perform these tests. Thus, it has not been established which clotting times represent the desired level of anticoagulation versus inadequate or excessive anticoagulation. A normal PT and PTT indicate that rivaroxaban and apixaban are no longer in the circulation, which could be vital in the preoperative period. The most reliable test to detect the presence or absence of dabigatran in the plasma is the thrombin time (TT). However, because TT is very sensitive to dabigatran, a prolonged thrombin time cannot be used to accurately determine the amount of circulating drug present. **Table 1** summarizes oral anticoagulants and their associated laboratory tests.

PERIPROCEDURAL MANAGEMENT OF WARFARIN-INDUCED ANTICOAGULATION IN PATIENTS WITH AF

The periprocedural management of anticoagulation in patients with AF must balance the competing goals of preventing thromboembolism (TE) and minimizing the risk from intraoperative or postoperative bleeding. A rational approach to this medical condition must weigh the risk of TE and the severity of its potential consequences, in particular the risk of embolic stroke, against the nature of the surgical procedure and other factors that could increase the risk of clinically significant bleeding. These factors determine whether anticoagulants need to be discontinued before surgery and the need for and timing of bridging therapy.

Table 1
Oral anticoagulants and laboratory tests

Drug	Half-life (h)	Test(s) Used to Monitor Anticoagulant Effect	Test(s) Affected by Anticoagulant but not Useful for Monitoring Anticoagulation Level	Reversal Agent(s)
Warfarin	20–60	PT and INR	PTT when INR supratherapeutic	Vitamin K and PCCs
Dabigatran	12–14	None	TT	None
Rivaroxaban	5–9[a]	None	PT, PTT, anti-Xa[b]	PCCs or activated
Apixaban	12[a]	None	PT, PTT, anti-Xa[b]	coagulation factors may be tried

Abbreviations: PCCs, prothrombin complex concentrates; PT, prothrombin time; PTT, partial thromboplastin time.
[a] Increases with incremental loss of renal function.
[b] The anti-Xa assay is very sensitive to rivaroxaban and apixaban.

For low-risk procedures, such as minor dental[6,7] or dermatologic[6] and some ophthalmologic procedures (including cataract extraction[8] and 25-gauge vitrectomy with peribulbar or retrobulbar block[9]), discontinuation of warfarin is not routinely required, but can be considered, depending on the type of procedure, the amount of bleeding expected, and the likelihood of difficulty with maintaining surgical hemostasis. For dental surgery, if warfarin therapy is continued, oral prohemostatic agents such as antifibrinolytics can be used to control procedure-associated bleeding.

If warfarin is to be discontinued, the 2012 American College of Chest Physicians (ACCP) guidelines recommend doing so 5 days before surgery,[6] which results in normalization of the INR in all but a minority of patients.[6,10,11] Because a small number of patients may still have INRs greater than 1.5, testing on the day of surgery is necessary, particularly when the adverse consequences of bleeding are potentially severe (eg, neurosurgery). Spyropoulos and Douketis[12] recommend measuring the INR on the day before surgery to provide the opportunity to hasten its normalization by the administration of a small dose of oral vitamin K (1.0–2.5 mg). This approach, although reasonable, is not always practical, because many patients arrive from far away on the evening before or on the day of the surgery.

Management for Urgent or Emergent Surgeries

Periprocedural anticoagulation management for urgent or emergent surgeries has a more compressed timeline. If a patient presents less than 24 hours before surgery, administration of frozen plasma and/or a prothrombin complex concentrate plus intravenous (IV) vitamin K can rapidly reverse the effect of warfarin. If the surgery is scheduled to take place more than 24 hours from presentation, then IV vitamin K alone is usually sufficient to correct the INR.[6]

Risk of TE

The use of unfractionated heparin (UFH) or LMWH as bridging therapy (**Table 2** shows dosages) during the period when warfarin is being withheld has become widespread. However, their efficacy and safety remain controversial, and additional studies are underway.[6,13–15] A means of determining the risk of periprocedural TE is necessary

Table 2 Commonly used anticoagulation bridging therapy regimens	
Drug	**Dose**
UFH	Target PTT to match anti-Xa of 0.3–0.7 units/mL[a]
Enoxaparin	1 mg/kg SC twice a day or 1.5 mg/kg SC daily[b]
Dalteparin	100 IU/kg SC twice a day or 200 IU/kg SC daily[c]
Tinzaparin	175 IU/kg daily[d]

Abbreviations: IU, international unit; SC, subcutaneously; UFH, unfractionated heparin.
[a] Because it is metabolized by the liver, no dose adjustment is needed for patients with renal dysfunction.
[b] For patients with creatinine clearance greater than 30 mL/min, no dose adjustment is necessary. For those with creatinine clearance less than 30 mL/min, the recommendation is a dose of 1 mg/kg SC every 24 hours.
[c] No standard dose adjustment for patients with renal dysfunction. Adjustments based on monitoring anti-Xa results.
[d] Caution is recommended, but no specific dose adjustment guidelines are available at this time.
Data from Douketis JD, Spyropoulos AC, Spencer FA, et al. Perioperative management of antithrombotic therapy: antithrombotic therapy and prevention of thrombosis, 9th ed: American College of Chest Physicians Evidence-Based Clinical Practice Guidelines. Chest 2012;141(Suppl 2):e326S–50S.

to guide decision making regarding the use of bridging therapy. In AF, several risk-stratification schemes have been developed for estimating the risk of arterial thromboembolism (**Table 3**).[16] The $CHADS_2$ (congestive heart failure, hypertension, age, diabetes, prior stroke) score includes 1 point each for congestive heart failure, hypertension, age greater than or equal to 75 years, and diabetes mellitus, and 2 points for history of either stroke or transient ischemic attack. The $CHADS_2$ score was used in the 2012 ACCP guidelines to risk stratify patients with AF undergoing elective surgery.[6] The CHA_2DS_2-VASc (congestive heart failure, hypertension, age $\geq$75 years, diabetes mellitus, stroke, vascular disease, age 65–74 years, sex category) score adds an additional point for a history of vascular disease (including coronary artery disease), age greater than or equal to 65 years, and female gender.[16] The CHA_2DS_2-VASc score seems to be better at assessing the risk of TE than the $CHADS_2$ score, especially for categorizing patients as low risk for TE and placing fewer patients in the nebulous intermediate-risk category.[16–18]

It is unknown whether the same factors that increase the risk of TE in the chronic outpatient setting contribute to the same degree in the periprocedural period. However, given that surgery and its associated inflammatory response induce a hypercoagulable state,[19–21] it is reasonable to assume that the risk of TE is greater in the periprocedural than in the outpatient setting. Kaatz and colleagues[22] showed in a retrospective study that perioperative stroke risk was higher in patients with chronic AF than in those without AF. In addition, the incidence of stroke observed in patients with AF in this study was higher than that predicted based on proration of the annual stroke risk in patients with chronic AF, supporting the hypothesis that risk of stroke is greater in the perioperative period. This study also found the $CHADS_2$ score to be predictive of postoperative stroke.[22] Because the CHA_2DS_2-VASc score is a refinement of the $CHADS_2$ score, it is likely to provide a valid stratification of periprocedural stroke (and other TE) risk in patients with chronic AF, although additional work needs to be done to confirm this. In this scoring system, a score of 0 is considered low risk, a score of 1 is intermediate, and a score of 2 or higher is considered high risk.[16] For patients receiving warfarin with a CHA_2DS_2-VASc score of 0 we recommend no bridging therapy, because warfarin is not recommended for these patients for the prevention of TE because of chronic AF (**Fig. 1**). We recommend bridging therapy (beginning 2 days

Table 3
The CHA_2DS_2-VASc score

Risk Factor	Points
Congestive heart failure or left ventricular dysfunction	1
Hypertension	1
Age $\geq$75 y	2
Diabetes mellitus	1
Stroke, TIA, or thromboembolism in past	2
Vascular disease (history of MI, PAD, or aortic plaque)	1
Age 65–74 y	1
Sex (ie, female gender)	1

Abbreviations: MI, myocardial infarction; PAD, peripheral arterial disease; TIA, transient ischemic attack.

Modified from Lip GY, Nieuwlaat R, Pisters R, et al. Refining clinical risk stratification for predicting stroke and thromboembolism in atrial fibrillation using a novel risk factor-based approach: the euro heart survey on atrial fibrillation. Chest 2010;137(2):263–72.

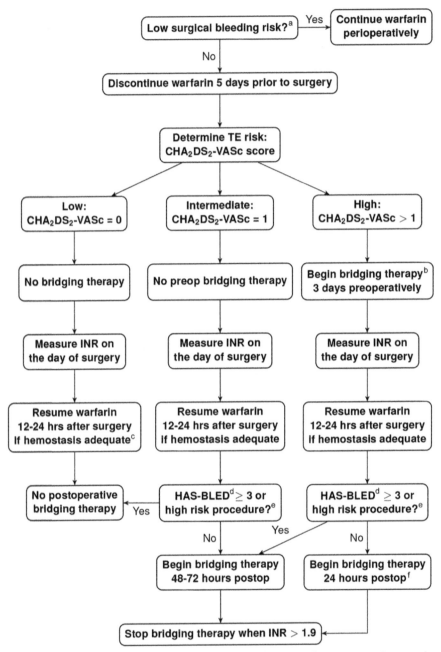

Fig. 1. Periprocedural management of warfarin in AF. [a] For example, cataract and some other eye surgeries, minor dental or dermatologic procedures. [b] See bridging regimens in **Table 2**. [c] Long-term anticoagulation for AF is not generally recommended in this group. Resumption of warfarin should be based on the patient's other indication(s) for warfarin. [d] See HAS-BLED table (**Table 4**). [e] Procedures with a high bleeding risk: cardiac surgery, carotid endarterectomy, craniotomy, spine surgery, major abdominal surgery, major orthopedic surgery. [f] As an alternative, start prophylactic dose of LMWH 24 hours after surgery followed by therapeutic dose 48 hours after surgery. postop, postoperatively; preop, preoperatively.

Table 4	
The HAS-BLED score	
Risk Factor	**Points**
Hypertension	1
Abnormal renal or hepatic function	1 point for each
Stroke	1
Bleeding history or predisposition	1
Labile INR	1
Elderly (age>75 y)	1
Drug (antiplatelet or NSAID) or alcohol use	1 point for each

Abbreviation: NSAID, nonsteroidal antiinflammatory drug.
  Modified from Pisters R, Lane DA, Nieuwlaat R, et al. A novel user-friendly score (HAS-BLED) to assess 1-year risk of major bleeding in patients with atrial fibrillation: the Euro Heart Survey. Chest 2010;138(5):1093–100.

after stopping warfarin) for those with a CHA_2DS_2-VASc score of 2 or more. For the intermediate-risk group (CHA_2DS_2-VASc score of 1), we advise against the use of preoperative bridging therapy. However, as with all clinical decisions, the patient-specific evaluation of the adverse effect of TE versus bleeding on quality of life should also influence this decision.

Bridging Therapy

Because bridging therapy is associated with an increased risk of intraprocedural and postprocedural bleeding,[23] there is also a rationale for stratifying patients according to their risk of morbidity and mortality from surgical bleeding when deciding on the use and timing of postprocedural bridging therapy. The HAS-BLED (hypertension, abnormal renal/liver function, stroke, bleeding history or predisposition, labile INR, elderly, drugs/alcohol concomitantly) score (see **Fig. 1**) has been used to predict risk of bleeding in patients receiving anticoagulants for chronic AF.[24–26] In a retrospective study by Omran and colleagues,[27] a HAS-BLED score of greater than or equal to 3 was also found to predict bleeding during bridging therapy. The bleeding risk associated with the surgical procedure must also be considered. Procedures considered to have a high bleeding risk include cardiac, carotid endarterectomy, major abdominal, craniotomy, spinal, major orthopedic, and some endoscopic and urologic surgery.[6,28,29] In patients with an intermediate risk of TE (CHA_2DS_2-VASc score of 1), we recommend not initiating or resuming bridging therapy after the procedure if there is an increased risk of bleeding, as indicated by a HAS-BLED score of greater than or equal to 3 or a high-risk surgical procedure. For those with a CHA_2DS_2-VASc score of 1, a HAS-BLED score of less than 3, and a lower-risk surgical procedure, we recommend beginning postoperative bridging therapy 48 to 72 hours after surgery. In patients at higher risk of TE (CHA_2DS_2-VASc score ≥2), we recommend resuming bridging therapy at least 24 hours after a procedure in those with a lower risk of bleeding (HAS-BLED<3) and delaying resumption of bridging therapy until 48 to 72 hours in those with a higher risk of bleeding (HAS-BLED ≥3 or high-risk procedure).

PERIPROCEDURAL MANAGEMENT OF WARFARIN-INDUCED ANTICOAGULATION IN PATIENTS WITH DVT AND VTE

The periprocedural management of patients with a history of DVT with or without VTE has recently changed. Most experts agree with discontinuation of warfarin 5 days before major surgery, and risk stratification delineates the patients who require bridging therapy with heparin before and/or after the procedure.

In the course of assessing the need for bridging therapy in patients with a history of DVT/VTE, much of the risk of recurrent thrombosis is determined by how much time has passed since the most recent DVT/VTE episode. If the hiatus is longer than 12 months, the patient has the lowest risk of recurrent thrombosis and does not require bridging therapy, whereas patients with a hiatus less than 3 months have the highest risk and should receive bridging therapy (**Fig. 2**). If the most recent DVT/VTE was between 3 and 12 months before the planned procedure, the requirement for bridging therapy is determined by the morbidity and mortality risk from bleeding associated with the surgical procedure, in conjunction with the underlying conditions of the patient that may predispose to thrombosis. Therefore, patients with a moderate risk of recurrent DVT/VTE are more likely to receive LMWH than those with a higher intraprocedure or postprocedure risk of bleeding.

PERIPROCEDURAL MANAGEMENT OF WARFARIN-INDUCED ANTICOAGULATION IN PATIENTS WITH MECHANICAL HEART VALVES

For patients with mechanical valves, risk stratification is based not only on the type of valve but also its location. In the 2012 ACCP guidelines,[6] a specific $CHADS_2$ score for risk is not given; however, the $CHADS_2$ score components all play a role in the risk category and the decision to bridge with heparin (**Fig. 3**). Otherwise, the algorithm is much the same as for patients with a history of DVT/VTE.

PERIPROCEDURAL MANAGEMENT OF PATIENTS ON ANTIPLATELET MEDICATIONS

As for oral anticoagulants, the number of antiplatelet medications available has increased steadily over the past 2 decades. Aspirin, the first commonly used antiplatelet drug, was initially marketed as an antipyretic and analgesic, but further studies elucidated its antiplatelet effect, and it has remained the mainstay of antiplatelet therapy for years.[30] However, in 1997, the US Food and Drug Administration (FDA) approved clopidogrel after the Clopidogrel versus Aspirin in Patients at Risk of Ischemic Events (CAPRIE) trial showed the superiority of clopidogrel compared with aspirin in reducing cardiovascular events in patients with history of a recent myocardial infarction (MI), stroke, or peripheral artery disease.[31] Since then, the approved indications for clopidogrel have increased, and at the same time the practice of dual antiplatelet therapy has become more commonplace, thus complicating management of this patient population. As with other anticoagulants, the periprocedural management of patients on antiplatelet drugs depends on a delicate balance between preventing thrombosis as well as periprocedural bleeding.[32]

PERIPROCEDURAL MANAGEMENT OF PATIENTS ON ASPIRIN

Aspirin's antiplatelet function is based on its irreversible inhibition of cyclooxygenase. It is rapidly absorbed and the half-life for low doses (<250 mg) is approximately 2 to 4.5 hours.[33] Therefore, platelets synthesized or transfused after the drug is eliminated are not inhibited. The 2012 ACCP guidelines recommend continuing aspirin in patients undergoing minor procedures, such as dental, dermatologic, or cataract surgery. This recommendation also holds for patients undergoing noncardiac surgeries that have a moderate to high risk for cardiovascular events. In patients at low risk for cardiovascular events, aspirin can be discontinued 7 to 10 days before surgery.[6] Although not

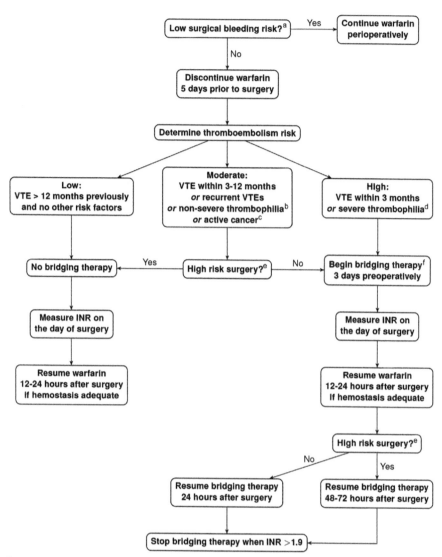

Fig. 2. Periprocedural management of warfarin in DVT/pulmonary embolism. [a] For example, cataract and some other eye surgeries, minor dental or dermatologic procedures. [b] Nonsevere thrombophilia is a heterozygous factor V Leiden or prothrombin gene mutation. [c] Treated in the last 6 months or in palliative care. [d] Severe thrombophilia is deficiency of protein C, protein S, or antithrombin; antiphospholipid antibodies; multiple abnormalities. [e] Procedures with a high bleeding risk: cardiac surgery, carotid endarterectomy, craniotomy, spine surgery, major abdominal surgery, major orthopedic surgery, or if additional risk factors for bleeding are present (thrombocytopenia, bleeding disorders) or previous major bleeding. [f] See **Table 2** for bridging regimens.

addressed in the 2012 ACCP guidelines, some investigators recommend discontinuing aspirin for procedures in which hemorrhage could prove detrimental to surgical outcomes, such as intracranial, middle ear, posterior eye, and intramedullary spinal surgeries.[34] Because of concerns over aspirin withdrawal syndrome, some guidelines

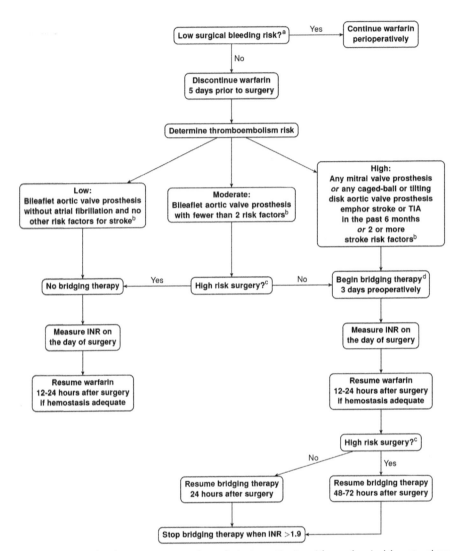

Fig. 3. Periprocedural management of warfarin in patients with mechanical heart valves.
[a] For example, cataract and some other eye surgeries, minor dental or dermatologic procedures. [b] Risk factors include congestive heart failure, hypertension, age greater than
75 years, diabetes mellitus, prior stroke, or AF. [c] Procedures with a high bleeding risk: cardiac
surgery, carotid endarterectomy, craniotomy, spine surgery, major abdominal surgery, major
orthopedic surgery, or if additional risk factors for bleeding are present (thrombocytopenia,
bleeding disorders) or previous major bleeding. [d] See **Table 2** for bridging regimens.

recommend resuming aspirin 24 hours after surgery, as long as adequate hemostasis
has been established.[6,34]

In patients undergoing coronary artery bypass graft surgery, aspirin should be
continued. However, as alluded to earlier, some patients are on dual antiplatelet therapy. In that case, aspirin should be continued, but the longer acting agents, such as
clopidogrel or prasugrel, should be discontinued 5 days before surgery.[6] Some agents,
discussed later, may require longer periods of discontinuation before the procedure.

For patients with coronary stents who are being treated with dual antiplatelet agents, the surgery should be delayed if possible to allow for the minimum duration of antiplatelet therapy after stent placement to prevent stent thrombosis. For bare-metal stents, at least 6 weeks of antiplatelet therapy is recommended, whereas at least 6 months and preferably 12 months of such therapy are recommended for drug-eluting stents. However, if surgery is required before this, dual antiplatelet therapy should be continued in the periprocedural period.[6,35,36]

PERIPROCEDURAL MANAGEMENT OF PATIENTS ON OTHER ANTIPLATELET DRUGS

Clopidogrel, prasugrel, ticagrelor, and ticlopidine exert their antiplatelet effect by blocking $P2Y_{12}$ receptors. Compared with aspirin, the half-lives of these medications are much longer. Thus, newly synthesized platelets or transfused platelets may be inhibited as long as the drug is still active. Hence, bleeding could ensue even in patients with a normal platelet count, because these platelets may be unable to participate in normal hemostasis.

The varying half-lives of these agents affect the recommendations for preprocedural discontinuation. Clopidogrel and prasugrel should be discontinued for at least 5 days,[37] whereas 7 days is recommended for ticagrelor.[38] Although no longer commonly used, recommendations for discontinuing ticlopidine range from 10 to 14 days because its half-life can be as long as 96 to 120 hours in chronic treatment.[39] After surgery, these antiplatelet agents can be restarted as soon as adequate hemostasis is achieved. Because they often take time to achieve a steady state, a loading dose can be given, if required.

APPROVED USES OF NEW ORAL ANTICOAGULANTS

Dabigatran, rivaroxaban, and apixaban are approved for prevention of strokes and embolic events in patients with nonvalvular AF. However, rivaroxaban is the only one of these agents approved by the FDA for the treatment of DVT/VTE. Although the periprocedural use of rivaroxaban has not been widely studied, it is of great interest because of its rapid onset of action and short half-life.

The RE-ALIGN (Randomized, Phase II Study to Evaluate the Safety and Pharmacokinetics of Oral Dabigatran Etexilate in Patients after Heart Valve Replacement) phase II trial evaluated the possible use of dabigatran in patients with mechanical heart valves.[40] However, the trial was abandoned prematurely after the dabigatran group had a significantly higher incidence of ischemic stroke, MI, and serious bleeding episodes compared with the warfarin group. The investigators speculated that dosing regimens may have played a role in the failure, but suggested that apixaban and rivaroxaban would produce similar results. Thus, the use of these agents in patients with mechanical heart valves has been abandoned at this time.[41]

PERIPROCEDURAL MANAGEMENT OF PATIENTS ON NEW ORAL ANTICOAGULANTS

The periprocedural management of anticoagulation induced by dabigatran, rivaroxaban, and apixaban is in some ways simpler than that of patients on warfarin. It is generally agreed that bridging therapy is not necessary because their anticoagulant effects dissipate more quickly than those of warfarin and their onset is much more rapid (within hours of the first dose) once reinitiated after the procedure.[12,42–44] The primary difficulties with these drugs in the preprocedural period are the lack of readily available tests to accurately determine residual anticoagulant activity and the inability to easily reverse their effects (see **Table 1**).

PREPROCEDURAL PERIOD

Insufficient data exist to determine the safety of continuing dabigatran, rivaroxaban, or apixaban for surgical procedures for which it is considered safe to continue warfarin before, during, or after the procedure. However, preliminary evidence suggests that dabigatran can be continued for catheter ablation of AF as well as for implantation of cardiac devices.[45,46] For other procedures, the goal is to discontinue anticoagulants early enough to ensure minimal effect at the time of the planned procedure. In order to meet this goal, their kinetics must be understood.

Half-life of Dabigatran

The apparent half-life of dabigatran varies with renal function, ranging from 12 to 14 hours in healthy subjects to 15 to 17 hours in patients with a creatinine clearance between 50 and 80 mL/min and 18 to 19 hours when the creatinine clearance is 30 to 50 mL/min.[44] In patients with creatinine clearance less than 30 mL/min, the terminal half-life of dabigatran is greater than 24 hours. Because there is no specific reversal agent for dabigatran and reliable methods to measure its anticoagulant effect are not widely available, it is prudent to withhold the drug for 5 half-lives, which can be accomplished in patients with creatinine clearance greater than 80 mL/min by withholding the drug for 2 days (ie, the last dose taken on the evening of the third day before surgery, at least 60 hours before the planned procedure). In patients with creatinine clearance of 50 to 80 mL/min, dabigatran should be held for 3 days, and in those with clearance between 30 and 50 mL/min for 4 to 5 days. If the consequences of a small increase in bleeding risk would be severe (eg, neurosurgery or neuraxial blockade), withholding an additional dose should be considered, especially in patients with poor renal function.

Half-lives of Rivaroxaban and Apixaban

The apparent half-life of rivaroxaban ranges from 5 to 9 hours in healthy subjects 20 to 45 years old, and from 11 to 13 hours in patients 45 years of age or older.[43,47] Because renal dysfunction also prolongs the effect of rivaroxaban, it is recommended to withhold it for 2 days before the planned procedure in patients with a creatinine clearance greater than 30 mL/min, and 3 days when the creatinine clearance is 15 to 30 mL/min.[12]

The elimination of apixaban also depends on renal function, but to a much lesser extent than for dabigatran and rivaroxaban. Apixaban has a short elimination half-life (6 hours), but is slowly absorbed, resulting in a longer-than-expected duration of effect after the last dose and an apparent half-life of 12 hours.[43,48] Apixaban should therefore be held for 2 days before the planned procedure in patients with normal creatinine clearance, and for 3 days in patients with creatinine clearance between 30 and 50 mL/min.[12]

POSTPROCEDURAL MANAGEMENT OF PATIENTS ON NEW ORAL ANTICOAGULANTS

Dabigatran, rivaroxaban, and apixaban all have rapid onset of anticoagulant activity.[42,43] Patients due to receive them after a procedure do not require postprocedural bridging therapy if the drug is restarted in the time frame recommended for resumption of bridging therapy. However, the rapidity of onset, duration of effect, and inability to easily reverse the effects of these drugs raises the question of the optimal time to resume administration. Our practice is to use LMWH (as described earlier for warfarin) until there is no longer any concern about bleeding risk or the patient is ready for discharge. Using LMWH allows more rapid reversal of anticoagulation should bleeding develop. The availability of more reliable testing for the anticoagulant effect of LMWH (ie, the anti-Xa assay) also facilitates management of this situation.

MANAGEMENT OF ANTICOAGULATION WITH NEURAXIAL ANESTHESIA OR ANALGESIA

The use of neuraxial (spinal or epidural) anesthesia or analgesia in patients on oral anticoagulants is associated with a significant risk of spinal hematoma, which may result in permanent neurologic injury, even with prompt recognition and treatment.[49] The use of UFH and LMWH in close temporal proximity to needle placement or catheter removal has also been associated with an increased risk of this complication, which is compounded by concomitant use of antiplatelet drugs.[49] It is currently recommended that coagulation status should be normal at the time of needle placement and at the time of catheter removal.[49,50] To achieve this goal, patient management is similar to the approach for surgical procedures with a high risk of bleeding: warfarin must be held for 5 days before the procedure, and dabigatran, rivaroxaban, and apixaban should be held based on the recommendations stated earlier. In addition, if bridging therapy is used, IV UFH should be discontinued 4 hours before needle placement, and the last dose of enoxaparin (if ≤ 1 mg/kg) must have been given at least 24 hours before needle placement.

Timing of initiation of anticoagulation in the postoperative period must take into account the presence and timing of removal of an epidural catheter and thus should be done in consultation with the anesthesiologist. Therapeutic anticoagulation should not be initiated while an epidural catheter is in place, with the exception of warfarin, which can be reintroduced when there is a plan to remove the catheter before the INR is greater than 1.5. Administration of UFH needs to be delayed by at least 1 hour following catheter removal. Therapeutic or twice-daily prophylactic enoxaparin should not be initiated until 4 hours after catheter removal, and administration of fondaparinux should be delayed by at least 12 hours.[49,50] There is limited published evidence on the risks of spinal hematoma with the new oral anticoagulants. Although some investigators have proposed guidelines for removal of epidural catheters in patients who have received these agents,[50,51] until more information is available it is prudent to withhold them while an epidural catheter is in place, and to delay initiation until at least 4 hours after catheter removal. If placement of the epidural block was traumatic, therapeutic anticoagulation should be delayed for at least 24 hours following needle placement.[51]

SUMMARY

The periprocedural management of patients on anticoagulants, both old and new, for AF, DVT/VTE, and mechanical heart valves continues to evolve, contributing to the confusion among practicing clinicians. Furthermore, there is often disagreement between anesthesiologists and surgeons about the risks of thromboembolic events versus risks from intraoperative and postoperative bleeding. Evidence-based, consensus guidelines on the periprocedural management of patients on anticoagulants have been promulgated by national organizations. Although intended to reduce variation and improve care, such conventional clinical practice guidelines have drawbacks that can limit clinician buy-in.[52] In contrast, standardized clinical assessment and management plans (SCAMPs) offer a clinician-designed and clinician-driven approach that accommodates patients' individual differences, respects local providers' clinical acumen, and keeps pace with the rapid growth of medical knowledge.[53] The algorithms presented in this article represent 3 examples of SCAMPs developed at our own institution, which are likely to be helpful even though they will undoubtedly undergo dynamic revisions as more data to guide clinical decision-making become available.

REFERENCES

1. Cushman M. Epidemiology and risk factors for venous thrombosis. Semin Hematol 2007;44(2):62–9.
2. Deitelzweig SB, Johnson BH, Lin J, et al. Prevalence of clinical venous thrombo-embolism in the USA: current trends and future projections. Am J Hematol 2011; 86(2):217–20.
3. Heit JA. The epidemiology of venous thromboembolism in the community. Arterioscler Thromb Vasc Biol 2008;28(3):370–2.
4. Go AS, Hylek EM, Phillips KA, et al. Prevalence of diagnosed atrial fibrillation in adults: national implications for rhythm management and stroke prevention: the AnTicoagulation and Risk Factors in Atrial Fibrillation (ATRIA) Study. JAMA 2001;285(18):2370–5.
5. Deviri E, Sareli P, Wisenbaugh T, et al. Obstruction of mechanical heart valve prostheses: clinical aspects and surgical management. J Am Coll Cardiol 1991;17(3):646–50.
6. Douketis JD, Spyropoulos AC, Spencer FA, et al. Perioperative management of antithrombotic therapy: antithrombotic therapy and prevention of thrombosis, 9th ed: American College of Chest Physicians evidence-based clinical practice guidelines. Chest 2012;141(2 Suppl):e326S–50S.
7. Nematullah A, Alabousi A, Blanas N, et al. Dental surgery for patients on anticoagulant therapy with warfarin: a systematic review and meta-analysis. J Can Dent Assoc 2009;75(1):41.
8. Jamula E, Anderson J, Douketis JD. Safety of continuing warfarin therapy during cataract surgery: a systematic review and meta-analysis. Thromb Res 2009; 124(3):292–9.
9. Mason JO 3rd, Gupta SR, Compton CJ, et al. Comparison of hemorrhagic complications of warfarin and clopidogrel bisulfate in 25-gauge vitrectomy versus a control group. Ophthalmology 2011;118(3):543–7.
10. Schulman S, Elbazi R, Zondag M, et al. Clinical factors influencing normalization of prothrombin time after stopping warfarin: a retrospective cohort study. Thromb J 2008;6:15.
11. White RH, McKittrick T, Hutchinson R, et al. Temporary discontinuation of warfarin therapy: changes in the international normalized ratio. Ann Intern Med 1995;122(1):40–2.
12. Spyropoulos AC, Douketis JD. How I treat anticoagulated patients undergoing an elective procedure or surgery. Blood 2012;120(15):2954–62.
13. Douketis JD. Contra: "Bridging anticoagulation is needed during warfarin interruption when patients require elective surgery". Thromb Haemost 2012;108(2): 210–2.
14. Spyropoulos AC. Pro: "Bridging anticoagulation is needed during warfarin interruption in patients who require elective surgery". Thromb Haemost 2012;108(2): 213–6.
15. Nutescu EA, Spinler SA, Wittkowsky A, et al. Low-molecular-weight heparins in renal impairment and obesity: available evidence and clinical practice recommendations across medical and surgical settings. Ann Pharmacother 2009; 43(6):1064–83.

16. Lip GY, Nieuwlaat R, Pisters R, et al. Refining clinical risk stratification for predicting stroke and thromboembolism in atrial fibrillation using a novel risk factor-based approach: the Euro Heart Survey on Atrial Fibrillation. Chest 2010; 137(2):263–72.

17. Chen JY, Zhang AD, Lu HY, et al. CHADS2 versus CHA2DS2-VASc score in assessing the stroke and thromboembolism risk stratification in patients with atrial fibrillation: a systematic review and meta-analysis. J Geriatr Cardiol 2013;10(3): 258–66.

18. Olesen JB, Lip GY, Hansen ML, et al. Validation of risk stratification schemes for predicting stroke and thromboembolism in patients with atrial fibrillation: nationwide cohort study. BMJ 2011;342:d124.

19. Heit JA. Risk factors for venous thromboembolism. Clin Chest Med 2003;24(1): 1–12.

20. Levi M, van der Poll T. Two-way interactions between inflammation and coagulation. Trends Cardiovasc Med 2005;15(7):254–9.

21. Alfirevic Z, Alfirevic I. Hypercoagulable state, pathophysiology, classification and epidemiology. Clin Chem Lab Med 2010;48(Suppl 1):S15–26.

22. Kaatz S, Douketis JD, Zhou H, et al. Risk of stroke after surgery in patients with and without chronic atrial fibrillation. J Thromb Haemost 2010;8(5):884–90.

23. Siegal D, Yudin J, Kaatz S, et al. Periprocedural heparin bridging in patients receiving vitamin K antagonists: systematic review and meta-analysis of bleeding and thromboembolic rates. Circulation 2012;126(13):1630–9.

24. Lip GY, Frison L, Halperin JL, et al. Comparative validation of a novel risk score for predicting bleeding risk in anticoagulated patients with atrial fibrillation: the HAS-BLED (Hypertension, Abnormal Renal/Liver Function, Stroke, Bleeding History or Predisposition, Labile INR, Elderly, Drugs/Alcohol Concomitantly) score. J Am Coll Cardiol 2011;57(2):173–80.

25. Pisters R, Lane DA, Nieuwlaat R, et al. A novel user-friendly score (HAS-BLED) to assess 1-year risk of major bleeding in patients with atrial fibrillation: the Euro Heart Survey. Chest 2010;138(5):1093–100.

26. European Heart Rhythm Association, European Association for Cardio-Thoracic Surgery, Camm AJ, et al. Guidelines for the management of atrial fibrillation: the Task Force for the Management of Atrial Fibrillation of the European Society of Cardiology (ESC). Eur Heart J 2010;31(19):2369–429.

27. Omran H, Bauersachs R, Rubenacker S, et al. The HAS-BLED score predicts bleedings during bridging of chronic oral anticoagulation. Results from the national multicentre BNK Online bRiDging REgistRy (BORDER). Thromb Haemost 2012;108(1):65–73.

28. Anderson MA, Ben-Menachem T, Gan SI, et al. Management of antithrombotic agents for endoscopic procedures. Gastrointest Endosc 2009;70(6):1060–70.

29. Wysokinski WE, McBane RD, Daniels PR, et al. Periprocedural anticoagulation management of patients with nonvalvular atrial fibrillation. Mayo Clin Proc 2008;83(6):639–45.

30. Willard JE, Lange RA, Hillis LD. The use of aspirin in ischemic heart disease. N Engl J Med 1992;327(3):175–81.

31. CAPRIE Steering Committee. A randomised, blinded, trial of clopidogrel versus aspirin in patients at risk of ischaemic events (CAPRIE). CAPRIE Steering Committee. Lancet 1996;348(9038):1329–39.

32. Peter K, Myles PS. Perioperative antiplatelet therapy: a knife-edged choice between thrombosis and bleeding still based on consensus rather than evidence. Thromb Haemost 2011;105(5):750–1.

33. Hartwig-Otto H. Pharmacokinetic considerations of common analgesics and antipyretics. Am J Med 1983;75(5A):30–7.

34. Gerstein NS, Schulman PM, Gerstein WH, et al. Should more patients continue aspirin therapy perioperatively?: clinical impact of aspirin withdrawal syndrome. Ann Surg 2012;255(5):811–9.

35. Chen TH, Matyal R. The management of antiplatelet therapy in patients with coronary stents undergoing noncardiac surgery. Semin Cardiothorac Vasc Anesth 2010;14(4):256–73.

36. Savonitto S, Caracciolo M, Cattaneo M, et al. Management of patients with recently implanted coronary stents on dual antiplatelet therapy who need to undergo major surgery. J Thromb Haemost 2011;9(11):2133–42.

37. Hall R, Mazer CD. Antiplatelet drugs: a review of their pharmacology and management in the perioperative period. Anesth Analg 2011;112(2):292–318.

38. Dweck MR, Cruden NL. Noncardiac surgery in patients with coronary artery stents. Arch Intern Med 2012;172(14):1054–5.

39. Oprea AD, Popescu WM. ADP-receptor inhibitors in the perioperative period: the good, the bad, and the ugly. J Cardiothorac Vasc Anesth 2013;27(4):779–95.

40. Eikelboom JW, Connolly SJ, Brueckmann M, et al. Dabigatran versus warfarin in patients with mechanical heart valves. N Engl J Med 2013;369(13):1206–14.

41. Hylek EM. Dabigatran and mechanical heart valves – not as easy as we hoped. N Engl J Med 2013;369(13):1264–6.

42. Kubitza D, Becka M, Roth A, et al. Dose-escalation study of the pharmacokinetics and pharmacodynamics of rivaroxaban in healthy elderly subjects. Curr Med Res Opin 2008;24(10):2757–65.

43. Mueck W, Schwers S, Stampfuss J. Rivaroxaban and other novel oral anticoagulants: pharmacokinetics in healthy subjects, specific patient populations and relevance of coagulation monitoring. Thromb J 2013;11(1):10.

44. Stangier J, Rathgen K, Stahle H, et al. Influence of renal impairment on the pharmacokinetics and pharmacodynamics of oral dabigatran etexilate: an open-label, parallel-group, single-centre study. Clin Pharmacokinet 2010;49(4):259–68.

45. Maddox W, Kay GN, Yamada T, et al. Dabigatran versus warfarin therapy for uninterrupted oral anticoagulation during atrial fibrillation ablation. J Cardiovasc Electrophysiol 2013;24(8):861–5.

46. Rowley CP, Bernard ML, Brabham WW, et al. Safety of continuous anticoagulation with dabigatran during implantation of cardiac rhythm devices. Am J Cardiol 2013;111(8):1165–8.

47. Xarelto prescribing information. Available at: http://www.xareltohcp.com/sites/default/files/pdf/xarelto_0.pdf. Accessed January 15, 2014.

48. Eliquis prescribing information. Available from: http://packageinserts.bms.com/pi/pi_eliquis.pdf. Accessed January 15, 2014.

49. Horlocker TT, Wedel DJ, Rowlingson JC, et al. Regional anesthesia in the patient receiving antithrombotic or thrombolytic therapy: American Society of Regional Anesthesia and Pain Medicine evidence-based guidelines (third edition). Reg Anesth Pain Med 2010;35(1):64–101.

50. Green L, Machin SJ. Managing anticoagulated patients during neuraxial anaesthesia. Br J Haematol 2010;149(2):195–208.

51. Llau JV, Ferrandis R. New anticoagulants and regional anesthesia. Curr Opin Anaesthesiol 2009;22(5):661–6.

52. Harrison MB, Legare F, Graham ID, et al. Adapting clinical practice guidelines to local context and assessing barriers to their use. CMAJ 2010;182(2):E78–84.
53. Farias M, Jenkins K, Lock J, et al. Standardized clinical assessment and management plans (SCAMPs) provide a better alternative to clinical practice guidelines. Health Aff (Millwood) 2013;32(5):911–20.

Four-Factor Prothrombin Complex Concentrate Versus Plasma for Urgent Vitamin K Antagonist Reversal

New Evidence

⊛ CrossMark

Ravi Sarode, MD

KEYWORDS

- Anticoagulants • Hemorrhage • Plasma • Prothrombin complex concentrates
- Vitamin K antagonist

KEY POINTS

- Vitamin K antagonist (VKA) therapy is a mainstay of treatment for patients at risk of thromboembolic events.
- Despite widespread use, a major limitation of VKA therapy is the substantial risk of serious bleeding complications, which often require rapid reversal of anticoagulation.
- A recent randomized, multicenter comparison between a 4-factor prothrombin complex concentrate (4F-PCC) and plasma in patients with acute major bleeding has provided important new evidence of the benefit of 4F-PCC over plasma for urgent VKA reversal.
- Compared with plasma, 4F-PCC provided significantly faster correction of the international normalized ratio due to rapid increase in vitamin K-dependent factors, comparable hemostatic efficacy, a shorter infusion time, and smaller infusion volume, the latter probably contributing to a lower risk of treatment-related fluid overload or similar cardiac events.

INTRODUCTION AND BACKGROUND

Long-term vitamin K antagonist (VKA) therapy is a mainstay of treatment for patients at risk of thromboembolic events despite use of target-specific new oral anticoagulants, with more than 4.2 million US patients receiving a prescription for warfarin in 2012.[1] However, a major limitation of VKA therapy is the substantial risk of serious bleeding

Conflict of Interest Statement: Dr R. Sarode has a working relationship (consulting and advisory) with CSL Behring, Marburg, Germany.
Division of Transfusion Medicine and Hemostasis, Department of Pathology, University of Texas Southwestern Medical Center, 5323 Harry Hines Boulevard, Dallas, TX 75390-9234, USA
E-mail address: ravi.sarode@utsouthwestern.edu

events. In a recent population-based cohort study of more than 125,000 Canadian patients with atrial fibrillation who were followed for 5 years, warfarin use was associated with an overall rate of major hemorrhage of 3.8% per person-year, with the risk being highest during the first 30 days of treatment, at 11.8% per person-year.[2] Moreover, during the 5-year follow-up period, 8.7% of patients visited the hospital because of major hemorrhage; of these, 18.1% died in the hospital or within 7 days of discharge.[2] Hospitalization data from the Canadian study are supported by data from the United States, where it is estimated that there are around 21,000 emergency hospitalizations annually for warfarin-related hemorrhages,[3] and more than 60,000 emergency room visits for warfarin-related bleeding.[4] Indeed, the clinical significance of the bleeding risk associated with warfarin resulted in the US Food and Drug Administration (FDA) mandating the addition of a boxed warning to the product labeling in 2006.[5]

Among warfarin-related serious bleeding events, intracerebral hemorrhage is potentially the most serious, requiring rapid reversal of the anticoagulant effect to stop hematoma growth.[6,7] In addition, anticoagulated patients requiring emergency surgery or invasive diagnostic procedures, or those with extremely elevated international normalized ratio (INR) values and at risk for bleeding are also candidates for urgent VKA reversal.[8] Therefore, clear strategies must be in place to swiftly and completely reverse oral anticoagulation, particularly in patients who experience serious bleeding.

While some management guidelines recommend vitamin K administration as a component of VKA-reversal therapy,[9–11] vitamin K monotherapy does not normalize INR and hemostasis sufficiently rapidly in an emergency situation.[12] Other therapy options include prothrombin complex concentrates (PCCs) and plasma.[12] Although plasma has been considered the standard of care for urgent VKA reversal in the United States, randomized, controlled trials of plasma have not been conducted to verify its effectiveness in this setting. In addition to the paucity of effectiveness data, the use of plasma is associated with a number of drawbacks, including the need for a large infusion volume, which increases the time taken to achieve hemostasis and puts patients at risk of fluid overload.[13,14] The latter is associated with prolongation of hospital stays and increased hospital costs.[15] Moreover, incomplete anticoagulation reversal,[16–18] the time needed to match blood group, and the time to thaw and transport plasma are significant limitations for the effective management of severe bleeding, where time is critical.

Several management guidelines recommend infusion of a PCC for urgent VKA reversal. The British Committee for Standards in Haematology and the American College of Chest Physicians recommend a combination of a 4-factor PCC (4F-PCC) and vitamin K for emergency anticoagulation reversal,[9,10] while the French clinical practice guidelines advocate a PCC and vitamin K.[11] The Board of the German Medical Association also recommends PCCs for the emergency reversal of anticoagulant effects.[19] In addition, PCC is recommended for the emergency reversal of vitamin K-dependent oral anticoagulants in the European guidelines on the management of perioperative bleeding[20] and bleeding following major trauma.[21] These recommendations reflect findings from a range of studies showing that PCCs are effective in lowering INR for prompt VKA reversal.[22–26]

Recently, 2 new studies have shed light on the comparative efficacy and safety of 2 4F-PCCs versus plasma in patients requiring urgent VKA reversal: a randomized, multicenter trial of Beriplex/Kcentra in patients with acute major bleeding[27] and a retrospective cohort study of Octaplex in emergency department patients.[28] This article provides an overview of these recent findings and considers additional issues that can be addressed with the availability of this randomized dataset and imminent data from further randomized, controlled trials of PCC administration.

RECENT DATA
Sarode and Colleagues

The efficacy and safety profile of 4F-PCC was compared with that of plasma in 216 VKA-treated patients with acute major bleeding who were enrolled in a randomized trial conducted at 36 centers located in the United States and Europe.[27] Eligible patients were at least18 years old, receiving VKA therapy, and had an INR of at least 2.0; they were randomly allocated (1:1) to receive an infusion of 4F-PCC at a dose comparable to the product's dosing recommendations (25–50 IU of Factor IX per kg, according to baseline INR)[29] or plasma (10–15 mL/kg, according to baseline INR). According to the protocol, all patients were to receive vitamin K by slow intravenous infusion. However, 4 patients in the 4F-PCC and 2 in the plasma group did not receive vitamin K during the study, and 8 and 3 patients, respectively, received vitamin K by a nonintravenous route. The coprimary efficacy endpoints were: INR correction (reduction to ≤1.3) 30 minutes after the end of infusion and 24-hour hemostatic efficacy from the start of infusion. The trial was conducted as a noninferiority study, with 4F-PCC deemed to be noninferior to plasma if the lower ends of the 95% confidence intervals (CIs) for the between-group differences were less than −10% for each coprimary endpoint. If noninferiority criterion was met, superiority for an endpoint could be demonstrated if the lower end of the 95% CI, for the between-group difference was greater than 0. Additional secondary endpoints included time to INR correction, plasma levels of factors II, VII, IX, and X, and plasma levels of natural anticoagulant proteins (proteins C and S).

The study showed that 4F-PCC was superior to plasma for rapid INR reduction, with 62.2% (95% CI: 52.6, 71.8) of patients in the 4F-PCC group achieving an INR of ≤ 1.3 within 30 minutes of the end of infusion, compared with 9.6% (95% CI: 3.9, 15.3) of patients in the plasma group (**Fig. 1**).[27] The difference in percentages for

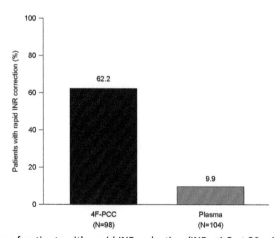

Fig. 1. Proportion of patients with rapid INR reduction (INR ≤1.3 at 30 min after the end of infusion): 4F-PCC versus plasma. (*Data from* Sarode R, Milling TJ Jr, Refaai MA, et al. Efficacy and safety of a 4-factor prothrombin complex concentrate in patients on vitamin K antagonists presenting with major bleeding: a randomized, plasma-controlled, phase IIIb study. Circulation 2013;128(11):1234–43.)

4F-PCC versus plasma was 52.6% (95% CI: 39.4, 65.9). INR correction occurred significantly faster with 4F-PCC, with more than two-thirds (69%) of 4F-PCC patients achieving an INR of ≤ 1.3 at 1 hour after the start of infusion, compared with no patients in the plasma group at this time point (**Fig. 2**A). The difference in median INR for 4F-PCC versus plasma was statistically significant through 12 hours after the start of infusion (see **Fig. 2**B).

4F-PCC was noninferior to plasma for hemostatic efficacy in the first 24 hours from the start of infusion. Effective hemostasis (rated by a blinded endpoint adjudication board as excellent or good) was achieved in 72.4% (95% CI: 63.6, 81.3) of 4F-PCC patients and 65.4% (95% CI: 56.2, 74.5) of plasma patients, with an intergroup difference of 7.1% in favor of 4F-PCC (95% CI: −5.8, 19.9).

The safety profile was generally similar between the 4F-PCC and plasma treatment groups, with 66 patients (64.1%) and 71 patients (65.1%) reporting at least 1 adverse

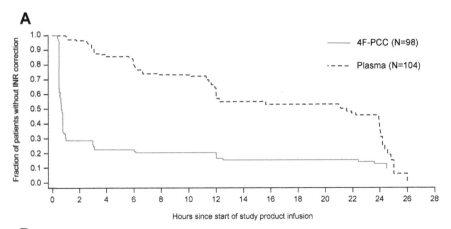

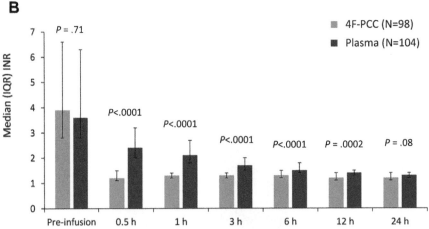

Fig. 2. Kinetics of INR correction: 4F-PCC versus plasma. (*A*) Time to INR correction. (*B*) Median INR by time point. IQR, Interquartile Range. (*From* Sarode R, Milling TJ Jr, Refaai MA, et al. Efficacy and safety of a 4-Factor prothrombin complex concentrate in patients on vitamin K antagonists presenting with major bleeding: a randomized, plasma-controlled, phase IIIb study. Circulation 2013;128(11):1234–43.)

event, respectively.[27] However, fluid overload occurred more frequently in the plasma group (12.8%) than in the 4F-PCC (4.9%) group. Fluid overload events were considered by the investigator to be treatment related in 7 patients (6.4%) who received plasma, but no such treatment-related events were reported in patients receiving 4F-PCC. Thromboembolic events occurred at comparable rates in the 2 treatment groups (4F-PCC: 7.8% [n = 8]; plasma: 6.4% [n = 7]); the blinded safety adjudication board judged that there were 2 treatment-related serious thromboembolic events in each study arm.[27]

Hickey and Colleagues

Another recent publication reported a retrospective cohort study of adverse event frequency following urgent warfarin reversal with a 4F-PCC (Octaplex) or plasma in 2 Canadian emergency departments.[28] This was a before–after study over consecutive 2-year periods, with data prior to and following the change from routine use of plasma to 4F-PCC being compared for the primary endpoint of serious adverse events (death, ischemic stroke, myocardial infarction, heart failure, venous thromboembolism, or peripheral arterial thromboembolism). Secondary endpoints included time to INR reversal, length of hospital stay, and 48-hour red blood cell transfusion. The study analyzed health record data from 314 warfarin-treated patients at least 18 years of age, with an INR of at least 1.5 and who had received plasma or 4F-PCC for active bleeding or prior to an emergency procedure. All patients treated with 4F-PCC received a fixed, standard dose of 1000 IU, except for patients with intracerebral hemorrhage, who received a fixed dose of 1500 IU.

The incidence of 7-day serious adverse events was significantly higher for plasma compared with 4F-PCC (19.5% vs 9.7%, relative risk = 2.0, 95% CI: 1.1, 3.5; $P =$ .0164), and this difference persisted on multivariate analysis. Of note, significantly more patients experienced heart failure possibly related to volume overload in the plasma group than in the 4F-PCC group, whereas there was no difference between groups in the rate of thromboembolic events. It was also found that the time to INR reversal was significantly shorter and the mean number of red blood cell transfusions significantly lower in the 4F-PCC treatment group compared with the plasma group.[28] However, this study has several drawbacks inherent to a retrospective analysis, as such chart reviews could have missed important observations.

Discussion of the Randomized Controlled Trial Data

In the study by Sarode and colleagues,[27] the use of coprimary endpoints (hemostatic efficacy and INR correction) was the most practical way to address the fact that many trials of bleeding disorders, mainly hemophilias, have used hemostatic efficacy as an outcome measure, whereas most clinicians rely on INR correction to guide treatment of bleeding caused by VKA therapy. Certain features of the trial design may explain the lack of superiority of 4F-PCC over plasma for hemostatic efficacy in this study. First, the study was only designed to show non-inferiority and was not intended to have statistical power to demonstrate superiority. Second, FDA-mandated assessment of hemostatic efficacy at 4 to 24 hours after the end of infusion may have limited the ability to demonstrate the importance of rapid coagulation-factor replacement and INR correction to hemostatic efficacy. In addition, the assessment of the hemostatic effect of study treatment at 24 hours is confounded by the contribution of intravenous vitamin K that was administered to both groups (vitamin K was administered in accordance with guidelines for the management of VKA-related bleeding). Interestingly, results for those bleeding types for which an early assessment was possible revealed a more pronounced clinical effect of 4F-PCC compared with plasma, suggesting the possibility of a difference between groups at early time points for this measure.[27] Because of the timing of the hemostatic assessments in this trial, for many of the most common types of bleeding, actual hemostasis may have been achieved earlier than the time of recording.

Data from the randomized comparison of 4F-PCC and plasma revealed additional benefits of 4F-PCC over plasma supplementary to those measured by the coprimary endpoints. The median infusion time for 4F-PCC was substantially shorter than for plasma (median 17.0 min vs 148.0 min), and the median infusion volume was considerably lower (median 99.4 mL vs 813.5 mL). The latter difference was reflected in the absence of cases of treatment-related fluid overload in 4F-PCC patients, compared with 7 such cases in the plasma arm. The risk of fluid overload in patients undergoing plasma transfusion has been noted previously.[14]

Several previous studies have reported thromboembolic events with different PCCs. However, these studies did not include a control group and were further limited by small sample sizes.[30] Despite the rapid increases in coagulation factor levels seen in the 4F-PCC arm of the randomized study, the risk of thromboembolic events associated with PCC used for urgent VKA reversal was low and comparable to that observed with plasma.[27] A previous prospective trial of Beriplex/Kcentra in patients requiring urgent VKA reversal for acute bleeding or emergency surgical intervention showed that rapid infusion of this product at 8 mL/min does not induce more adverse events than slower infusion rates.[22,31] In addition, the low risk of thromboembolic events with PCC treatment is supported by data from the large retrospective analysis by Hickey and colleagues.[28]

4F- VERSUS 3F-PCCS

There is existing evidence that treatment with 3F-PCCs, which contain relatively low levels of Factor VII and insufficient amounts of natural anticoagulant proteins C and S, does not result in complete INR correction and might not be able to restore hemostasis adequately in patients receiving VKA therapy. In a study of 40 patients with supratherapeutic INR who presented with bleeding or were at high risk of bleeding, treatment with 3F-PCC reduced INR to less than 3.0 in only 43% to 50% of cases, compared with 63% of historical controls who received plasma.[32] Furthermore, no randomized, controlled trials have compared the efficacy of 4F- and 3F-PCCs for urgent VKA reversal. Therefore, the emergence of this new evidence for the efficacy of 4F-PCCs combined with the paucity of evidence supporting the effectiveness of 3F-PCCs for VKA reversal suggests that 4F-PCCs should be the PCCs of choice for urgent VKA reversal.

FUTURE RESEARCH QUESTIONS

The availability of this randomized, controlled dataset will enable further research questions to be investigated (eg, characterization of the thromboembolic events in the 4F-PCC and plasma treatment arms and characterization of the correction of INR and coagulation factor levels in urgent VKA reversal). In addition, 2 forthcoming randomized, controlled trials of 4F-PCC (one each for Beriplex/Kcentra and Octaplex) in patients requiring an urgent surgical intervention will provide further data on the comparative efficacy and safety of 4F-PCC and plasma. Together, these trials will allow pooled analyses to address issues such as efficacy in patient subgroups (eg, hemostasis by dose, initial INR, age), and the risk and predictors of fluid overload in plasma-treated patients.

There are few published data on the cost-effectiveness of 4F-PCC or plasma for urgent VKA reversal. Although the cost per unit of plasma is lower than that of 4F-PCC, the use of plasma may be associated with a substantial economic burden due to increased health care resource utilization and plasma-related adverse reactions such as fluid overload.[15] Indeed, a single modeling study comparing 4F-PCC (Beriplex) with fresh frozen plasma for emergency warfarin reversal in patients with acute bleeding in the United Kingdom found 4F-PCC to be more cost-effective,[33] although there are few real-world economic data to confirm this model estimate. Future studies should aim to investigate not only the efficacy and safety profiles of PCC and plasma, but also the relative total cost of health care following each intervention.

SUMMARY

Results from the first randomized, controlled trial of a 4F-PCC (Beriplex/Kcentra) versus plasma in VKA-treated patients with acute major bleeding demonstrate the noninferiority to plasma through a clinical endpoint and show superiority through bioanalytical endpoints such as INR correction and rapid factors increments. The benefits of 4F-PCC therapy were obtained with an acceptable safety profile. Despite the rapid increases in coagulation factor levels seen in the 4F-PCC arm of this study, the incidence of thromboembolic events remained low. Further insights into the efficacy of this 4F-PCC for VKA reversal will come from secondary analyses of this randomized dataset, from a forthcoming randomized, controlled trial in patients requiring urgent surgical intervention for hemostasis, and from pooled analyses of these 2 trials.

ACKNOWLEDGEMENTS

Medical writing and editorial assistance was provided by Rianne Stacey at Fishawack Communications Ltd, Abingdon, Oxon, United Kingdom.

REFERENCES

1. IMS data US national prescription audit; MAT (moving annual total) 2011–2012. Avaiable at: http://www.imshealth.com/ims/Global/Content/Insights/IMS%20Institute%20for%20Healthcare%20Informatics/IHII_Medicines_in_U.S_Report_2011.pdf.
2. Gomes T, Mamdani MM, Holbrook AM, et al. Rates of hemorrhage during warfarin therapy for atrial fibrillation. CMAJ 2013;185(2):E121–7.
3. Budnitz DS, Lovegrove MC, Shehab N, et al. Emergency hospitalizations for adverse drug events in older Americans. N Engl J Med 2011;365(21):2002–12.
4. Shehab N, Sperling LS, Kegler SR, et al. National estimates of emergency department visits for hemorrhage-related adverse events from clopidogrel plus aspirin and from warfarin. Arch Intern Med 2010;170(21):1926–33.
5. Wysowski DK, Nourjah P, Swartz L. Bleeding complications with warfarin use: a prevalent adverse effect resulting in regulatory action. Arch Intern Med 2007; 167(13):1414–9.
6. Goldstein JN, Thomas SH, Frontiero V, et al. Timing of fresh frozen plasma administration and rapid correction of coagulopathy in warfarin-related intracerebral hemorrhage. Stroke 2006;37(1):151–5.
7. Aguilar MI, Hart RG, Kase CS, et al. Treatment of warfarin-associated intracerebral hemorrhage: literature review and expert opinion. Mayo Clin Proc 2007;82(1):82–92.
8. Hirsh J, Fuster V, Ansell J, et al. American Heart Association/American College of Cardiology Foundation guide to warfarin therapy. Circulation 2003;107(12):1692–711.

9. Keeling D, Baglin T, Tait C, et al. Guidelines on oral anticoagulation with warfarin—fourth edition. Br J Haematol 2011;154(3):311–24.

10. Holbrook A, Schulman S, Witt DM, et al. Evidence-based management of antico-agulant therapy: antithrombotic therapy and prevention of thrombosis, 9th ed: American College of Chest Physicians evidence-based clinical practice guide-lines. Chest 2012;141(Suppl 2):e152S–84S.

11. Pernod G, Godier A, Gozalo C, et al. French clinical practice guidelines on the management of patients on vitamin K antagonists in at-risk situations (overdose, risk of bleeding, and active bleeding). Thromb Res 2010;126(3):e167–74.

12. Levy JH, Tanaka KA, Dietrich W. Perioperative hemostatic management of pa-tients treated with vitamin K antagonists. Anesthesiology 2008;109(5):918–26.

13. Ageno W, Gallus AS, Wittkowsky A, et al. Oral anticoagulant therapy: antithrom-botic therapy and prevention of thrombosis, 9th ed: American College of Chest Physicians evidence-based clinical practice guidelines. Chest 2012;141(Suppl 2):e44S–88S.

14. Narick C, Triulzi DJ, Yazer MH. Transfusion-associated circulatory overload after plasma transfusion. Transfusion 2012;52(1):160–5.

15. Magee G, Zbrozek A. Fluid overload is associated with increases in length of stay and hospital costs: pooled analysis of data from more than 600 US hospitals. Clinicoecon Outcomes Res 2013;5:289–96.

16. Fredriksson K, Norrving B, Stromblad LG. Emergency reversal of anticoagulation after intracerebral hemorrhage. Stroke 1992;23(7):972–7.

17. Makris M, Greaves M, Phillips WS, et al. Emergency oral anticoagulant reversal: the relative efficacy of infusions of fresh frozen plasma and clotting factor concen-trate on correction of the coagulopathy. Thromb Haemost 1997;77(3):477–80.

18. Hanley JP. Warfarin reversal. J Clin Pathol 2004;57(11):1132–9.

19. 4 Plasma for therapeutic use. Transfus Med Hemother 2009;36(6):388–97.

20. Kozek-Langenecker SA, Afshari A, Albaladejo P, et al. Management of severe perioperative bleeding: guidelines from the European Society of Anaesthesiol-ogy. Eur J Anaesthesiol 2013;30(6):270–382.

21. Spahn DR, Bouillon B, Cerny V, et al. Management of bleeding and coagulopathy following major trauma: an updated European guideline. Crit Care 2013;17(2): R76.

22. Pabinger I, Brenner B, Kalina U, et al. Prothrombin complex concentrate (Beriplex P/N) for emergency anticoagulation reversal: a prospective multinational clinical trial. J Thromb Haemost 2008;6(4):622–31.

23. Kalina M, Tinkoff G, Gbadebo A, et al. A protocol for the rapid normalization of INR in trauma patients with intracranial hemorrhage on prescribed warfarin ther-apy. Am Surg 2008;74(9):858–61.

24. Khorsand N, Veeger NJ, van Hest RM, et al. An observational, prospective, two-cohort comparison of a fixed versus variable dosing strategy of prothrombin complex concentrate to counteract vitamin K antagonists in 240 bleeding emer-gencies. Haematologica 2012;97(10):1501–6.

25. Bruce D, Nokes TJ. Prothrombin complex concentrate (Beriplex P/N) in severe bleeding: experience in a large tertiary hospital. Crit Care 2008;12(4):R105.

26. Scott LJ. Prothrombin complex concentrate (Beriplex P/N). Drugs 2009;69(14): 1977–84.

27. Sarode R, Milling TJ Jr, Refaai MA, et al. Efficacy and safety of a 4-Factor pro-thrombin complex concentrate in patients on vitamin K antagonists presenting with major bleeding: a randomized, plasma-controlled, phase IIIb study. Circula-tion 2013;128(11):1234–43.

28. Hickey M, Gatien M, Taljaard M, et al. Outcomes of urgent warfarin reversal with frozen plasma versus prothrombin complex concentrate in the emergency department. Circulation 2013;128(4):360–4.

29. Kcentra US prescribing information. 2013. Available at: http://www.kcentra.com/docs/Kcentra_Prescribing_Information.pdf.

30. Dentali F, Marchesi C, Pierfranceschi MG, et al. Safety of prothrombin complex concentrates for rapid anticoagulation reversal of vitamin K antagonists. A meta-analysis. Thromb Haemost 2011;106(3):429–38.

31. Pabinger I, Tiede A, Kalina U, et al. Impact of infusion speed on the safety and effectiveness of prothrombin complex concentrate: a prospective clinical trial of emergency anticoagulation reversal. Ann Hematol 2010;89(3):309–16.

32. Holland L, Warkentin TE, Refaai M, et al. Suboptimal effect of a three-factor prothrombin complex concentrate (Profilnine-SD) in correcting supratherapeutic international normalized ratio due to warfarin overdose. Transfusion 2009;49(6): 1171–7.

33. Guest JF, Watson HG, Limaye S. Modeling the cost-effectiveness of prothrombin complex concentrate compared with fresh frozen plasma in emergency warfarin reversal in the United Kingdom. Clin Ther 2010;32(14):2478–93.

Prothrombin Complex Concentrates as Reversal Agents for New Oral Anticoagulants

Lessons from Preclinical Studies with Beriplex

Gerhard Dickneite, PhD

KEYWORDS

- Beriplex • Prothrombin complex concentrate • New oral anticoagulants
- Anticoagulant reversal

KEY POINTS

- The preclinical study results obtained with Beriplex have demonstrated consistent reversal of new oral anticoagulant (NOAC)-associated bleeding and provide encouraging evidence for the use of this nonactivated 4-factor prothrombin complex concentrate for NOAC reversal.
- There is a need for clinical data, particularly in bleeding patients, to further validate this reversal strategy.
- The lack of correlation between coagulation parameters and hemostasis observed in some of the studies needs to be explored further to help guide clinician diagnostics.

INTRODUCTION

New oral anticoagulants (NOACs) represent an effective anticoagulation therapy option and have several advantages over warfarin and other vitamin K antagonists (VKAs), including a low potential for food and drug interactions, a relatively short half-life, and a rapid and reliable onset of action.[1–4] NOACs include the activated factor II (FIIa), or thrombin, inhibitor (dabigatran etexilate [Pradaxa, Prazaxa]) and FXa inhibitors (rivaroxaban [Xarelto], apixaban [Eliquis], and edoxaban [Lixiana]).[5,6] These agents specifically inhibit important elements in the coagulation cascade, unlike

Conflict of Interest Statements: Prof. Dr G. Dickneite is an employee of CSL Behring and owns CSL Behring stock.
Editorial assistance was provided by Alan Saltzman at Fishawack Communications Ltd, with a grant from CSL Behring, Marburg, Germany.
CSL Behring, Preclinical R&D, PO Box 1230, Marburg 35002, Germany
E-mail address: Gerhard.Dickneite@cslbehring.com

Clin Lab Med 34 (2014) 623–635
http://dx.doi.org/10.1016/j.cll.2014.06.001
0272-2712/14/$ – see front matter © 2014 Elsevier Inc. All rights reserved.

VKAs, which interfere with the synthesis of multiple vitamin K-dependent factors (VKDFs; eg, FII, FVII, FIX, and FX) (**Fig. 1**).

Clinical trials of NOACs have demonstrated their noninferiority or superiority over VKAs for the prevention of thrombotic events.[5] Nevertheless, NOAC therapy is still associated with a risk for bleeding complications.[5] Although this risk is apparently lower than that for VKAs,[5] it is still a significant issue, as bleeding in patients on anticoagulants has been associated with poorer outcomes.[7–11] This is further compounded by the fact that no validated strategy for NOAC reversal is yet available. Presently, the treatment of choice for VKA reversal is prothrombin complex concentrate (PCC), coadministered with vitamin K.[12] PCCs contain significant quantities of VKDFs II, IX, and X, with either low (3-factor [3F]-PCC) or therapeutic levels (4-factor [4F]-PCC) of FVII, and replace the VKDFs that are deficient as a result of VKA therapy.[13] The efficacy of PCCs for urgent VKA reversal was demonstrated in a recent phase IIIb clinical trial in which treatment with a nonactivated 4F-PCC (Beriplex) was shown to be at least as good as plasma for urgent VKA reversal in patients with acute major bleeding.[14] Further details on this trial and other studies that have evaluated the effectiveness of 4F-PCC for VKA reversal can be found elsewhere in this supplement.[15]

Currently, only preclinical and early clinical results have been published on NOAC reversal, including the use of VKA reversal agents, such as PCCs. Theoretically, PCCs could overcome the anticoagulant effects of FIIa and FXa inhibitors by enhancing thrombin generation.[16] However, because the reversal of the anticoagulant effect would be mechanistically different from that for VKAs, procedures for the use of PCCs in the reversal of NOAC-associated bleeding would need to be validated. Interestingly, in one recent report of reversal of dabigatran-associated intestinal bleeding, treatment with the 4F-PCC Octaplex resulted in control of hemorrhagic complications in 4 of the 5 patients included in the study.[17]

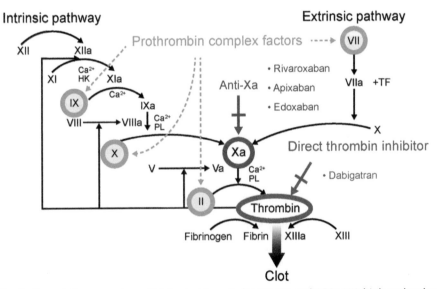

Fig. 1. Coagulation cascade and biological targets for NOACs and PCCs. HK, high molecular weight kininogen; PL, platelet membrane phospholipid; TF, tissue factor.

This article summarizes the current published preclinical data for the reversal of NOACs with Beriplex, a nonactivated 4F-PCC. This agent has been the most extensively studied PCC for NOAC reversal and has demonstrated efficacy for VKA reversal.[14,18] We also aim to put the findings presented on NOAC reversal with Beriplex into context with results obtained with other reversal agents (eg, other PCCs, activated and nonactivated, and recombinant activated FVII [rFVIIa]).

PRECLINICAL STUDIES OF NOAC REVERSAL WITH BERIPLEX
FIIa Inhibitors: Dabigatran

In vivo rabbit model combined with in vitro/ex vivo studies

Inconsistencies have been observed between PCC-mediated reversal of dabigatran-induced anticoagulation and reversal of dabigatran-associated hemorrhage.[19] A rabbit study was performed to study the effect of Beriplex on both dabigatran-modulated thrombin generation activity (TGA) and bleeding in one set of experiments.[20] This included (1) TGA measurements after in vitro spiking with dabigatran and Beriplex in platelet-poor plasma (PPP) from untreated rabbits, (2) spiking experiments with Beriplex in PPP obtained from rabbits treated with dabigatran, and (3) evaluation of TGA in PPP from rabbits treated with both dabigatran and Beriplex in vivo, combined with assessment of hemorrhage.

The study demonstrated a dose-dependent decrease of peak thrombin and endogenous thrombin potential (ETP), as well as a prolonged lag time, when rabbit PPP was spiked with dabigatran 200 to 800 ng/mL (**Fig. 2**A; CSL Behring data on file). Addition of Beriplex 0.156 to 0.625 U/mL to PPP treated with dabigatran 400 ng/mL resulted in a dose-dependent increase in peak thrombin and ETP, leading to normalization of both parameters (see **Fig. 2**B; CSL Behring data on file). However, there was only a slight effect on the lag time. In the in vivo part of the study, the administration of dabigatran 0.4 mg/kg led to a marked impairment of thrombin generation (see **Fig. 2**C; CSL Behring data on file) and a strong bleeding signal in a kidney incision wound model.[20] Addition of Beriplex (0.156–0.94 U/mL) to PPP from dabigatran-treated animals resulted in normalization of ETP and peak thrombin, although the lag time was only slightly reduced (see **Fig. 2**C). To evaluate the ability of Beriplex to normalize TGA and reverse dabigatran-mediated bleeding, 20, 35, or 50 IU/kg doses of Beriplex were administered to rabbits treated with dabigatran 0.4 mg/kg.[20] Increased blood loss due to dabigatran administration was significantly reduced with Beriplex in a dose-dependent manner, with normal levels obtained at the highest dose (50 IU/kg) and a significant reduction seen at 35 IU/kg.[20] Similarly, time to hemostasis, which increased with dabigatran treatment, decreased with increasing doses of Beriplex, and was returned to values close to the normal range at the highest dose.[20] Thrombin generation was normalized over time, as demonstrated in **Fig. 2**D for a representative animal treated with Beriplex 35 IU/kg (data on file). In contrast, dabigatran-induced activated partial thromboplastin time (aPTT) prolongation remained unaffected with Beriplex treatment, whereas prothrombin time (PT) remained elevated in 2 of 5 animals receiving Beriplex 50 IU/kg.[20] This study demonstrates that thrombin generation parameters correlate with Beriplex-mediated bleeding reversal, with peak thrombin level being the most sensitive parameter.

In vitro reversal studies

The reversal of dabigatran-mediated inhibition of thrombin generation by Beriplex was evaluated in a cell-based model that used freshly prepared platelet-rich human plasma and activated macrophages as a tissue factor source.[21] In accordance with the rabbit model described previously,[20] this human cell-based model demonstrated that Beriplex was able to reverse dabigatran-induced inhibitory effects on the rate,

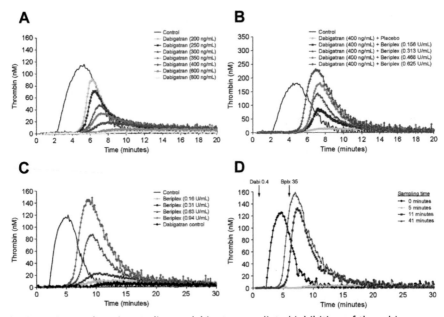

Fig. 2. In vitro and ex vivo studies on dabigatran-mediated inhibition of thrombin generation and its reversal by Beriplex. Thrombin generation induced by the extrinsic pathway was performed in rabbit PPP. Samples were measured using calibrated automated thrombinography (CAT; Thrombinoscope B.V., Maastricht, the Netherlands) and the Thrombinoscope software version 3.0.0.29. The concentration of recombinant relipidated tissue factor was 5 pM (picomolar) and of phospholipids 4 μM. (*A*) Inhibition of thrombin generation by dabigatran in vitro. (*B*) Reversal of dabigatran-mediated thrombin generation inhibition by Beriplex in vitro. (*C*) Beriplex-mediated ex vivo reversal of thrombin generation inhibition in PPP from dabigatran-treated (0.4 mg/kg) rabbits. (*D*) Time course of Beriplex-mediated reversal of dabigatran-induced inhibition of thrombin generation in vivo (data from one representative rabbit). TGA was measured at baseline (t = 0). Dabigatran (0.4 mg/kg; Dabi 0.4) was given 1 minute later (t = 1) and TGA was measured 4 minutes after dabigatran treatment (t = 5). Beriplex (35 IU/kg; Bplx 35) was administered 5 minutes after dabigatran treatment (t = 6) and the TGA was measured 5 minutes (t = 11) and 35 minutes (t = 41) after Beriplex treatment (all data on file).

peak, and area under the thrombin generation curve, and increase these parameters to levels at or above control. However, the dabigatran-induced increase in the lag period before thrombin generation was not reversed by Beriplex.

Ex vivo reversal studies

Two ex vivo studies have reported on the efficacy of Beriplex in the reversal of dabigatran-induced anticoagulant effects.[22–24] These studies showed contrasting effects with regard to both the anticoagulant and the reversal agent effects, which limits interpretation.

In one study, the potential of Beriplex to reverse the dabigatran-induced inhibition of thrombin generation was assessed using blood from healthy human subjects who had received the anticoagulant 2 hours prior.[22] Dabigatran administration only significantly affected the lag time (the ETP was only marginally inhibited and dabigatran had no effect on peak thrombin), and Beriplex was able to reduce the dabigatran-induced lag time prolongation only slightly.

In a second study, blood samples from healthy individuals treated with dabigatran for 5 days were used to evaluate the ability of Beriplex (50 IU/kg) to reverse dabigatran-induced effects on standard coagulation parameters.[23,24] In contrast with the previous study,[22] dabigatran administration had a significant impact on parameters of thrombin generation (eg, peak thrombin) in this study. Addition of Beriplex was able to at least partially reverse the changes in thrombin generation parameters associated with dabigatran treatment. Although Beriplex administration was able to partially reverse dabigatran effects on clot firmness, the effect of dabigatran on other visco-elastic parameters and fibrin formation was not modified by Beriplex.

In vivo reversal studies
Four in vivo studies, performed in mice, rats, and rabbits, have evaluated Beriplex for the reversal of bleeding mediated by dabigatran.[20,25–28] These studies have demonstrated the ability of Beriplex to reverse dabigatran-induced effects on bleeding time (BT) and time to hemostasis, although this did not always correlate with reversal of coagulation assay parameters, a finding similar to that reported in studies with other PCCs.[26,29]

In a murine intracerebral hemorrhage (ICH) model, dabigatran, injected 1 hour before ICH induction, doubled hematoma size, and this increase was significantly reversed with Beriplex treatment.[25] The reversal of dabigatran effect on hematoma size was dose dependent, and all 3 doses of Beriplex (25, 50, and 100 IU/kg) were efficacious. In contrast, the increase in tail vein BT with dabigatran treatment, assessed in the same study, was significantly reduced only at the highest concentration.

In a rat tail vein model, Beriplex restored dabigatran-elevated BT to baseline levels within 5 minutes of administration, an effect that was maintained for at least 2 hours.[26] However, thrombin time (TT), aPTT, and ecarin clotting time (ECT) remained prolonged, despite normalization of bleeding and PT.

Finally, 2 in vivo studies were performed in rabbits to assess dabigatran reversal by Beriplex,[20,27,28] one of which has been described previously. Herzog and colleagues[27,28] evaluated anticoagulation reversal using an arterial-venous (AV) shunt model and bleeding reversal using a kidney incision model. In the AV shunt model, anticoagulation induced by dabigatran doses of 200 µg/kg or more was not fully reversed by the administration of Beriplex. In contrast, 200 µg/kg dabigatran-stimulated bleeding, as evaluated by time to hemostasis and blood loss in the kidney incision model, was reduced to normal values in a dose-dependent manner.

FXa Inhibitors: Rivaroxaban

In vitro reversal studies
In an in vitro study using blood samples from healthy volunteers treated with rivaroxaban, Beriplex 50 IU/kg was able to reverse alterations in thrombin generation (eg, rivaroxaban-induced prolongation of the lag-phase and reduction of the maximal peak).[30] Some effect also was seen in modifying the rivaroxaban-induced reduction in platelet and fibrin interactions.

Ex vivo reversal studies
Two ex vivo studies, previously discussed in the dabigatran reversal section, have also evaluated the efficacy of Beriplex to reverse the anticoagulant effects induced by rivaroxaban.[22–24] As with dabigatran, these studies showed contrasting effects with regard to both the anticoagulant and the reversal agent effects, and should be interpreted with caution.

In the first study, which assessed rivaroxaban reversal using blood from healthy volunteers who had received the anticoagulant 2 hours prior, rivaroxaban showed pronounced inhibitory effects on thrombin generation parameters.[22] In this model, rivaroxaban-induced inhibition of the ETP and peak thrombin, and prolongation of the lag time, were not corrected by Beriplex.

In the second study, which used blood samples from healthy volunteers treated with rivaroxaban for 5 days, rivaroxaban had only a modest inhibitory effect on thrombin generation.[23,24] Addition of Beriplex 50 IU/kg was able to partially reverse the effects of rivaroxaban on peak thrombin and corrected rivaroxaban-mediated changes in clot viscoelasticity, while also significantly improving fibrin formation.

In vivo reversal studies

Three published studies in mice, rats, and healthy human volunteers have evaluated the reversal of rivaroxaban with Beriplex.[31–33] Although the study in human subjects assessed only coagulation parameters, and demonstrated variable results for Beriplex depending on the parameter being considered,[33] the 2 animal studies demonstrated that administration of Beriplex was able to reverse rivaroxaban-induced prolongation of BT and prevent intracerebral hematoma expansion.[31,32]

In the murine ICH model, rivaroxaban treatment nearly doubled hematoma volume, and this effect could be significantly reversed by administration of Beriplex (50 or 100 IU/kg).[31] The Beriplex 25-IU/kg dose, although not as effective as the higher doses in reducing hematoma expansion in rivaroxaban-treated mice, substantially improved neurologic defects. Beriplex did not have any effect on rivaroxaban-induced PT prolongation in this model.

In the rat bleeding model, administration of Beriplex 50 IU/kg was able to significantly reduce BT in rivaroxaban-treated animals, although the lower (25 IU/kg) dose of Beriplex was not effective in this model.[32] In contrast to the previous study,[31] Beriplex treatment was able to partially reverse rivaroxaban effects on PT and on thrombin generation as measured by the thrombin–antithrombin (TAT) levels.

In the study conducted in healthy volunteers, rivaroxaban was given for 4 days to attain steady-state levels before Beriplex administration (50 IU/kg).[33] The PT was shortened to within 30 minutes of Beriplex treatment, but effects on ETP were less pronounced.

FXa Inhibitors: Apixaban

In vitro reversal studies

Reversal of apixaban-mediated changes in coagulation parameters with Beriplex 50 IU/kg was evaluated in thrombin-generation assays, thromboelastometry studies, and perfusion studies using human whole blood.[34] In thrombin-generation assays, addition of Beriplex was able to partially reverse some of the apixaban-mediated effects on thrombin generation (eg, reduced peak thrombin).[34] In thromboelastometry studies, addition of Beriplex partially reversed apixaban-induced reduction of maximum clot firmness, but had less of an impact on clotting time altered by apixaban treatment.[34] Finally, in perfusion studies, addition of Beriplex also was able to reverse the apixaban-mediated reduction in fibrin generation, although it had minimal effects on the reduction of platelet interactions.[34]

FXa Inhibitors: Edoxaban

In vivo reversal studies

A dose-dependent reversal of bleeding induced by a high intravenous dose of edoxaban (1200 µg/kg) was achieved with Beriplex treatment (25–75 IU/kg) in a rabbit kidney injury model, with significant reductions in both time to hemostasis and blood loss seen after administration of the 50 IU/kg dose of Beriplex.[35] Reversal of bleeding was best correlated with the following biomarkers: PT, whole blood clotting time, and ETP.

DISCUSSION

Although NOACs are at least as efficacious as VKAs for the prevention of thrombotic events, with advantages such as reduced laboratory monitoring requirements, more predictable pharmacodynamic and pharmacokinetic properties, and simpler dosing regimens, the risk of bleeding complications remains a concern, particularly considering the lack of validated reversal strategies.[1–6] Therefore, there is an urgent need to identify validated treatments for the reversal of the effects of NOACs during such bleeding events or when the possibility for bleeding exists, such as with surgery.

One potential strategy for NOAC reversal is the use of therapies currently used for VKA reversal, including PCCs, activated PCCs (eg, Factor VIII Inhibitor Bypassing Activity [FEIBA]) and rFVIIa. This article has focused on the potential for the use of PCCs for NOAC reversal, reviewing the available preclinical data for Beriplex, the PCC most studied for this application.

Overall, the studies reviewed here have shown that Beriplex treatment consistently improved hemostasis in animals treated with either dabigatran, rivaroxaban, or edoxaban (**Table 1**).[20,25–28,32,33,35] Efficacy was shown in various animal models, including a murine ICH model, rat artery and tail vein models, and a rabbit kidney incision model.[20,25–28,32,33,35] Reversal of NOAC bleeding, or prevention of NOAC-induced hematoma expansion, was observed despite variable results on coagulation parameters, such as TT, PT, and aPTT.[20,26–28,32,33,35] Although these results are encouraging, additional studies, particularly in bleeding patients, are warranted to confirm these preclinical findings.

One of the potential complications of reversal therapy with these agents is thromboembolic risk, which has historically been associated with treatment with (activated) PCCs.[36] However, pharmacovigilance data obtained with Beriplex have demonstrated no proven cases of treatment-related thromboembolism.[36] Results obtained in reversal studies that also assessed the prothrombotic risk of PCCs are consistent with this finding. For example, in the study that evaluated dabigatran reversal with Beriplex in rabbits, histopathological analysis did not reveal any evidence of thrombosis in the treated animals.[27,28] Furthermore, Levi and colleagues[33] also reported that no signs of prothrombotic response were observed in their study of rivaroxaban-induced anticoagulation reversal in healthy volunteers.

When comparing the different and sometimes discrepant reversal results obtained in in vitro studies, it is important to remember that standard laboratory assays were not originally developed to measure reversal of new oral anticoagulants. In addition, different assay measures vary considerably in their sensitivity to new oral anticoagulants.[37,38] Therefore, absence of or only partial reversal of NOAC-induced changes in in vitro assay parameters does not necessarily mean there will be no reversal of bleeding in an in vivo study or in the clinical setting. There is a need for in vitro assays that are calibrated for use with NOACs. In the absence of such assays, effect on bleeding is a much more reliable demonstration of reversal of NOACs. Reversal of NOAC anticoagulation in standard laboratory assays needs to be analyzed in detail and results should be interpreted with caution, especially if no bleeding data were presented.

In this regard, variability of the effect of Beriplex on the NOAC-modulated coagulation assay parameters, despite efficacy in vivo, indicates there is a need to identify a

Table 1
Summary of study results for new oral anticoagulant reversal with Beriplex

Study	Model	Results Coagulation Parameters	Bleeding
Dabigatran			
Hoffman et al,[21] 2012	Cellular in vitro coagulation, human	↑ rate, peak, and total amount of thrombin generation; no effect on lag time	No data
Pillitteri et al,[22] 2013	Cellular ex vivo coagulation, human	Slight reduction in lag time	No data
Galan et al,[23] 2012; Galan et al,[24] 2013	Cellular ex vivo coagulation, human	↑ velocity index, time to peak and peak of thrombin generation. Partial effect on clot firmness, but no effect on other viscoelastic parameters or fibrin formation	No data
Zhou et al,[25] 2011	Intracerebral hemorrhage model, mouse	No data	↓
van Ryn et al,[26] 2011	Tail cut model/ coagulation, rat	No change in TT, aPTT, or ECT, but PT reversed to baseline	↓
Herzog et al,[27,28] 2013	Arterial venous shunt/ coagulation, rabbit	Improvements in thrombin generation parameters, but no change in PT or dilute PT	↓
Pragst et al,[20] 2012	Kidney bleeding/ coagulation, rabbit	↓ PT and normalization of peak amount of thrombin generation, ETP, and V_{max} for thrombus formation, but no change in aPTT and only slight effect on lag time	↓
Rivaroxaban			
Arellano-Rodrigo et al,[30] 2013	Cellular in vitro coagulation, human	↑ peak and ↓ lag phase of thrombin generation. ↑ platelet/fibrin interactions	No data
Pillitteri et al,[22] 2013	Cellular ex vivo coagulation, human	No effect on ETP, peak, and lag time of thrombin generation	No data
Galan et al,[23] 2012; Galan et al,[24] 2013	Cellular ex vivo coagulation, human	Modest ↑ in peak of thrombin generation. Reversal of rivaroxaban-induced effects on clot viscoelastic properties. ↑ fibrin formation	No data
Zhou et al,[31] 2013	Intracerebral hemorrhage model, mouse	No change in PT, but ↑ in plasma activity of FII, FIX, FX and proteins C and S	↓ (hematoma volume)
Perzborn et al,[32] 2013	Mesenteric bleeding/ coagulation, rat	↑ TAT; ↓ PT, but reversal was partial	↓
Levi et al,[33] 2013	In vivo coagulation, human	↓ PT; ↑ ETP	No data

(continued on next page)

		Results	
Study	Model	Coagulation Parameters	Bleeding
Apixaban			
Escolar et al,[34] 2013	Cellular in vitro coagulation, human	↑ peak of thrombin generation; ↑ clot firmness but minimal effect on velocity index; ↑ fibrin generation but minimal effect on platelet accumulation	No data
Edoxaban			
Herzog et al,[35] 2013	Kidney bleeding/ coagulation, rabbit	↓ PT; ↑ ETP; ↓ WBCT	↓

Table 1 (continued)

↑, increase; ↓, decrease.

Abbreviations: aPTT, activated partial thromboplastin time; ECT, ecarin clotting time; ETP, endogenous thrombin potential; F, factor; PT, prothrombin time; TAT, thrombin–antithrombin; TT, thrombin time; WBCT, whole blood clotting time.

relevant monitoring tool for NOAC-induced anticoagulation. Patient studies have shown that aPTT, TT, and ECT are sensitive to dabigatran concentration, whereas thrombin generation and PT were variable or unresponsive.[37] However, some in vivo studies of NOAC reversal have failed to demonstrate a correlation between reversal of bleeding and reversal of dabigatran-sensitive coagulation assay parameters.[20,26] Regarding rivaroxaban monitoring, it has been suggested that PT and anti-FXa assays are sensitive to rivaroxaban levels.[37] However, observations from preclinical studies have shown little correlation between reversal of rivaroxaban-associated bleeding and reversal of PT prolongation.[31]

Other nonactivated PCCs have also been studied for NOAC reversal, and variable results on their effect on reversal of NOAC-mediated bleeding have been reported, although limited information is available. Administration of the 4F-PCC Octaplex was able to successfully reverse dabigatran-induced prolongation of BT in a rat tail vein model,[26] but did not significantly reduce blood loss in dabigatran-treated mice.[39] A rat tail vein model also was used to assess the efficacy of the 3F-PCCs Profilnine and Bebulin, and both agents were shown to reduce the dabigatran-induced prolongation of BT to baseline levels.[29] However, it should be noted that the effect of the 3F-PCCs lasted for only 30 minutes,[29] rather than the 2 hours reported for 4F-PCCs in the same model,[26] a finding that is consistent with previous reports of suboptimal efficacy of 3F-PCCs for VKA reversal.[40] The 4F-PCC Kaskadil was evaluated in a rabbit model of rivaroxaban-mediated bleeding reversal, and was found to be ineffective in reducing blood loss, despite partial correction of thrombin-generation parameters.[41] The wide variation in the amount of coagulation factors, and proteins C and S, that PCCs contain[13,19] makes comparisons between PCCs difficult, and caution should be advised when contrasting these study results.

Activated PCC (FEIBA) and rFVIIa also have been studied for NOAC reversal and have proven effective in reversing NOAC-stimulated bleeding in some animal studies.[25,26,31,32] In a rat tail bleeding model, these agents had comparable efficacy to Beriplex in reversing dabigatran-enhanced bleeding.[26] Similar efficacy was also reported for the reversal of rivaroxaban-enhanced bleeding with FEIBA or rFVIIa, as compared with Beriplex, in murine ICH and rat mesenteric bleeding models.[31,32]

However, in a murine ICH model, dabigatran-enhanced hematoma expansion was not lessened by rFVIIa, although Beriplex was efficacious.[25] Although these agents have proven efficacious for the reversal of NOAC-associated bleeding, they may pose a greater risk of thrombosis and some guidelines recommend the use of nonactivated PCCs as the first choice for reversal of NOAC effects.[42]

In addition to the previously mentioned reversal strategies, selective agents are also currently in development for NOAC reversal.[43–45] Dabigatran antibody fragments have shown efficacy in in vitro and ex vivo models, and for the reversal of dabigatran-associated bleeding in a rat tail vein model.[45,46] Administration of the specific FXa inhibitor antidote PRT064445 was associated with dose-dependent reversal of rivaroxaban-associated blood loss in rats.[44] Although these agents may have advantages due to their selectivity, efficacy data are still limited to preclinical studies and nonselective reversal agents are still likely to be clinically useful.[19]

In conclusion, the preclinical study results obtained with Beriplex have demonstrated consistent reversal of NOAC-induced bleeding and provide encouraging evidence for the use of this nonactivated 4F-PCC for NOAC reversal. However, there is a need for clinical data, particularly in bleeding patients, to further validate this reversal strategy. In addition, the lack of correlation between coagulation parameters and hemostasis observed in some of the studies needs to be explored further to help guide clinician diagnostics.

REFERENCES

1. Nutescu EA, Shapiro NL, Chevalier A, et al. A pharmacologic overview of current and emerging anticoagulants. Cleve Clin J Med 2005;72(Suppl 1):S2–6.
2. Ahrens I, Peter K, Lip GY, et al. Development and clinical applications of novel oral anticoagulants. Part II. Drugs under clinical investigation. Discov Med 2012;13(73):445–50.
3. Moser M, Bode C. Anticoagulation in atrial fibrillation: a new era has begun. Hamostaseologie 2012;32(1):37–9 [in German].
4. Eriksson BI, Quinlan DJ, Eikelboom JW. Novel oral factor Xa and thrombin inhibitors in the management of thromboembolism. Annu Rev Med 2011;62:41–57.
5. Ahrens I, Peter K, Lip GY, et al. Development and clinical applications of novel oral anticoagulants. Part I. Clinically approved drugs. Discov Med 2012;13(73): 433–43.
6. Samama MM. The mechanism of action of rivaroxaban—an oral, direct factor Xa inhibitor—compared with other anticoagulants. Thromb Res 2011;127(6):497–504.
7. Budnitz DS, Lovegrove MC, Shehab N, et al. Emergency hospitalizations for adverse drug events in older Americans. N Engl J Med 2011;365(21):2002–12.
8. Budnitz DS, Shehab N, Kegler SR, et al. Medication use leading to emergency department visits for adverse drug events in older adults. Ann Intern Med 2007;147(11):755–65.
9. Huhtakangas J, Tetri S, Juvela S, et al. Effect of increased warfarin use on warfarin-related cerebral hemorrhage: a longitudinal population-based study. Stroke 2011;42(9):2431–5.
10. Rosand J, Eckman MH, Knudsen KA, et al. The effect of warfarin and intensity of anticoagulation on outcome of intracerebral hemorrhage. Arch Intern Med 2004; 164(8):880–4.
11. Wysowski DK, Nourjah P, Swartz L. Bleeding complications with warfarin use: a prevalent adverse effect resulting in regulatory action. Arch Intern Med 2007; 167(13):1414–9.

12. Holbrook A, Schulman S, Witt DM, et al. Evidence-based management of antico-agulant therapy: Antithrombotic Therapy and Prevention of Thrombosis, 9th ed: American College of Chest Physicians Evidence-Based Clinical Practice Guide-lines. Chest 2012;141(2 Suppl):e152S–84S.
13. Kalina U, Bickhard H, Schulte S. Biochemical comparison of seven commercially available prothrombin complex concentrates. Int J Clin Pract 2008;62(10):1614–22.
14. Sarode R, Milling TJ Jr, Refaai MA, et al. Efficacy and safety of a 4-factor pro-thrombin complex concentrate in patients on vitamin K antagonists presenting with major bleeding: a randomized, plasma-controlled, phase IIIb study. Circula-tion 2013;128(11):1234–43.
15. Sarode R. Four-factor prothrombin complex concentrate versus plasma for urgent VKA reversal: what's new? Clin Lab Med, in press.
16. Eerenberg ES, Kamphuisen PW, Sijpkens MK, et al. Reversal of rivaroxaban and da-bigatran by prothrombin complex concentrate: a randomized, placebo-controlled, crossover study in healthy subjects. Circulation 2011;124(14):1573–9.
17. Diaz MQ, Borobia AM, Nunez MA, et al. Use of prothrombin complex concen-trates for urgent reversal of dabigatran in the emergency department. Haemato-logica 2013;98(11):e143–4.
18. Pabinger I, Brenner B, Kalina U, et al. Prothrombin complex concentrate (Beriplex P/N) for emergency anticoagulation reversal: a prospective multinational clinical trial. J Thromb Haemost 2008;6(4):622–31.
19. Dickneite G, Hoffman M. Reversing the new oral anticoagulants with prothrombin complex concentrates (PCCs): what is the evidence? Thromb Haemost 2013; 111(2):189–98 Availabe at: http://www.ncbi.nlm.nih.gov/pubmed/24136202.
20. Pragst I, Zeitler SH, Doerr B, et al. Reversal of dabigatran anticoagulation by pro-thrombin complex concentrate (Beriplex P/N) in a rabbit model. J Thromb Hae-most 2012;10(9):1841–8.
21. Hoffman M, Volovyk Z, Monroe D. Partial reversal of dabigatran effect by a pro-thrombin complex concentrate in a model of thrombin generation (2012 ASH ab-stracts). Blood 2012;120:3420.
22. Pillitteri D, Pilgrimm-Thorp AK, Krause M, et al. Antidotal effects of non-specific reversal agents on anticoagulant-induced inhibition of thrombin generation (2013 ISTH abstracts). J Thromb Haemost 2013;11(Suppl s2):562–3.
23. Galan AM, Arellano-Rodrigo E, Sanz V, et al. Reversal of the antithrombotic action of rivaroxaban and dabigatran: a clinical study in healthy volunteers. (2012 ASH abstracts). Blood 2012;120(21):2261.
24. Galan AM, Arellano-Rodrigo E, Sanz V, et al. Effects of rivaroxaban and dabiga-tran on hemostasis and reversion of their antithrombotic effects by different coag-ulation factors. Evidence raised from a clinical study in healthy volunteers (2013 ISTH abstracts). J Thromb Haemost 2013;11(Suppl s2):418–9.
25. Zhou W, Schwarting S, Illanes S, et al. Hemostatic therapy in experimental intra-cerebral hemorrhage associated with the direct thrombin inhibitor dabigatran. Stroke 2011;42(12):3594–9.
26. van Ryn J, Schurer J, Kink-Eiband M, et al. The successful reversal of dabigatran-induced bleeding by coagulation factor concentrates in a rat tail bleeding model do not correlate with ex vivo markers of anticoagulation (2011 ASH abstracts). Blood 2011;118:2316.
27. Herzog E, Kaspereit F, Krege W, et al. Pre-clinical safety aspects on the use of Beriplex P/N for reversal of Dabigatran anticoagulation [abstract P5-1]. Paper presented at: 57th Annual Meeting of the German Thrombosis and Haemostasis Research Society. Munich, Germany, February 20–23, 2013.

28. Herzog E, Kaspereit F, Krege W, et al. Non-clinical safety and efficacy of prothrombin complex concentrates (PCC) for the reversal of dabigatran mediated anticoagulation (2013 ISTH abstracts). J Thromb Haemost 2013;11(Suppl s2):693.

29. van Ryn J, Schurer J, Kink-Eiband M, et al. Successful reversal of dabigatran-induced bleeding by 3-factor coagulation concentrates in a rat tail bleeding model: lack of correlation with ex vivo markers of anticoagulation. Paper presented at: AHA Scientific Sessions and Resuscitation Science Symposium. Los Angeles, USA, November 3–5, 2012.

30. Arellano-Rodrigo E, Galan AM, Sanz V, et al. Alterations induced by rivaroxaban on hemostasis can be reversed by different coagulation factor concentrates: in vitro experimental studies with steady and circulating human blood (2013 ISTH abstracts). J Thromb Haemost 2013;11(Suppl s2):953–4.

31. Zhou W, Zorn M, Nawroth P, et al. Hemostatic therapy in experimental intracerebral hemorrhage associated with rivaroxaban. Stroke 2013;44(3):771–8.

32. Perzborn E, Gruber A, Tinel H, et al. Reversal of rivaroxaban anticoagulation by haemostatic agents in rats and primates. Thromb Haemost 2013;110(1):162–72.

33. Levi M, Moore T, Castillejos CF, et al. Effects of three-factor and four-factor prothrombin complex concentrates on the pharmacodynamics of rivaroxaban (2013 ISTH abstracts). J Thromb Haemost 2013;11(Suppl s2):167.

34. Escolar G, Fernandez-Gallego V, Arellano-Rodrigo E, et al. Reversal of apixaban induced alterations in hemostasis by different coagulation factor concentrates: significance of studies in vitro with circulating human blood. PLoS One 2013; 8(11):e78696.

35. Herzog E, Kaspereit F, Krege W, et al. Four-factor prothrombin complex concentrate (4-PCC) effectively reverses edoxaban induced bleeding in a rabbit model of acute injury (2013 ASH abstracts). Blood 2013;122:1133.

36. Sorensen B, Spahn DR, Innerhofer P, et al. Clinical review: prothrombin complex concentrates—evaluation of safety and thrombogenicity. Crit Care 2011;15(1): 201.

37. Baglin T, Hillarp A, Tripodi A, et al. Measuring Oral Direct Inhibitors (ODIs) of thrombin and factor Xa: a recommendation from the Subcommittee on Control of Anticoagulation of the Scientific and Standardisation Committee of the International Society on Thrombosis and Haemostasis. J Thromb Haemost 2013;11(4): 756–60.

38. Samama MM, Mendell J, Guinet C, et al. In vitro study of the anticoagulant effects of edoxaban and its effect on thrombin generation in comparison to fondaparinux. Thromb Res 2012;129(4):e77–82.

39. Lambourne MD, Eltringham-Smith LJ, Gataiance S, et al. Prothrombin complex concentrates reduce blood loss in murine coagulopathy induced by warfarin, but not in that induced by dabigatran etexilate. J Thromb Haemost 2012;10(9): 1830–40.

40. Holland L, Warkentin TE, Refaai M, et al. Suboptimal effect of a three-factor prothrombin complex concentrate (Profilnine-SD) in correcting supratherapeutic international normalized ratio due to warfarin overdose. Transfusion 2009;49(6): 1171–7.

41. Godier A, Miclot A, Le Bonniec B, et al. Evaluation of prothrombin complex concentrate and recombinant activated factor VII to reverse rivaroxaban in a rabbit model. Anesthesiology 2012;116(1):94–102.

42. Turpie AG, Kreutz R, Llau J, et al. Management consensus guidance for the use of rivaroxaban—an oral, direct factor Xa inhibitor. Thromb Haemost 2012;108(5): 876–86.

43. Ahmad Y, Lip GY. Anticoagulation in atrial fibrillation. Arrhythmia & Electrophysiology Review 2012;1:12–6.
44. Lu G, DeGuzman FR, Hollenbach SJ, et al. A specific antidote for reversal of anticoagulation by direct and indirect inhibitors of coagulation factor Xa. Nat Med 2013;19(4):446–51.
45. van Ryn J, Litzenburger T, Waterman A, et al. An antibody selective to dabigatran safely neutralizes both dabigatran-induced anticoagulant and bleeding activity in in vitro and in vivo models [Abstract P-MO-166]. Paper presented at: 57th Annual Meeting of the International Society on Thrombosis and Haemostasis. Kyoto, Japan, July 23–28, 2011.
46. van Ryn J, Litzenburger T, Schurer J. Reversal of anticoagulant activity of dabigatran and dabigatran-induced bleeding in rats by a specific antidote (antibody fragment) [abstract 9928]. Paper presented at: American Heart Association Scientific Sessions and Resuscitation Science Symposium. Los Angeles, USA, November 3–7, 2012.

Perioperative Management of Patients Receiving New Oral Anticoagulants

An International Survey

David Faraoni, MD[a],*, Charles Marc Samama, MD, PhD[b],
Marco Ranucci, MD, FESC[c], Wulf Dietrich, MD, PhD[d],
Jerrold H. Levy, MD, FAHA, FCCM[e]

KEYWORDS

• New oral anticoagulants • Survey • Guidelines • Recommendation

KEY POINTS

• New oral anticoagulants (NOACs) are increasingly replacing standard anticoagulants.
• These new drugs have recently been introduced into clinical practice, and specific knowledge regarding preoperative interruption, anticoagulation assessment, and reversal therapies is needed. In this international survey, it was observed that physicians had limited knowledge about the perioperative management of patients treated with NOACs and the management of emergency procedures.
• This situation has arisen from the lack of published experience, guidelines, widely available strategies to monitor NOAC effects, and clinically effective reversal strategies.
• Robust prospective studies are urgently needed to define guidelines and improve perioperative management.

The Society of Cardiovascular Anesthesiologists (SCA, http://www.scahq.org) and the European Association of Cardiothoracic Anaesthesiologists (EACTA, http://www.eacta.org) both endorsed this international survey.
Conflict of Interest Statements: Dr Samama received Speaker's fee from Bayer, BMS, Boehringer-Ingelheim, CSL Behring, Daichii, GSK, LFB, Octapharma, Pfizer, Rovi, Sanofi; Advisory committees, Bayer, BMS, Boehringer-Ingelheim, Daichii-Sankyo, GSK, Pfizer, Roche, Sanofi; Primary Investigator, Bayer, BMS, Boehringer-Ingelheim, LFB, GSK, Sanofi. Prof. J.H. Levy serves on steering committees for Boehringer Ingelheim, CSL Behring AG, Grifols, Janssen Pharmaceuticals, and The Medicines Company.
[a] Department of Anesthesiology, Queen Fabiola Children's University Hospital, 15 JJ Crocq Avenue, Brussels B-1020, Belgium; [b] Department of Anesthesia and Intensive Care, Cochin Hotel-Dieu University Hospitals, Place du Parvis Notre-Dame, 1, Paris 75181, France; [c] Department of Cardiothoracic and Vascular Anesthesia and Intensive Care, IRCCS Policlinico San Donato, Via Morandi, 30, San Donato Milanese, Milan 20097, Italy; [d] Institute for Research in Cardiac Anesthesia, Winthirstr 4, Munich 80639, Germany; [e] Duke University School of Medicine, Divisions of Cardiothoracic Anesthesiology and Critical Care, Duke University Hospital, 2301 Erwin Road, Durham, NC 27710, USA
* Corresponding author.
E-mail address: davidfaraoni@icloud.com

Clin Lab Med 34 (2014) 637–654
http://dx.doi.org/10.1016/j.cll.2014.06.006
0272-2712/14/$ – see front matter © 2014 Elsevier Inc. All rights reserved.

INTRODUCTION

The direct thrombin inhibitor dabigatran etexilate (Pradaxa [Boehringer-Ingelheim Pharma GmbH, Ingelheim am Rhein, Germany]) and direct factor Xa inhibitors rivaroxaban (Xarelto [Johnson and Johnson/Bayer HealthCare AG, Leverkusen, Germany]) and apixaban (Eliquis [Bristol Myers Squibb/Pfizer, Brystol-Myers Squibb House, Uxbridge, United Kingdom]) are increasingly used to prevent stroke in patients with nonvalvular atrial fibrillation,[1] for the treatment of venous thromboembolic diseases,[2] and for post-orthopedic surgery thromboprophylaxis.[3] In addition, rivaroxaban is indicated for the prevention of atherothrombotic events in adults after an acute coronary syndrome.[4]

The main objective of the present study is, therefore, to assess (1) physicians' current level of knowledge about perioperative management of patients treated with NOACs, (2) the current practices, and (3) the perspectives needed to improve the management of patients treated with NOACs. The study was performed both in Europe and in the United States using a self-reported Web-based survey. The results from this study will help to determine the potential need for future educational tools and practice guidelines for the perioperative management of patients treated with NOACs.

METHODS

A survey comprising 31 questions was developed to assess physicians' current knowledge about perioperative management of patients treated with NOACs, current practices, and perspectives needed to improve patient management. The survey was divided into 5 sections: demographic data (6 questions), the use of guidelines (7 questions), practices in case of scheduled surgery (12 questions), practices in case of emergent procedures (4 questions), and perspectives (2 questions). The survey questionnaire is available in the supplementary material (Appendix 1).

An invitation to participate in the survey was sent by e-mail to all members of the Society of Cardiovascular Anesthesiologists (SCA) and the European Association of Cardiothoracic Anaesthesiologists (EACTA). The survey was open from October 1, 2012 to December 31, 2012. To maximize response rate, 2 sequential e-mails were sent to the society members during the study period. All regular members of the 2 societies were invited without restriction. The responder's region of origin, type of practice (academic, private, government), and principal field of activity (anesthesia, intensive care, emergency department) were recorded in the demographic section. Data obtained in each section were recorded and analyzed separately.

Statistical Analysis

Data are presented as number and proportion (%), or median and range (percentile 25 to percentile 75). Analyses were performed according to the number of responses obtained for each question. Categorical variables were compared using χ^2 analysis. Subanalyses were performed to compare practices by region of origin. A one-way analysis of variance (ANOVA) was used to compare the means between regions of origin. In all cases, a 2-tailed P value less than .05 was considered statistically significant. Statistical analyses were performed with Prism 6 for Mac OS (version 6.0a; GraphPad Software, San Diego, CA; http://www.graphpad.com).

RESULTS
Questionnaire Responses

A total of 450 responses were received from 5262 invited members (9%); 117/450 physicians (26%) completed the questionnaire in full. All 450 responders (100%)

completed the section demographic data, 390 of 450 (87%) completed the section regarding NOACs and guidelines, 135 of 450 (30%) completed the questions about preoperative management in case of scheduled surgery, 117 of 450 (26%) completed the section regarding emergent procedures and 117 of 450 (26%) completed the section regarding perspectives (**Fig. 1**).

Responder Profile

Sixty-one percent of responders listed their region of origin as North America, 30% as Europe, 3% as South America, 3% as Asia, and 3% as Africa. They worked mostly in university hospitals (48%) or private practice (43%); 12% of responders were government workers. Eighty-three percent of the responders worked as anesthesiologists (15% in intensive care units and 2% in emergency rooms). The responders were mostly (94%) staff physicians; only 6% were residents or fellows. The median number of years in practice was 18 (10–25). Demographic data by region of origin are presented in **Table 1**. Of the responders, 59% declared that they are confronted several times a month with patients treated with NOACs (**Fig. 2**).

Guideline Use

In response to the questions on guidelines on NOAC reversal, of 450 responders, 132 (29%) declared that no guidelines are used in their institution; 126 (28%) used local guidelines, 158 (35%) referred to national guidelines, and 65 (14%) used international guidelines. However, most of the physicians (46%) declared that no consensus was established at their institution for using guidelines, and 18% believed that no guidelines had been established because of the lack of relevant literature. Ninety-seven percent of responders declared that guidelines are needed to improve perioperative management of patients treated with NOACs, as well as new data regarding monitoring (69%) and reversal therapies (73%).

NOAC Reversal Strategies

To define the preoperative interruption strategy, most physicians considered the risk of bleeding based on the type of surgery (53%) and the NOACs received (51%). However, only 27% considered the pharmacokinetic properties of the NOAC received to guide preoperative management. Marked variation in the duration of NOAC interruption was observed in case of low-risk surgery (**Fig. 3**A), with a median interruption

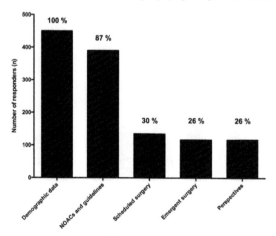

Fig. 1. Response rate obtained in the different sections of the survey.

Table 1
Demographic data by region of origin

	Overall (N = 450)	North America (n = 275)	Europe (n = 134)	Other (n = 41)	P Value
Survey completed	117 (26)	67 (24)	41 (30)	9 (22)	NS
Type of Practice[a]					
Academic	217 (48)	119 (43)	84 (63)	14 (34)	<.001
Private	194 (43)	151 (55)	23 (17)	20 (49)	<.001
Government	54 (12)	13 (4)	31 (23)	10 (24)	<.001
Staff	423 (94)	266 (97)	116 (86)	41 (100)	<.001
Years in practice	18 (10–25)	17 (8–25)	20 (12–25)	18 (12–25)	NS
Specialty[a]					
Anesthesiologist	433 (96)	270 (98)	124 (92)	39 (95)	NS
Intensive care unit physician	79 (17)	19 (7)	56 (42)	4 (10)	<.05

Data are expressed as number (percentage) or median (percentile 25 to percentile 75).
Abbreviation: NS, not significant.
[a] The total exceeds 100% because more than 1 answer was allowed.

period of 2 days for all drugs but ranges varying from 0 to 7 days for apixaban and rivaroxaban and 0 to 15 days for dabigatran. Similar observations were made for high-risk surgery (see **Fig. 3**B), with a median interruption period of 3 days for all drugs but ranges varying from 0 to 10 days for apixaban and rivaroxaban, and 0 to 15 days for dabigatran. Preoperative bridging was considered by 77% of responders in high-risk patients, by 12% of responders in all patients; 11% of responders never considered preoperative bridging. Low-molecular-weight heparin (LMWH) was preferred by 75% of the responders compared with 37% for unfractionated heparin (UFH).

Table 2 highlights the diverse range of tests that were used to assess coagulation status in an emergent situation. In the same situation, no relevant conclusion could be drawn from the therapeutic approach responses when physicians were asked to rank different therapeutic approaches (recombinant activated factor VII [rFVIIa], fresh frozen plasma [FFP], prothrombin complex concentrates [PCCs], hemodialysis, and

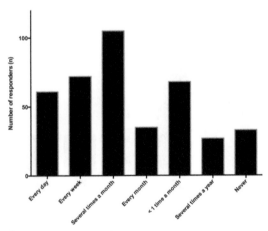

Fig. 2. Frequency of exposition to NOACs.

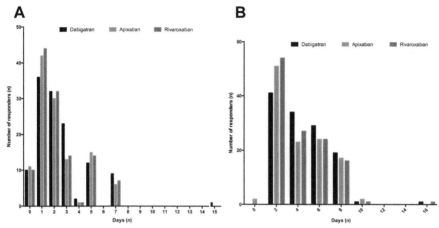

Fig. 3. Histogram of the interruption delay before (*A*) low-risk procedure, (*B*) high-risk procedure.

charcoal) in order of preference (**Fig. 4**). Each therapy was used with the same proportion in each position regardless of the NOAC that had been administered.

DISCUSSION

The main finding of this international survey of the members of the SCA and EACTA is that responders (principally anesthesiologists) had little knowledge about perioperative management of patients treated with NOACs, either for scheduled surgery or emergent procedures. Although almost 60% of the responders declared that they managed patients treated with NOACs several times a month, marked divergence in the practices used for NOAC reversal was observed.

Compared with warfarin, advantages of NOACs include their relatively rapid onset and offset of action and relatively predictable anticoagulant effect; routine coagulation

Table 2			
Tests used to assess coagulation status in a bleeding patient treated with a new oral anticoagulant			
Monitoring	**Dabigatran**	**Apixaban**	**Rivaroxaban**
aPTT	36 (32.1)	27 (24.1)	26 (23.2)
PT	19 (17)	29 (25.9)	32 (28.6)
INR	22 (19.6)	23 (20.5)	22 (19.6)
ACT	11 (9.8)	8 (7.1)	8 (7.1)
ECT	28 (25.0)	5 (4.5)	6 (5.3)
Factor Xa activity	16 (14.3)	**42 (37.5)**	**47 (41.9)**
Thrombin time	**35 (31.2)**	13 (11.6)	12 (10.7)
Diluted thrombin time (Hemoclot)	14 (12.5)	2 (1.8)	2 (1.8)
None	**33 (29.5)**	**34 (30.4)**	32 (28.6)

Results are expressed as number of responses and percentage (%) for each test, calculated for each drug.

The values in bold indicate the test(s) most commonly used for each of the NOACs.

Abbreviations: ACT, activated clotting time; aPTT, activated partial thromboplastin time; ECT, ecarin clotting time; INR, international normalized ratio; PT, prothrombin time.

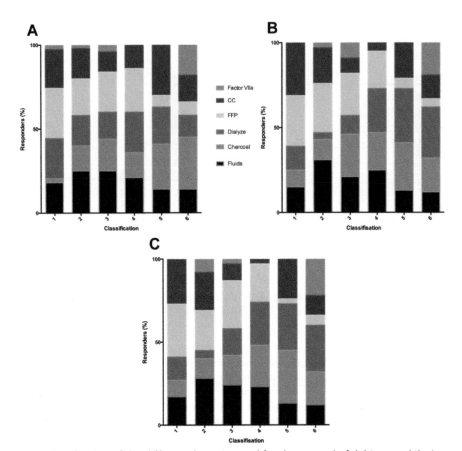

Fig. 4. Classification of the different therapies used for the reversal of dabigatran (A), rivaroxaban (B), and apixaban (C). The numbers (1, 2, 3, 4, 5, 6) correspond to the repartition of first choice, second choice, and so forth. CC, complex concentrate; FFP, fresh frozen plasma.

monitoring is not required but is possible in patients, for whom it is important to have information on coagulation status.[5] In certain clinical settings such as emergency surgery, trauma, acute bleeding, and suspected overdose, tests to measure coagulation are needed.[6] Dabigatran, a direct thrombin inhibitor, and rivaroxaban and apixaban, 2 factor Xa inhibitors, can be routinely monitored in patients. Anti-Xa measurement and Hemoclot (HYPHEN BioMed, Neuville sur-Oise, France), a thrombin diluted clotting assay, are specific assays, which have been proposed for rivaroxaban and dabigatran, respectively.[7] In case of emergent procedures or bleeding situations, management cannot be standardized, because no antidote has been developed. Furthermore, the efficacy of standard reversal therapies (eg, FFP, 3-factor or 4-factor PCCs, and rFVIIa) has not been adequately studied in these settings.[8] The limited experience regarding manipulation of NOACs and the higher costs should also be considered as a major drawback.

Data on perioperative management of patients receiving NOACs are sparse, and relevant recommendations are based only on expert opinions[9–11] or guidelines published by working groups or international societies (**Table 3**).[12–17] In 2011, the Working Group on Perioperative Hemostasis proposed guidelines for the management of

Table 3
Articles on recommendations for the perioperative management of patients treated with NOACs

Author, Year	Endorsed	Comments
Rosencher et al,[29] 2007		Regional anesthesia
Llau & Ferrandis,[28] 2009		Regional anesthesia
Gogarten et al,[27] 2010	ESA	Regional anesthesia
Horlocker et al,[26] 2010	ASRA	Regional anesthesia
Levy et al,[25] 2010		Review article
Sie et al,[12] 2011	GIHP	Perioperative recommendations
Vandermeulen et al,[24] 2011	BARA	Regional anesthesia
Spyropoulos et al,[9] 2012		Review article with recommendations
Levy et al,[10] 2013		Review article with recommendations
Kozek-Langenecker et al,[13] 2013	ESA	ESA guidelines
Spahn et al,[14] 2013		Updated European trauma guidelines
Steiner et al,[15] 2013	DKG	Emergency management
Fawole et al,[11] 2013		Review article with recommendations
Ferrandis et al,[16] 2013	WGSFAA	Review article with recommendations
Pernod et al,[17] 2013	GIHP	Bleeding complications and emergency surgery

Abbreviations: ASRA, American Society of Regional Anesthesia and Pain Medicine; BARA, Belgian Association for Regional Anesthesia; DKG, German Society of Cardiology; ESA, European Society of Anaesthesiology; GIHP, Working Group on Perioperative Hemostasis; WGSFAA, Working Group of Spanish Forum on Anticoagulation and Anesthesia.

patients treated with NOACs scheduled for an invasive procedure or surgery.[12] Based on the pharmacokinetic properties of each drug, these investigators proposed interruption of NOACs 2 days before surgery without bridging in case of low-risk procedures, and a 5-day interruption in case of high-risk surgery. In this situation, bridging with LMWH or UFH should be considered in case of high thromboembolic risk. The same group recently completed their recommendations for the management of major bleeding complications and emergency surgery in patients receiving long-term NOAC treatment.[17] The investigators noted that because of the lack of relevant data, only proposals could be formulated rather than recommendations. Similarly, in the European Society of Anaesthesiology's (ESA) recently published guidelines on the management of severe perioperative bleeding,[13] only weak recommendations were formulated because of the lack of relevant data. The ESA recommends the assessment of creatinine clearance in patients receiving NOACs who are scheduled for surgery (grade 1B). The ESA suggests that NOACs should not be interrupted (grade 2C) for superficial surgeries (skin, dental, eyes), and that NOACs can be discontinued 5 days before surgery without bridging in patients with low-risk thromboembolic complications (grade 1C). In patients with high-risk thromboembolic complications, the ESA guidelines recommend interruption 5 days before surgery without bridging if creatinine clearance is less than 50 mL/min, or with UFH bridging therapy if renal function is normal (grade 2C). In the recent version of the European guidelines for the management of bleeding and coagulopathy after trauma, the investigators suggest the measurement of substrate-specific anti–factor Xa activity in patients treated or suspected of being treated with rivaroxaban and apixaban (grade 2C).[14] The administration of high-dose (25–50 IU/kg) PCC is recommended in case of life-threatening bleeding (grade 2C). However, the investigators do not recommend the administration of PCCs in patients being treated or suspected of being treated with dabigatran (grade 2B). No alternative is proposed. These weak recommendations also highlight the lack of useful monitoring techniques to assess the anticoagulation level obtained with NOACs. This confusion was clearly shown by the marked variation in the tests used to assess coagulation status for each of the NOACs that was observed in our international survey (see **Table 2**).

The Grading of Recommendations Assessment, Development and Evaluation system used by the investigators of the different guidelines should be considered before NOAC reversal strategies are applied in clinical practice.[18] Only grade 1A and 1B recommendations are based on data from prospective randomized trials in which benefits seem to overweigh risks. Grade 1C comes from observational or low-quality randomized controlled trials. In contrast, trials in which the benefits were closely balanced with risks are classified as grade 2. In light of this system, the recommendations formulated in these 2 guidelines should be considered with caution, and further studies are needed to better inform guidelines.

A recent study has suggested that an activated PCC (FEIBA [factor 8 inhibitor bypassing activity]) may be effective in reversing the anticoagulant effect of both rivaroxaban and dabigatran[19]; however, the study was performed in healthy volunteers, and the results need to be confirmed in the clinical setting.

Healey and colleagues[20] performed a subanalysis of the Randomized Evaluation of Long-Term Anticoagulation Therapy trial, with the aim of assessing the incidence of periprocedural bleeding and thromboembolic events with dabigatran compared with warfarin. These investigators observed that dabigatran and warfarin were associated with similar rates of periprocedural bleeding, a result that was observed in the subset of patients who underwent urgent surgery. The investigators concluded that dabigatran facilitated a shorter interruption of oral anticoagulation compared with warfarin. However, the study was not designed to study this end point, and a higher incidence of bleeding complications could be expected in the general population than in the selected participants in a clinical trial. Further large prospective trials are needed to better assess the incidence of bleeding with NOACs compared with standard therapies. In addition, because of the lack of antidote, further studies should also assess the severity of complications observed with NOACs.

The present international survey has certain limitations. The accuracy of the results may have been affected by nonresponse bias, because only 9% of the invited members participated in the survey. This low response rate is a common limitation of online or e-mail surveys and has been well documented.[21–23] However, the possibility could not be excluded that the appropriate population was not targeted (lack of interest regarding this topic) or that a lack of knowledge in the nonresponder population led to nonparticipation in the survey. Physicians with a particular interest in cardiovascular anesthesia were targeted in the 2 societies, and a more general population would be preferable. In addition, only 26% of the responders completed the survey in full. Technical issues, the large number of questions, or a lack of relevant knowledge could explain this low response rate. Although these limitations should be kept in mind, the results of the survey could be used in future to assess the effects of guidelines on clinical practice and knowledge.

The results of this survey highlight the lack of knowledge and standardized practices concerning the perioperative management of patients treated with NOACs. These results could be explained by a lack of guidelines, a lack of experience in this setting, and a lack of data regarding safety, monitoring, and NOAC reversal therapy. Large randomized controlled trials should be performed to better study the incidence of perioperative bleeding with NOACs and to better inform treatment algorithms and guidelines. Until the results of such large trials are available, all institutions should implement local guidelines on when to use each test or intervention. Learning tools should be implemented through international societies to educate physicians and improve the management of patients treated with NOACs.

REFERENCES

1. Heidbuchel H, Verhamme P, Alings M, et al. EHRA practical guide on the use of new oral anticoagulants in patients with non-valvular atrial fibrillation: executive summary. Eur Heart J 2013;34:2094–106.
2. Gallego P, Roldan V, Lip GY. Conventional and new oral anticoagulants in the treatment of chest disease and its complications. Am J Respir Crit Care Med 2013;188(4):413–21.
3. Kwok CS, Pradhan S, Yeong JK, et al. Relative effects of two different enoxaparin regimens as comparators against newer oral anticoagulants: meta-analysis and adjusted indirect comparison. Chest 2013;144:593–600.
4. Bayer Pharma AG. Rivaroxaban summary of product characteristics. Available at: http://www.ema.europa.eu/docs/en_GB/document_library/EPAR_-_Product_Information/human/000944/WC500057108.pdf. Accessed December 9, 2013.
5. Eikelboom JW, Weitz JI. New anticoagulants. Circulation 2010;121:1523–32.
6. Samama MM, Amiral J, Guinet C, et al. Monitoring plasma levels of factor Xa inhibitors: how, why and when? Expert Rev Hematol 2013;6:155–64.
7. Samama MM, Guinet C, Le Flem L, et al. Measurement of dabigatran and rivaroxaban in primary prevention of venous thromboembolism in 106 patients, who have undergone major orthopedic surgery: an observational study. J Thromb Thrombolysis 2013;35:140–6.
8. Kaatz S, Crowther M. Reversal of target-specific oral anticoagulants. J Thromb Thrombolysis 2013;36:195–202.
9. Spyropoulos AC, Douketis JD. How I treat anticoagulated patients undergoing an elective procedure or surgery. Blood 2012;120:2954–62.
10. Levy JH, Faraoni D, Spring JL, et al. Managing new oral anticoagulants in the perioperative and intensive care unit setting. Anesthesiology 2013;118:1466–74.
11. Fawole A, Daw HA, Crowther MA. Practical management of bleeding due to the anticoagulants dabigatran, rivaroxaban, and apixaban. Cleve Clin J Med 2013; 80:443–51.
12. Sie P, Samama CM, Godier A, et al. Surgery and invasive procedures in patients on long-term treatment with direct oral anticoagulants: thrombin or factor-Xa inhibitors. Recommendations of the Working Group on Perioperative Haemostasis and the French Study Group on Thrombosis and Haemostasis. Arch Cardiovasc Dis 2011;104:669–76.
13. Kozek-Langenecker SA, Afshari A, Albaladejo P, et al. Management of severe perioperative bleeding: guidelines from the European Society of Anaesthesiology. Eur J Anaesthesiol 2013;30:270–382.
14. Spahn DR, Bouillon B, Cerny V, et al. Management of bleeding and coagulopathy following major trauma: an updated European guideline. Crit Care 2013;17:R76.
15. Steiner T, Bohm M, Dichgans M, et al. Recommendations for the emergency management of complications associated with the new direct oral anticoagulants (DOACs), apixaban, dabigatran and rivaroxaban. Clin Res Cardiol 2013;102:399–412.
16. Ferrandis R, Castillo J, de Andres J, et al. The perioperative management of new direct oral anticoagulants: a question without answers. Thromb Haemost 2013; 110(3):515–22.

17. Pernod G, Albaladejo P, Godier A, et al. Management of major bleeding complications and emergency surgery in patients on long-term treatment with direct oral anticoagulants, thrombin or factor-Xa inhibitors: proposals of the Working Group on Perioperative Haemostasis (GIHP). Arch Cardiovasc Dis 2013;106:382–93.

18. Guyatt G, Eikelboom JW, Akl EA, et al. A guide to GRADE guidelines for the readers of JTH. J Thromb Haemost 2013;11(8):1603–8.

19. Marlu R, Hodaj E, Paris A, et al. Effect of non-specific reversal agents on anticoagulant activity of dabigatran and rivaroxaban: a randomised crossover ex vivo study in healthy volunteers. Thromb Haemost 2012;108:217–24.

20. Healey JS, Eikelboom J, Douketis J, et al. Periprocedural bleeding and thromboembolic events with dabigatran compared with warfarin: results from the randomized evaluation of long-term anticoagulation therapy (RE-LY) randomized trial. Circulation 2012;126:343–8.

21. Braithwaite D, Emery J, De Lusignan S, et al. Using the Internet to conduct surveys of health professionals: a valid alternative? Fam Pract 2003;20:545–51.

22. Mavis BE, Brocato JJ. Postal surveys versus electronic mail surveys. The tortoise and the hare revisited. Eval Health Prof 1998;21:395–408.

23. Cannesson M, Pestel G, Ricks C, et al. Hemodynamic monitoring and management in patients undergoing high risk surgery: a survey among North American and European anesthesiologists. Crit Care 2011;15:R197.

24. Vandermeulen E, Decoster J, Dewandre PY, et al. Central neural blockade in patients with a drug-induced alteration of coagulation. Third edition of the Belgian Association for Regional Anaesthesia (BARA) Guidelines. Acta Anaesthesiol Belg 2011;62:175–91.

25. Levy JH, Key NS, Azran MS. Novel oral anticoagulants: implications in the perioperative setting. Anesthesiology 2010;113:726–45.

26. Horlocker TT, Wedel DJ, Rowlingson JC, et al. Executive summary: regional anesthesia in the patient receiving antithrombotic or thrombolytic therapy: American Society of Regional Anesthesia and Pain Medicine Evidence-Based Guidelines (Third Edition). Reg Anesth Pain Med 2010;35:102–5.

27. Gogarten W, Vandermeulen E, Van Aken H, et al. Regional anaesthesia and antithrombotic agents: recommendations of the European Society of Anaesthesiology. Eur J Anaesthesiol 2010;27:999–1015.

28. Llau JV, Ferrandis R. New anticoagulants and regional anesthesia. Curr Opin Anaesthesiol 2009;22:661–6.

29. Rosencher N, Bonnet MP, Sessler DI. Selected new antithrombotic agents and neuraxial anaesthesia for major orthopaedic surgery: management strategies. Anaesthesia 2007;62:1154–60.

APPENDIX 1: THE SURVEY QUESTIONNAIRE

Background:

New oral anticoagulants (NOAs) include the direct thrombin inhibitor, dabigatran etexilate, and the direct factor Xa inhibitors, rivaroxaban and apixiban.
As these agents will increasingly replace older parenteral agents and vitamin K antagonists (VKAs) in clinical practice, it is important to consider that patients treated with NOAs will be exposed to different clinical situations (spontaneous or postoperative bleeding, overdose, trauma, scheduled or emergent surgical procedures) that require targeted interventions. Different articles, national or international guidelines were recently published. The primary objective of this international survey is the evaluation of physician's knowledge about published recommendations. Second, we would like to evaluate local practices in different clinical situations.

David Faraoni, MD
Charles Marc Samama, MD, PhD, FCCP
Wulf Dietrich, MD, PhD
Jerrold H. Levy, MD, FAHA

Demographic data

1. Name of the hospital you currently work in:

[   ]

2. City

[   ]

3. Country

[   ]

4. Type of practice

☐ University

☐ Private

☐ Government

☐ Other

[   ]

5. Status

○ Resident/Fellow

○ Staff

Years in training/practice

[   ]

6. Principal activity

☐ Anesthesiology

☐ Intensive Care

☐ Emergency department

☐ Other

[   ]

New oral anticoagulants (NOAs) and guidelines:

1. How did you hear about NOA's

☐ Literature

☐ Meeting

☐ Society

☐ Pharmaceutical literature

☐ News

☐ Colleagues

☐ Other

[   ]

2. In your clinical practice, you manage patients treated with NOAs

◯ Every day

◯ Every weeks

◯ Several times per month

◯ Every month

◯ Less then once a month

◯ Several times a year

◯ Never

3. In your institution, you used

☐ Local guideline

☐ National guideline

☐ International guideline

☐ No guideline

Reference

[   ]

4. If local guideline exists, it was set up by

☐ Anesthesiologists

☐ ICU doctors

☐ Cardiologists

☐ Hematologists

☐ Multidisciplinary

Describe the multidisciplinary approach

5. Do you think that guideline is needed to improve patient's outcome?

◯ Yes

◯ No

6. If yes

☐ Local guideline

☐ National guideline

☐ International guideline

7. If you do not have local guideline, why?

☐ No enough literature

☐ No consensus

☐ Time consuming

☐ Will not improve patient outcomes

☐ Other

In case of scheduled surgery

1. NOAs must be stopped

☐ The day before

☐ Two days before

☐ Several days: how much

☐ Depending on the drug

☐ Depend on the pharmacokinetic properties

☐ Depend of the type of surgery and the risk of bleeding

☐ No interruption

☐ None

2. Specific management for procedures with low risk of bleeding

Dabigatran will be
stopped ... day(s) before [   ]

Apixaban will be
stopped ... day(s) before [   ]

Rivaroxaban will be
stopped ... day(s) before [   ]

3. Specific management for procedure with moderate or high risk of bleeding

You stop dabigatran ......
day(s) before [   ]

You stop apixaban ......
day(s) before [   ]

You stop rivaroxaban ......
day(s) before [   ]

4. Specific management for procedure with low risk of bleeding

You restart dabigatran ......
day(s) after the procedure [   ]

You restart apixaban ......
day(s) after the procedure [   ]

You restart rivaroxaban
...... day(s) after the
procedure [   ]

5. Specific management for procedure with moderate or high risk of bleeding

You restart dabigatran ......
day(s) after the procedure [   ]

You restart apixaban ......
day(s) after the procedure [   ]

You restart rivaroxaban
...... day(s) after the
procedure [   ]

6. What test(s) do you consider to assess the degree of anticoagulation?

	Dabigatran	Apixaban	Rivaroxaban
aPTT	☐	☐	☐
PT	☐	☐	☐
INR	☐	☐	☐
ACT	☐	☐	☐
Ecarin Clotting Time	☐	☐	☐
Factor Xa activity	☐	☐	☐
Thrombin Time	☐	☐	☐
Diluted Thrombin Time (Haemoclot®)	☐	☐	☐
None	☐	☐	☐

7. What delay do you consider safe in these different clinical situations?

	Dabigatran	Apixaban	Rivaroxaban
Spinal Anesthesia	▾	▾	▾
Epidural Anesthesia	▾	▾	▾
Catheter withdrawal	▾	▾	▾
Next dose after withdrawal	▾	▾	▾

8. When do you consider bridging therapy?

☐ Never

☐ Always

☐ High risk thromboembolic complication

Other (please specify)

[   ]

9. How many hours before surgery do start bridging therapy?

[▾]

10. What agent do you use for bridging therapy?

☐ LMWH

☐ UFH

Other (please specify)

[   ]

11. The indication for NOA is quite different. It makes a difference, whether a patient has a prosthetic valve or is under prophylactic treatment. Is this difference considered in regard to stopping or postoperative commencement of therapy?

[▾]

12. If yes, explain

[   ]

4. In case of emergency procedure, bleeding, trauma, overdose

1. What test do you consider to assess the degree of anticoagulation?

	Dabigatran	Apixaban	Rivaroxaban
aPTT	☐	☐	☐
PT	☐	☐	☐
INR	☐	☐	☐
ACT	☐	☐	☐
Ecarin Clotting Time	☐	☐	☐
Factor Xa activity	☐	☐	☐
Thrombin Time	☐	☐	☐
Diluted Thrombin Time (Haemoclot®)	☐	☐	☐
None	☐	☐	☐

2. If you want to reverse dabigatran, you will use:

[▼] Fluid/PRBC

[▼] Charcoal

[▼] Dialyze

[▼] FFP

[▼] PCC

[▼] Factor VIIa

3. If you want to reverse apixaban, you will use

[▼] Fluid/PRBC

[▼] Charcoal

[▼] Dialyze

[▼] FFP

[▼] PCC

[▼] Factor VIIa

4. 4.2. If you want to reverse rivaroxaban, you will use:

[▼] Fluid/PRBC

[▼] Charcoal

[▼] Dialyze

[▼] FFP

[▼] PCC

[▼] Factor VIIa

The future

1. What changes do you expect, in a near future, for the management of new oral anticoagulants in perioperative period and critical care settings:

☐ New clear guidelines

☐ New monitoring

☐ New reversal agents

☐ Other

2. General comments:

The End

On the behalf of my collaborators, I thank you very much for your time and your consideration. If you have additional comments or if you want to receive more details about this survey, do not hesitate to contact me.

David Faraoni, MD
davidfaraoni@me.com

Management of Anticoagulation and Hemostasis for Pediatric Extracorporeal Membrane Oxygenation

Arun Saini, MD, Philip C. Spinella, MD*

KEYWORDS

- Anticoagulation • Congenital heart defect • Extracorporeal membrane oxygenation
- Heparin • Platelet function • Thromboelastography

KEY POINTS

- Extracorporeal membrane oxygenation (ECMO) circuit causes activation of multiple systems, including thrombin generation, inflammation, platelet activation and endothelial dysfunction. Prolonged hemostatic activation can lead to consumption of coagulation factors and reduced platelet aggregation. Commonly used medications may also inhibit platelets.
- A delicate balance between the use of antihemostatic agents to reduce thrombotic events in the circuit and patient and the preservation of hemostatic potential to prevent severe bleeding in the patient is required.
- Unfractionated heparin is the most common anticoagulation agent used.
- Activated clot time is the most common monitoring test, but may not be an accurate measure of anticoagulation for children on ECMO.
- A comprehensive evaluation of relational hemostasis is required to optimize antihemostatic therapy and blood product administration to improve outcomes for children requiring ECMO.

INTRODUCTION

The use of anticoagulation/antihemostatic agents in children, for either prevention or treatment of thrombotic complications, is increasing, although their use is still relatively rare when compared with adults.[1] There are many challenges to the use of anticoagulants in children, as listed in **Box 1**.[2] These challenges become apparent in the

Disclosures: Partially supported by National Institutes of Health (U54 HL112303).
Division of Critical Care Medicine, Department of Pediatrics, Washington School of Medicine in St Louis, 8th floor, Northwest Towers, One Children's Place, St Louis, MO 63110, USA
* Corresponding author.
E-mail address: spinella_p@kids.wustl.edu

Clin Lab Med 34 (2014) 655–673
http://dx.doi.org/10.1016/j.cll.2014.06.014
0272-2712/14/$ – see front matter © 2014 Elsevier Inc. All rights reserved.

labmed.theclinics.com

Box 1
Challenges to use of anticoagulation agents in children

- Developmental hemostasis
- Limited pharmacokinetic and pharmacodynamics data for anticoagulation agents
- Different epidemiology of thromboembolism and risks of anticoagulation therapy
- Fewer pediatric formulations of common anticoagulation agents
- Restricted diagnostic evaluation due to need of sedation for diagnostic studies
- Irregular anticoagulation therapy monitoring due to difficult vascular access
- Inadequate validation of current diagnostic and treatment algorithms
- Lack of widespread experience and limited expertise
- Required collaborative approach with a multidisciplinary team
- Compliance concerns with high reliance on caregivers

Adapted from Monagle P, Newall F, Campbell J. Anticoagulation in neonates and children: pitfalls and dilemmas. Blood Rev 2010;24:151–62.

---

management of extracorporeal membrane oxygenation (ECMO), one of the most complex clinical scenarios in children. In this article, anticoagulation management, hemostatic adjuncts, and blood products transfusion in children requiring ECMO are the focal point. Antihemostatic agents to include all therapeutics that reduce thrombin formation or inhibit platelet aggregation are defined. Anticoagulants are medications that specifically reduce thrombin formation. Medications that inhibit platelets are antiplatelet agents.

Approximately 1500 to 2000 children (neonatal and pediatric) are placed on ECMO every year according to data collected at the Extracorporeal Life Support Organization (ELSO) centers.[3] Despite wider use and growing expertise, the survival rate has remained static since 2006 to 2012 at 66% to 70% (neonatal respiratory ECMO), 53% to 61% (pediatric respiratory ECMO), 41% to 46% (<30 days, cardiac ECMO), 48% to 62% (30 days to <1 year of age, cardiac ECMO), and 57% to 69% (>1 year to <16 years, cardiac ECMO).[3] Deaths are frequently related to severe hemorrhagic and thromboembolic complications and range between 30% and 40%.[3,4] Hemorrhagic and thromboembolic complications occur in this population because of alterations in hemostasis. The causes of these complications are in part due to the nonendothelial surface of extracorporeal circuit that activates both coagulation and inflammation and the use of anticoagulants to prevent thrombotic events. Also important is the underlying illness that may contribute to either a hypercoagulable or a hypocoagulable state due to immune and endothelial dysfunction as well as consumption of hemostatic factors.[5–8] Last, although uncommon, heparin-induced thrombocytopenia (HIT) or severe allergy to heparin can increase the risk of thrombotic events. Here, **ECMO-induced coagulopathy (EIC)** is defined as a pathophysiologic state of hemostasis for children on ECMO that can result in varying manifestations that range from a hypercoagulable to a hypocoagulable manifestation.

ECMO-INDUCED COAGULOPATHY
The ECMO Circuit

A typical ECMO circuit consists of cannulas, polyvinyl tubing with or without heparin coating, a roller or centrifugal pump, and a silicone membrane oxygenator. These components of the ECMO circuit are artificial and lead to activation of multiple hemostatic systems, including platelets, factor XII and kallikrein-kinin system, tissue factor and von Willebrand factor, fibrinolysis, and inflammation.[5-9] The initial contact of blood on the circuit leads to the cleavage of XII to XIIa and prekallikrein to kallikrein. Activated factor XII (XIIa) triggers the "intrinsic" pathway, whereas kallikrein activates inflammatory responses, fibrinolysis, and positive feedback to factor XIIa[8] and leads to a complex interaction of the inflammatory and hemostasis systems that activates cellular, complement, cytokine, hemostatic, and fibrinolytic pathways (**Fig. 1**).[6,8,9]

Inflammation

Patients on ECMO have increased both pro-inflammatory and anti-inflammatory cytokines[10-12] from the inflammatory response secondary to the patient's illness and the ECMO circuit. This inflammatory response may also contribute to ECMO-related multiorgan dysfunction as noted by increased levels of interleukin-6 (IL-6) in association with increased mortality in neonates on ECMO.[11] There is some evidence that soluble cytokines (such as IL-6, IL-1, IL-8, and tumor necrosis factor-α) and direct leukocyte-endothelial interaction might impair endothelial integrity.[12]

Thrombin Generation

Thrombin has diverse actions including cleavage of fibrinogen to fibrin, activation of factor XIII, activation of platelets via protease-activated receptor (PAR)-1 and PAR-4, and stimulation of endothelium to release tissue factor and von Willebrand factor.[8,9] The generation of thrombin on the circuit surface is partially counterbalanced by fibrinolysis-mediated by plasmin. The use of anticoagulation agents, primarily unfractionated heparin (UFH), prevents clot formation, but it does not halt low-grade thrombin generation and coagulation within the circuit.[9]

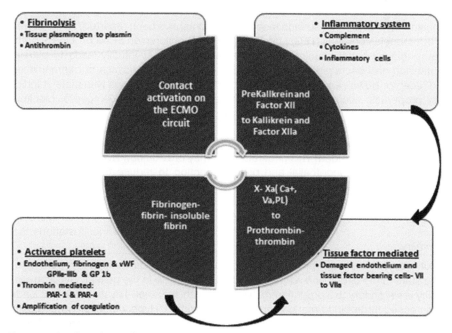

Fig. 1. Pathophysiology of EIC.

Endothelial Dysfunction

Coagulation activation on damaged endothelium via expression of tissue factor contributes to EIC[6,8,9,13,14] and is potentially responsible for thromboembolic events and disseminated intravascular coagulation (DIC). Biomarkers available to evaluate various endothelial functions include (1) integrity of endothelial glycocalyx (von Willebrand factor, tissue factor, syndecans, s-E-Selection), (2) production of endothelial reactive oxygen species (superoxide dismutase), (3) production of nitric oxide on endothelium (endothelial nitric oxide synthase), and (4) vascular endothelial junctions stability (s-Intercellular adhesion molecule-1).[15–17] The endothelium has multiple functions, and as a result, assessing endothelial dysfunction cannot be simply determined by measuring of 1 or 2 biomarkers. Further studies, perhaps using a system's biology approach to the endothelial dysfunction, are important to evaluate the role of endothelial dysfunction in ECMO better.

Platelet Dysfunction

The ECMO circuit also activates platelets, which amplifies thrombin generation on the surface of platelets. Activated platelets adhere to the ECMO circuit oxygenator and to damaged endothelium, further causing thrombocytopenia and increasing the risk of thrombotic events. Evidence for increased markers of platelet activation and degranulation, including platelet factor 4, thrombospondin, β-thromboglobulin, and adenosine diphosphate, is well documented for patients on ECMO.[6,18–21] Cheung and colleagues[18] described an increase in markers of platelet activation (P-selectin and matrix metalloproteinase -2 activity) with concurrent thrombocytopenia for neonates on ECMO. Fibrinogen deposition on the ECMO circuit activates and aggregates platelets via glycoprotein IIb/IIIa binding.[19] Straub and colleagues[19] report blocking glycoprotein IIb/IIIa receptors with tirofiban and a novel platelet phosphoinositide-3-kinase inhibitor (TGX-211) can decrease platelet aggregates on the circuit and adenosine diphosphate–induced platelet aggregation. Increased adenosine diphosphate and arachidonic acid platelet surface receptor inhibition have been reported, as measured by thromboelastography (TEG) platelet mapping, in children on ECMO.[21] One hypothesis is that repeated platelet stimulation on the circuit eventually leads to platelet exhaustion and decreased platelet aggregation over time because of degranulation and receptor down-regulation or inhibition.[18–21] In addition, drugs with platelet inhibitory properties, such as nitric oxide, milrinone, and histamine-2-receptor blockers that are commonly used in children on ECMO, may also influence platelet function.[22–24]

A better understanding of the interaction of endothelial dysfunction and activated platelets in EIC is needed. This understanding may provide new avenues for intervention to manipulate endothelial and platelet function to reduce the risk of adverse thrombotic events and severe bleeding for children on ECMO. Incorporation of point-of-care laboratory devices to measure endothelial, platelet, and immune function may enhance the feasibility of achieving this goal.

Summary

In summary, EIC is a complex and dynamic condition that can lead to a hypercoagulable state in the circuit and a mixed coagulopathic state in the patient. Hypercoagulability is secondary to a pro-inflammatory state with endothelial dysfunction that leads to increased thrombin formation and platelet activation. Hypocoagulability occurs via consumption of coagulation factors and platelet exhaustion and reduction of platelet aggregation potential. The differential effects on thrombin formation and platelet function may allow for the common clinical scenario of significant thrombotic events within the circuit with simultaneous bleeding in the patient.

ANTICOAGULATION MONITORING

A recent survey conducted between November 2010 and May 2011 indicated substantial variability in anticoagulation management policies and blood product administration in ECMO centers throughout the world.[25] This survey also highlighted that activated clotting time (ACT) remains the preferred anticoagulation monitoring tool (97% of respondents), although many centers have been incorporating a variety of additional anticoagulation monitoring tools, including antithrombin III activity (ATIII) (82%), anti-factor Xa concentration (65%), and TEG (43%).[25]

ACT Values and its Limitations

ACT is a whole blood point-of-care assay, which measures the time to fibrin clot formation after adding an activator of contact activation (celite or kaolin) that catalyzes the conversion of factor XII to XIIa. Anticoagulants increase the time for clot formation to occur, thus prolonging the ACT. Heparin binds to ATIII, inactivating thrombin and other proteases involved in blood clotting, most notably factor Xa. However, ACT values are increased by factors other than heparin, including hemodilution, hypothermia, decreased coagulation factor levels, and platelet dysfunction, which suggest that ACT has a tendency to overestimate the effect of heparin, limiting its accuracy.[26–29] Conversely, often ACT appears to underestimate the effect of heparin when simultaneous anti-Xa concentrations and TEG values are obtained. Possible reasons for these observations can be (1) instrument error in calibration, (2) use of aprotinin, but newer instruments are not affected, and (3) ACT is less sensitive at lower doses of heparin that are used in ECMO than the higher doses used for cardiopulmonary bypass.

Developmental hemostasis effects may also contribute to discrepancies between ACT values and actual heparin effect. Owings and colleagues[26] have demonstrated higher ACT values despite lower heparin concentrations in children for similar heparin dosing when compared with adults undergoing cardiopulmonary bypass. Also, there was persistent and increased thrombin generation in children compared with adults undergoing cardiopulmonary bypass despite ACT values between 400 and 800 seconds.[26]

The practice of using ACT to direct heparin dosing for ECMO occurred as a result of its use in cardiopulmonary bypass and the familiarity perfusionists had with this approach. There is no evidence that ACT use in ECMO is the most accurate method to titrate heparin or that its use is associated with improved outcomes. Heparin doses are higher during cardiopulmonary bypass and at these doses there is a stronger correlation between ACT and heparin serum concentrations.[27–29] In ECMO, where the heparin doses are much lower, there is a poor correlation between ACT values and heparin serum concentrations.[30–32] Other differences between the use of ACT for heparin dosing in cardiopulmonary bypass (CPB) versus ECMO are that the duration of ECMO is days to weeks versus hours in CPB; some patients requiring ECMO have multisystem organ failure with significant inflammation, whereas CPB patients typically have single-organ failure and are not in a persistent hyperinflammatory state. Prolonged activation of inflammation on ECMO affects ATIII and platelet function, which may weaken the correlation between ACT and fibrin formation. Each of these differences may affect the accuracy and therefore applicability of ACT in guiding heparin dosing for children on ECMO. The most commonly reported and recommended goal ACT range for nonbleeding children on ECMO is 180 to 220 seconds.[25,33] However, there is no evidence that this practice provides adequate anticoagulation in children on ECMO. The data from a retrospective single-centered study of 604 consecutive pediatric ECMO patients indicated that each increase of 10 U/kg/h in heparin dose up to 70 U/kg/h was predictive of increased odd of survival (odds ratio [OR] 1.27, confidence interval [CI] 1.03–1.42, $P<.001$), instead of ACT values (OR 0.996, CI 0.991–1.011, $P = .096$) on multivariate logistic regression.[34]

Anti-Xa Concentration Assays

The above concerns regarding the validity of ACT in the setting of ECMO has led many centers to use anti-Xa concentration assays to titrate heparin dosing for anticoagulation during ECMO in children. Anti-Xa concentration assays are based on the ability of heparin-ATIII complexes to inhibit a predetermined amount of factor Xa in the sample. They measure residual factor Xa activity by using either chromogenic or clotting-based methods.[35] The residual factor Xa activity is inversely proportional to the heparin concentration in the sample.[35,36] These assays have certain advantages: (1) they are a direct measure of heparin effect and (2) they are not affected by acute phase reactants such as factor VIII and fibrinogen.[36] However, they underestimate the concentration of heparin in the presence of ATIII deficiency in the sample,[37] which is especially important in neonates and children on ECMO, who have lower levels of ATIII than adults. In some centers, ATIII is supplemented within these assays, which causes overestimation of the heparin effect, but provides more accurate measure of heparin concentration in the sample.[37] If the physiologic effect of a heparinoid is more clinically relevant than a heparin concentration, then the anti-Xa assay used should not supplement with ATIII. Results from these assays will reflect the heparinoids effect on Xa more accurately. These factors should be considered while interpreting anti-Xa concentration assay results. Studies comparing anti-Xa concentration, ACT values, and heparin dosing or plasma concentrations are limited. Nankervis and colleagues[30] have reported a better correlation ($r = 0.75$) between anti-factor Xa concentration and heparin dose than between ACT and heparin dose ($r = 0.21$). Bembea and colleagues[31] have reported poor agreement between target anti-Xa concentration and target ACT (42%).[28] However, in their cohort, they reported a weak correlation between anti-Xa and heparin dose ($r = 0.33$). These correlation studies are difficult to interpret because there is no gold standard for a laboratory test that measures fibrin formation and hemostatic potential. Anti-Xa concentration is a direct measure of heparin effect, but many other factors influence overall hemostatic potential, including thrombin generation, fibrinogen and platelet function, and fibrinolysis. Using any individual parameter to estimate overall hemostatic potential should be avoided because no method has been developed to combine each of these functional properties of hemostasis accurately.

Anti-Xa Range

The most commonly reported goal anti-Xa range for heparin effect during ECMO is 0.3 to 0.7 IU/mL.[25,33] This range is mostly based on extrapolations from historic experience of heparin concentration on CPB and is considered to be adequate on ECMO. There is no direct evidence if the currently recommended anti-Xa range to titrate heparin dose is adequate to minimize thrombin generation in a child on ECMO. Studies are needed to measure and compare markers of thrombin generation (thrombin-antithrombin complex levels, prothrombin fragments 1 and 2, thrombin generation assays) to heparin concentration and clinical outcomes to determine the appropriate anti-Xa target during ECMO.

Activated Partial Thromboplastin Time

Activated partial thromboplastin time (aPTT) is commonly used to titrate heparin dosing in the treatment of a thrombus and correlates better than ACT to heparin plasma concentration within the low to medium range of 0.1 to 1 U/mL.[8,38] At higher heparin plasma concentrations greater than 1 U/mL, aPTT values are markedly prolonged (>150 seconds) and lack predictive change to heparin concentration. There is no recommended range of aPTT values in children on ECMO. However, the aPTT values corresponding to anti-Xa between 0.3 and 0.7 IU/mL had a median of 89 seconds (interquartile range: 69–122 seconds, range: 37–200 seconds) in a single-center study, but the correlation was weak ($r = 0.17$).[31]

Because ECMO can affect each phase of hemostasis due to its effect on thrombin/fibrin formation, fibrinogen and platelet function, and fibrinolysis, it is logical that global functional assays of hemostasis may assist in monitoring hemostasis in this population. Currently available global functional assays of hemostasis include both TEG with platelet mapping and rotational thromboelastometry (ROTEM).[39,40] These devices, which examine the viscoelastic properties of whole blood, have existed for decades, but have only recently gained increased attention because of digitization and standardization of methods.[40] These devices provide information regarding clot initiation (time to fibrin formation), clot kinetics (primarily fibrinogen function), clot strength (primarily platelet function), and fibrinolysis (**Fig. 2**A).[8,40] Various TEG parameters and their reference values for healthy pediatric patients are available.[41] Healthy infants demonstrate normal clot kinetics and clot strength despite lower levels of coagulation factors compared with adults.[22] To titrate heparin by using TEG/ROTEM, the reaction time (r-time) or clotting time is the most important parameter because it reflects fibrin formation (see **Fig. 2**B).[8,41] Heparinase TEG or ROTEM HEPTEM testing removes heparin effect from the sample, allowing for the analysis of the underlying or baseline hemostatic state of the patient. This information can be used to "normalize" hemostasis to allow for the prescribed anticoagulation to have a more predictable effect. The comparison of samples with and without heparinase can help in determining the magnitude of the effect of heparin, which may be valuable information when attempting to determine if a patient is resistant to heparin and if antithrombin should be given. TEG platelet mapping, a modification of TEG, measures a specific platelet surface receptors agonist mediated platelet aggregation and clot strength (see **Fig. 2**C). Platelet dysfunction occurs during ECMO, but is seldom considered in antihemostatic management. Preliminary data suggest that reduced platelet aggregation measured by TEG platelet mapping may be associated with bleeding complications and mortality.[21]

TEG or ROTEM-Guided Algorithms

The use of TEG-guided or ROTEM-guided algorithms in adults undergoing CPB has been shown to be associated with decreased blood product administration and mortality.[42–44] Weber and colleagues[42] have shown decreased blood product administration, better outcomes and cost effectiveness of point-of-care ROTEM, and platelet aggregometry assays of hemostasis. Although there are scant data regarding TEG/ROTEM use in ECMO patients, there is considerable experience with it in the pediatric ventricular assist device (VAD) population in guiding anticoagulation and antiplatelet therapy initiation and titration of dosing.[45,46] Currently, the predominant use of TEG/ROTEM for patients on ECMO is to assist with blood product indication for patients with active bleeding, but there is interest in determining how it can be used to assist with anticoagulation. The difficulty with incorporating TEG/ROTEM for

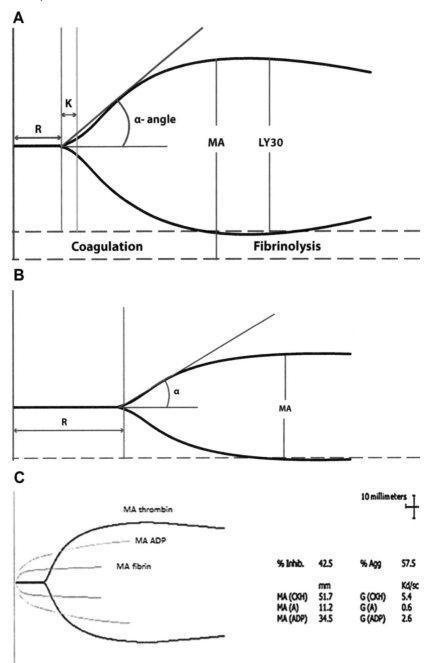

Fig. 2. (A) An hTEG of the patient on ECMO. Reaction time (r-time) is time to the initial clot formation and it reflects coagulation factor level. K-time is time to 20 mm of clot amplitude and it reflects fibrin cross-linking. Alpha angle (α) is another measure of clot kinetics. Maximum amplitude (MA) is the maximum clot strength, which depends on fibrinogen activity and platelet function. Percent lysis at 30 minutes (LY 30) is a measure of fibrinolytic activity. (B) Kaolin-activated citrated thromboelastrography tracing of the same patients. It shows heparin effect by prolongation of the r-time, decreased α angle, and low MA. (C) TEG platelet mapping tracing of the same patients. It shows the percentage platelet inhibition on ADP receptors.

ECMO anticoagulation management is defining threshold parameters for treatment indications and therapeutic range goals for the therapies that reduce fibrin formation or platelet activation.

Summary

Because of the complexity of hemostasis and heterogeneity of patients requiring ECMO, it is unlikely that one parameter will be adequate to monitor hemostasis and guide anticoagulation or ATIII replacement. Relational hemostasis is a concept whereby a composite of hemostasis variables is interpreted together in the context of the patient's underlying illness. The relationship between functional and quantitative parameters is likely to provide a more accurate estimation of hemostatic potential than just one parameter, and as a result, be more informative in guiding anticoagulation therapy. The in vitro assessment of in vivo hemostasis, a complex biologic system, will never be precise because current methods do not incorporate endothelial effects nor flow dynamics. Studies are needed to compare each method of coagulation monitoring directly (ACT, Anti-Xa, PTT, TEG, and ATIII) to determine which combination of parameters should be used to provide goal-directed antihemostatic management and improve clinical outcomes. Before this can be achieved, an evidence-based therapeutic target range for each parameter needs to be established in multiple patient cohorts. This evidence-based therapeutic target range can likely only be achieved in large comparative effectiveness trials.

ANTICOAGULATION AGENTS

Most anticoagulants have not been well studied in children on ECMO except UFH. UFH with varying dosages remains the most common anticoagulation agent used for ECMO.[25] UFH binds to ATIII to form a UFH-ATIII complex that results in conformational change in ATIII and increases its activity by 2000-fold to 3000-fold.[46,47] These UFH and ATIII complexes inactivate thrombin and prevent further thrombin generation. UFH exerts direct, but weak inhibition of factor Xa. Its biological activity depends on initial dosage, age of the patient, clearance by the kidneys and reticulo-endothelial system, size of circuit, and maintenance dose.[38,47–49] UFH has many advantages: being inexpensive, fast acting, reversible, and familiar in the pediatric population. However, there are some pharmacokinetic and biochemical limitations of UFH use. UFH-ATIII complexes can only inactivate free thrombin and thrombin bound to fibrin or subendothelial matrix remains unaffected by UFH-ATIII complexes. The bound thrombin serves as a pool of active thrombin that continues to stimulate multiple hemostatic systems. Similarly, UFH is ineffective in inhibiting the factor Xa bound to platelets. Activated platelets at the site of a thrombus secrete platelet factor 4, which directly inhibits UFH. UFH also binds to other plasma proteins and varying levels of these proteins from one patient to another or in a patient over time can change UFH dose effect.[46,47] Despite its vast experience, data on pharmacokinetics and pharmacodynamics of UFH in pediatric patients on ECMO are scant.[38] Anti-Xa concentration, which is reflective of heparin effect, of 0.3 to 0.7 IU/mL is considered adequate for ECMO based on anecdotal experience in patients requiring cardiopulmonary bypass. Relative heparin resistance in neonates and infants compared with adults is a matter of debate. As discussed above, low baseline level of ATIII may attenuate UFH action in neonates. However, neonates and infants have a low concentration of both procoagulation and anticoagulation factors, but functional assays reflect normal clot formation and fibrinolysis in this population.[8]

Direct Thrombin Inhibitors

Direct thrombin inhibitors, such as bivalirudin, agratroban, and lepirudin, can potentially overcome some of the UFH limitations as they (1) inhibit both free and bound thrombin, (2) have ATIII-independent thrombin inhibition, (3) have more predictable dose effect because they do not bind to plasma proteins, (4) are not inhibited by platelet factor-4, and (5) can be used in cases with HIT or severe allergy to UFH.[50] Use of direct thrombin inhibitors may permit more complete inhibition of thrombin generation than UFH, further attenuating thrombin-mediated activation of hemostasis and subsequent consumption of various coagulation factors. Data provided by Ranucci and colleagues[51] and Pieri and colleagues,[52] who compared use of UFH versus bivalirudin in adult patients on ECMO, appear to support this concept. Ranucci and colleagues[51] reported less blood loss and decreased blood product administration in the bivalirudin group compared with the UFH group despite significantly longer ACT, aPTT, and r-times at TEG. Pieri and colleagues[52] have reported no difference in bleeding, thromboembolic complications, and mortality, but found decreased variation in aPTT (defined as >20% of the previous value) in bivalirudin versus the UFH group (24 vs 52, $P<.001$). Use of non-UFH agents is currently limited to specific situations in children on ECMO, such as HIT or severe allergy to UFH due to lack of efficacy, safety, and cost-effectiveness data for these agents (**Table 1**).[50–55,57–62] In **Table 2** listed are some of the non-UFH agents with their reported dosing in patients on ECMO.

ATIII Activity

ATIII activity is essential for heparin-based anticoagulation as described above. It decreases the activity of coagulation serine proteases, especially thrombin and factor Xa. ATIII activity often decreases over time in children on ECMO, which reduces the efficacy of heparin.[63–65] Many centers frequently measure and supplement ATIII.[25] ELSO guidelines have suggested a target value of 80% to 120% of control.[33] The American Heart Association (AHA) recommends correction of ATIII deficiency in a situation of subtherapeutic ACT despite increasing heparin infusion (level of evidence IC).[66] Neonates and infants have low baseline ATIII (>40% considered normal).

Table 1
List of case reports of use of non-UFH antihemostatic agents in children on ECMO

Study	Age/Weight	Drug/Dose	Monitoring	Outcomes
Ranucci et al,[51] 2011, n = 5	Newborn child Weight 3.3–45 kg	Bivalirudin 0.03–0.05 mg/kg/h infusion	ACT 160–200 or aPTT 50–70	2 died on ECMO; 2 weaned off ECMO, but died; 1 survived
Hursting et al,[53] 2006, n = 12	Newborn to 16 y Weight not reported	Argatroban 15–50 µg/kg bolus in 2 cases 0.1–10 µg/kg/h infusion	ACT 160–200 in 8 cases aPTT 2 × baseline in 4 cases	2 cases had circuit clotting 1 case had DIC
Scott et al,[54] 2006, n = 1	17 mo Weight not reported	Argatroban Dose not reported	ACT 180–200	None
Deitcher et al,[55] 2002, n = 1	4 y Weight 12 kg	Lepirudin 0.4 mg/kg IV and 0.15 mg/kg/h infusion	aPTT 1.5 × baseline	Severe postoperative bleed and died

Data from Refs.[51,53–56]

Table 2
Newer antihemostatic agents and antithrombin III

Drug	Mechanism of Action	Half-Life	Excretion	Dosage and Monitoring	Special Considerations
Direct thrombin inhibitors					
Bivalirudin	Irreversible direct inhibition of thrombin; Also inhibits thrombin mediated platelet aggregation	25 min	Proteolysis 75% Renal 25%	0.125 mg/kg IV bolus followed by 0.05–0.125 mg/kg/h IV continuous infusion; aPTT	No antidote; action not dependent on ATIII activity
Argatroban		40 min	Liver	0.1–10 µg/kg/min IV continuous infusion; aPTT	No antidote; action not dependent on ATIII activity
Lepirudin		80 min	Renal	0.1–0.15 mg/kg/h IV continuous infusion; aPTT	No antidote; action not dependent on ATIII activity
Factor Xa inhibitors					
Fondaparinux	Synthetic pentasaccharide molecule that binds to ATIII and potentiates its anti-Xa activity	17 h	Renal	0.1 mg/kg once daily; anti-Xa concentration	No antidote, action dependent on ATIII activity
Danaparoid	Nonheparin low-molecular-weight sulfated glycosamino-glycuronans. Higher antifactor Xa/anti-IIa ratio (>1:20)	25 h	Renal	30 IU/kg IV bolus followed by infusion of 1.2–2.0 IU/kg/h; anti-Xa concentration	Not available in the US, possibility of cross-reactivity with anti-PF4/heparin antibodies
ATIII (Thrombate)	Serine protease inhibitor, primarily inhibits thrombin and factor Xa	11.6–17.7 h	—	A single dose of AT of 50 units/kg or based on the formula below: AT dose in units (IU) $= \dfrac{[\text{Desired} - \text{current}] \times \text{weight (kg)}}{1.4}$ Some suggest accounting for the circuit volume (400–600 mL) when calculating the dose. Every 75 mL circuit volume $\cong$ 1 kg of body weight.	Increase risk of hemorrhagic events

Therefore most neonates and infants would require ATIII supplementation to achieve ELSO and AHA target goal values.

There are conflicting data regarding effectiveness of ATIII administration in neonatal and pediatric ECMO. Byrnes and colleagues[64] have shown frequent circuit failure and no change in heparin dosing in an ATIII supplemented group. On the contrary, Perry and colleagues[65] in a cohort of neonates with congenital diaphragmatic hernia, who received ATIII, have shown decreased blood product administration during the first 3 days on ECMO.

Although it may seem reasonable to normalize ATIII activity in the pediatric population, this practice may put patients at risk of bleeding if procoagulant factors are also decreased. The authors suggest caution in the routine replacement of ATIII based on activity values alone before more data emerge regarding efficacy, cost, risk, and limitations of such practice. Research is needed to determine if functional measures of thrombin formation with assays that can incorporate heparinase, such as TEG or ROTEM, in conjunction with ATIII activity can provide more accurate information regarding the need for ATIII supplementation.

ANTIPLATELET AGENTS

Activation of platelets on the ECMO circuit has been described. However, the use of antiplatelet agents (aspirin, dipyridamole, clopidogrel, pentoxifylline, and abciximab) is extremely rare on ECMO as compared with pediatric VAD patients.[38] A recent survey reported an increase from 21.4% in 2000 to 2002 to 67.2% of patients receiving an antiplatelet agent in pediatric VAD patients.[56] Although experience from pediatric VAD patients may suggest utility of antiplatelet agents in ECMO (despite very different pathophysiology), further studies are required to assess the use of antiplatelet agents in children on ECMO and whether the current point-of-care (POC) platelet function assays can be used efficiently to monitor platelet function and to guide antiplatelet agent therapy.

HEMOSTATIC ADJUNCTS

Hemostatic adjuncts in bleeding patients, such as antifibrinolytic agents ε-aminocaproic acid and tranexamic acid, recombinant factor VIIa (FVIIa), and prothrombin complex concentrates, are sparingly used during ECMO because of the concern for severe thrombotic events (**Table 3**).[67–75]

Antifibrinolytic Agents

There are limited data regarding antifibrinolytic agents use in neonatal and pediatric ECMO (class IIb, level of evidence C).[66] There is some evidence that fibrinolysis occurs more frequently in pediatric patients (14%) compared with adults (1%).[8] The use of ε-aminocaproic acid or tranexamic acid is variable. Downard and colleagues[69] reported in 298 pediatric ECMO patients that aminocaproic acid administration of 100 mg/kg bolus before or immediately after beginning ECMO followed by 30 mg/kg/h for 72 hours resulted in decreased surgical site bleeding, which was most evident in cardiac surgery patients with no decrease in intracranial hemorrhages (ICH) or increase in thrombotic complications. In a multicenter trial, there was no difference in the incidence of ICH or thrombotic complications between the placebo and ε-aminocaproic acid groups.[70] Lack of dosing strategies and an increased risk of life-threatening thrombosis on antifibrinolytic agents preclude their routine use on pediatric ECMO patients. Research is needed to determine if the ROTEM-based APTEM test or the TEG-based

Table 3
List of hemostatic adjuncts and antiplatelet agent sparingly used in children on ECMO

Drug	Mechanism of Action	Half Life	Excretion	Dosing/Monitoring	Special Considerations
Recombinant Factor VII (NovaSeven)	It forms complexes with tissue factor and binds to platelet surface, which leads to X-Xa mediated activation of hemostasis	2–3 h	—	50–175 µg/kg (most often 90 µg/kg) IV, 1–4 doses per bleeding episode, can be repeated at every 1–4 h	Increased risk of thromboembolic events
Prothrombin complex concentrate	It is a combination of blood clotting factors II, VII, IX, and X, one type includes protein C and S	Varying half life 6–72 h		20–50 IU/kg or 1–2 mL/kg	Replacement of vitamin K-dependent coagulation factors, can cause allergic reactions and HIT, increase risk of thromboembolic events
Antifibrinolytics agents					
Tranexamic acid	Competitively inhibits the activation of plasminogen to plasmin, 8–10 times more active than ε-aminocaproic acid	2–4 h	Renal	10–50 mg/kg bolus IV followed by 1–2 mg/kg continuous infusion TEG-Clot lysis	Increased risk of thromboembolic events, renal injury, seizures, and other neurologic events
ε-aminocaproic acid (Amicar)	Competitively inhibits the activation of plasminogen to plasmin	2–4 h	Renal	50–100 mg/kg bolus IV over 1 h and then followed by continuous infusion of 25 mg/kg/h for 6–12 h, 48–72 h, or during the entire ECLS run. TEG-Clot lysis	Increased risk of thromboembolic events
Antiplatelet agents					
Aspirin	Inhibits cyclo-oxygenase-1 to block thromboxane A^2 production	20–40 min	Renal	4–10 mg/kg/d orally; TEG-platelet mapping or impedance aggregometry	Gastritis, gastrointestinal bleeding
Dipyridamole	Inhibits phosphodiesterase to increase intracellular cAMP and decreased adenosine uptake	2–3 h	Hepatic	2–5 mg/kg/d orally; TEG-platelet mapping or impedance aggregometry	Headache, vasodilation, bleeding
Clopidogrel	Irreversible blockade of the ADP receptor	8 h	Hepatic	0.1–0.7 mg/kg/d orally, TEG-platelet mapping or impedance aggregometry	Bleeding, decrease in white cell count

LY30% test can determine which children on ECMO would benefit from the initiation of an antifibrinolytic.

Recombinant Activated Factor VII

The off-label use of recombinant FVIIa on ECMO should be limited to control refractory bleeding. FVIIa forms a complex with tissue factor locally at the site of vascular injury that leads to the factor Xa-mediated activation of hemostasis, enhances thrombin generation, and binds to the surface of activated platelet to further generate thrombin.[72] Limited data from case reports and few case series suggest that FVIIa administration may decrease bleeding and blood transfusion requirement, but can increase the risk of patient-related or circuit-related thrombotic events.[71–75] Because of limited data regarding its efficacy and potential risk of thrombotic complications, its use on ECMO remains off-label. There are no recommendations of its use in children on ECMO.[33,66]

BLOOD PRODUCTS TRANSFUSION

Blood products are frequently administered on neonatal and pediatric ECMO to maintain normal hemostasis.[76–78] Stiller and colleagues[77] reported that pediatric ECMO patients on an average received 25 mL of platelet concentrate (PC), 60 mL of packed red blood cells (pRBCs), and 50 mL of fresh frozen plasma (FFP) transfusions for each kilogram body weight every day on ECMO. PC, cryoprecipitate, and FFP transfusion threshold are based on patient age, coagulation deficiencies, ongoing bleeding, or thrombotic complications. Thrombocytopenia and significant platelet dysfunction occur early in the course of ECMO. Low platelet counts are associated with bleeding complications and mortality. The incorporation of POC assays of platelet function, such as TEG-platelet mapping and whole blood impedance aggregometry in adults undergoing cardiopulmonary bypass, has been shown to decrease PC transfusions and mortality. In the authors' center, based on anecdotal experience, they have recently incorporated heparinase TEG (hTEG) parameters in addition to conventional measures (international normalized ratio [INR], platelet count, and fibrinogen level) to guide PC, cryoprecipitate, and FFP transfusion. In patients with significant bleeding, the authors target a platelet count of greater than $100,000/mm^3$, fibrinogen concentration greater than 200 mg/dL, and an INR less than 1.7 (class 1, level of evidence C).[66] Also, the authors correct hTEG of G <5, K >3, and R >12 by transfusing PC, cryoprecipitate, and FFP, respectively, in the patient with significant bleeding. There is need for larger pediatric studies to determine the appropriate thresholds for blood product indication as well as goal targets. The appropriate thresholds for blood product indication and goal targets will decrease blood product transfusion while minimizing hemorrhagic and thromboembolic complications and other transfusion-related adverse events (transfusion-related acute lung injury, transfusion-related immunosuppression, and transfusion-associated cardiac overload) in children on ECMO.

Red blood cells (RBCs) are commonly transfused to keep hemoglobin higher than 10 g/dL or hematocrit higher than 30% across all patients in the most centers. There is evidence that pRBC transfusion may augment inflammatory response and impede oxygen delivery to microcirculation.[78–81] In a single-center retrospective cohort, each RBC transfusion volume of 10 mL/kg/d on ECMO was associated with a 24% increase in the odds of in-hospital mortality (OR 1.024, 95% CI 1.004–1.046, $P = .018$).[78] It seems rational to define the critical hemoglobin level for each individual patient by considering various factors including ECMO flow, cyanotic or acyanotic heart defect, neurologic status, hemodynamics, and markers of oxygen delivery (such as lactic acid, near infrared spectroscopy, and mixed venous saturations).[78] Studies comparing the restrictive transfusion practice to the current practice are needed.

SUMMARY

Anticoagulation and hemostatic management of pediatric ECMO patients have many unique challenges. To overcome these challenges and improve outcomes on ECMO, several measures are required. First, a multidisciplinary team, including surgeons, intensivists, hematologists, anesthesiologists, perfusionists, respiratory therapists, pharmacists, and specialized ECMO nurses, is needed to provide optimal care and cohesive implementation of antihemostatic guidelines. The second measure a comprehensive evaluation of the hemostasis using a combination of tests to include functional measures, is required to provide a global assessment of each aspect of hemostasis that may contribute to the risk of adverse thrombotic or hemorrhagic events. The third measure is to conduct pediatric studies to determine which combination of tests is optimal to determine the indication and therapeutic target for anti-hemostatic agents, blood transfusions, and hemostatic agents. The fourth measure is to develop advanced point-of-care methods to measure inflammation, thrombin generation, fibrinogen, platelet and endothelial function, and fibrinolysis. These point-of-care methods would provide insight into pathophysiology of EIC and potential therapeutic targets. Finally, advances in biologically inert circuits may obviate anticoagulation.

REFERENCES

1. Monagle P, Newall F. Anticoagulation in children. Thromb Res 2012;130:142–6.
2. Monagle P, Newall F, Campbell J. Anticoagulation in neonates and children: pitfalls and dilemmas. Blood Rev 2010;24:151–62.
3. International summary, extracorporeal life support organization registry report. 2013. Available at: elsonet.org. Accessed January 20, 2014.
4. Paden ML, Conrad SA, Rycus PT, et al. Extracorporeal life support organization registry report 2012. ASAIO J 2013;59:202–10.
5. Hoffman M, Monroe DM 3rd. A cell-based model of hemostasis. Thromb Haemost 2001;85:965–8.
6. Despotis GJ, Avidan MS, Hogue CW Jr. Mechanisms and attenuation of hemostatic activation during extracorporeal circulation. Ann Thorac Surg 2001;72:S1821–31.
7. Eaton MP, Lannoli EM. Coagulation considerations for infants and children undergoing cardiopulmonary bypass. Paediatr Anaesth 2011;21:31–42.
8. Oliver WC. Anticoagulation and coagulation management for ECMO. Semin Cardiothorac Vasc Anesth 2009;13:154–75.
9. Edmunds LH Jr, Colman RW. Thrombin during cardiopulmonary bypass. Ann Thorac Surg 2006;82:2315–22.
10. Seghaye MC, Duchateau J, Grabitz RG, et al. Complement activation during cardiopulmonary bypass in infants and children. Relation to postoperative multiple system organ failure. J Thorac Cardiovasc Surg 1993;106:978–87.
11. Risnes I, Wagner K, Ueland T, et al. Interleukin-6 may predict survival in extracorporeal membrane oxygenation treatment. Perfusion 2008;23:173–8.
12. Peek GJ, Firmin RK. The inflammatory and coagulative response to prolonged extracorporeal membrane oxygenation. ASAIO J 1999;45:250–63.
13. Butenas S, Orfeo T, Mann KG. Tissue factor activity and function in blood coagulation. Thromb Res 2008;122(Suppl 1):S42–6.

14. De Somer F, Van Belleghem Y, Caes F, et al. Tissue factor as the main activator of the coagulation system during cardiopulmonary bypass. J Thorac Cardiovasc Surg 2002;123:951–8.

15. Peng Z, Pati S, Potter D, et al. Fresh frozen plasma lessens pulmonary endothelial inflammation and hyperpermeability after hemorrhagic shock and is associated with loss of syndecan 1. Shock 2013;40:195–202.

16. Pati S, Matijevic N, Doursout MF, et al. Protective effects of fresh frozen plasma on vascular endothelial permeability, coagulation, and resuscitation after hemorrhagic shock are time dependent and diminish between days 0 and 5 after thaw. J Trauma 2010;69:S55–63.

17. Kozar RA, Peng Z, Zhang R, et al. Plasma restoration of endothelial glycocalyx in a rodent model of hemorrhagic shock. Anesth Analg 2011;112:1289–95.

18. Cheung PY, Sawicki G, Salas E, et al. The mechanisms of platelet dysfunction during extracorporeal membrane oxygenation in critically ill neonates. Crit Care Med 2000;28:2584–90.

19. Straub A, Wendel HP, Dietz K, et al. Selective inhibition of the platelet phosphoinositide 3-kinase p110beta as promising new strategy for platelet protection during extracorporeal circulation. Thromb Haemost 2008;99:609–15.

20. Michelson AD. Thrombin-induced down-regulation of the platelet membrane glycoprotein Ib-XI complex. Semin Thromb Hemost 1992;18:18–27.

21. Saini A, Doctor A, Gazit A, et al. Platelet inhibition is associated with severe bleeding and mortality in children on ECLS. Crit Care Med 2013;41(Suppl):760.

22. Chung A, Wildhirt SM, Wang S, et al. Combined administration of nitric oxide gas and iloprost during cardiopulmonary bypass reduces platelet dysfunction: a pilot clinical study. J Thorac Cardiovasc Surg 2005;129:782–90.

23. Wesley MC, McGowan FX, Castro RA, et al. The effect of milrinone on platelet activation as determined by TEG platelet mapping. Anesth Analg 2009;108:1425–9.

24. Reilly TM, Forsythe MS, Racanelli AL, et al. Recombinant plasminogen activator inhibitor-1 protects platelets against the inhibitory effects of plasmin. Thromb Res 1993;71:61–8.

25. Bembea MM, Annich G, Rycus P, et al. Variability in anticoagulation management of patients on extracorporeal membrane oxygenation: an international survey. Pediatr Crit Care Med 2013;14:e77–84.

26. Owings JT, Pollock ME, Gosselin RC, et al. Anticoagulation of children undergoing cardiopulmonary bypass is overestimated by current monitoring techniques. Arch Surg 2000;135:1042–7.

27. Despotis GJ, Summerfield AL, Joist JH, et al. Comparison of activated coagulation time and whole blood heparin measurements with laboratory plasma anti-Xa heparin concentration in patients having cardiac operations. J Thorac Cardiovasc Surg 1994;108:1076–82.

28. Martindale SJ, Shayevitz JR, D'Errico C. The activated coagulation time: suitability for monitoring heparin effect and neutralization during pediatric cardiac surgery. J Cardiothorac Vasc Anesth 1996;10:458–63.

29. Guzzetta NA, Baja T, Fazlollah T, et al. A comparison of heparin management strategies in infants undergoing cardiopulmonary bypass. Anesth Analg 2008;106:419–25.

30. Nankervis CA, Preston TJ, Dysart KC, et al. Assessing heparin dosing in neonates on venoarterial extracorporeal membrane oxygenation. ASAIO J 2007;53:111–4.

31. Bembea MM, Schwartz JM, Shah N, et al. Anticoagulation monitoring during pediatric extracorporeal membrane oxygenation. ASAIO J 2013;59:63–8.

32. Muntean W. Coagulation and anticoagulation in extracorporeal membrane oxygenation. Artif Organs 1999;23:979–83.
33. ELSO Guidelines for Cardiopulmonary Extracorporeal Life Support Extracorporeal Life Support Organization, Version 1.3. Ann Arbor (MI): 2013. p. 13. Anticoagulation. Available at: www.elsonet.org. Accessed January 24, 2014.
34. Baired CW, Zurakowski D, Robinson B, et al. Anticoagulation and pediatric extracorporeal membrane oxygenation: impact of activated clotting time and heparin dosing on survival. Ann Thorac Surg 2007;83:912–9.
35. Ignjatovic V, Summerhayes R, Gan A, et al. Monitoring unfractioned heparin therapy: which anti-factor Xa assay is appropriate? Thromb Res 2007;120: 347–51.
36. Lehman CM, Rettmann JA, Wilson LW, et al. Comparative performance of three anti-factor Xa heparin assays in patients in a medical intensive care unit receiving intravenous, unfractionated heparin. Am J Clin Pathol 2006;126:416–21.
37. Krulder JW, Strebus AF, Meinders AE, et al. Anticoagulant effect of unfractionated heparin in antithrombin-depleted plasma in vitro. Haemostasis 1996;26:85–9.
38. Hirsh J, Rascheke R, Warkentin TE, et al. Heparin: mechanism of action, pharmacokinetics, dosing considerations, monitoring, efficacy, and safety. Chest 1995;108(Suppl 4):258S–75S.
39. Chen A, Teruya J. Global hemostasis testing thromboelastography: old technology, new applications. Clin Lab Med 2009;29:391–407.
40. Whiting D, Dinardo JA. TEG and ROTEM: technology and clinical application. Am J Hematol 2014. http://dx.doi.org/10.1002/ajh.23599.
41. Chan KL, Summerhayes RG, Ignjatovic V, et al. Reference values for kaolin-activated thromboelastography in healthy children. Anesth Analg 2007;105: 1610–3.
42. Weber CF, Görlinger K, Meininger D, et al. Point-of-care testing: a prospective, randomized clinical trial of efficacy in coagulopathic cardiac surgery patients. Anesthesiology 2012;117:531–47.
43. Westbrook AJ, Olsen J, Bailey M, et al. Protocol based on thromboelastograph (TEG) outperforms physician preference using laboratory coagulation tests to guide blood replacement during and after cardiac surgery: a pilot study. Heart Lung Circ 2009;18:277–88.
44. Girdauskas E, Kempfert J, Kuntze T, et al. Thromboelastometrically guided transfusion protocol during aortic surgery with circulatory arrest: a prospective, randomized trial. J Thorac Cardiovasc Surg 2010;140:1117–24.
45. Grölinger K, Bergmann L, Dirkmann D. Coagulation management in patients undergoing mechanical circulatory support. Best Pract Res Clin Anaesthesiol 2012;26:179–98.
46. Rutledge JM, Chakravarti S, Massicotte MP, et al. Antithrombotic strategies in children receiving long-term Berlin Heart EXCOR ventricular assist device therapy. J Heart Lung Transplant 2013;32:569–73.
47. Griffith MJ. Kinetics of the heparin-enhanced antithrombin III/thrombin reaction. Evidence for a template model for the mechanism of action of heparin. J Biol Chem 1982;257:7360–5.
48. Newall F, Ignjatovic V, Johnston L, et al. Age is a determinant factors for measures of concentration and effect in children requiring unfractionated heparin. Thromb Haemost 2010;103:1085–90.
49. Yee DL, O'Brien SH, Young G. Pharmacokinetics and pharmacodynamics of anticoagulants in paediatric patients. Clin Pharmacokinet 2013;52:967–80.
50. Weitz JI, Crowther M. Direct thrombin inhibitors. Thromb Res 2002;106:275–84.

51. Ranucci M, Ballotta A, Kandil H, et al. Bivalirudin-based versus conventional heparin anticoagulation for postcardiotomy extracorporeal membrane oxygenation. Crit Care 2011;15:R275. http://dx.doi.org/10.1186/cc10556.
52. Pieri M, Agracheva N, Bonaveglio E, et al. Bivalirudin versus heparin as an anticoagulant during extracorporeal membrane oxygenation: a case-control study. J Cardiothorac Vasc Anesth 2013;27:30–4.
53. Hursting MJ, Dubb J, Verme-Gibboney CN. Argatroban anticoagulation in pediatric patients: a literature analysis. J Pediatr Hematol Oncol 2006;28:4–10.
54. Scott KL, Grier LR, Conrad SA. Heparin-induced thrombocytopenia in a pediatric patient receiving extracorporeal support and treated with argatroban. Pediatr Crit Care Med 2006;7:255–7.
55. Deitcher SR, Topoulos AP, Bartholomew JR, et al. Lepirudin anticoagulation for heparin-induced thrombocytopenia. J Pediatr 2002;140:264–6.
56. Moffett BS, Cabrera AG, Teruva J, et al. Anticoagulation therapy trends in children supported by ventricular assist devices: a multi-institutional study. ASAIO J 2014. http://dx.doi.org/10.1097/MAT. 0000000000000037.
57. Bidlingmaier C, Magnani H, Girisch M, et al. Safety and efficacy of danaparoid (Orgaran) use in children. Acta Haematol 2006;115:237–47.
58. Malherbe S, Tsui BC, Stobart K, et al. Argatroban as anticoagulant in cardiopulmonary bypass in an infant and attempted reversal with recombinant activated factor VII. Anesthesiology 2004;100:443–5.
59. Ciccolo ML, Bernstein J, Collazos JC, et al. Argatroban anticoagulation for cardiac surgery with cardiopulmonary bypass in an infant with double outlet right ventricle and a history of heparin-induced thrombocytopenia. Congenit Heart Dis 2008;3:299–302.
60. Bauer C, Vlchova Z, Ffrench P, et al. Extracorporeal membrane oxygenation with danaparoid sodium after massive pulmonary embolism. Anesth Analg 2008; 106:1101–3.
61. Beiderlinden M, Treschan T, Gorlinger K, et al. Argatroban in extracorporeal membrane oxygenation. Artif Organs 2007;31:461–5.
62. Knoderer CA, Knoderer HM, Turrentine MW, et al. Lepirudin anticoagulation for heparin-induced thrombocytopenia after cardiac surgery in a pediatric patient. Pharmacotherapy 2006;26:709–12.
63. Agati S, Ciccarello G, Salvo D, et al. Use of a novel anticoagulation strategy during ECMO in a pediatric population: single-center experience. ASAIO J 2006; 52:513–6.
64. Byrnes JW, Swearingen CJ, Prodhan P, et al. Antithrombin III supplementation on extracorporeal membrane oxygenation: impact on heparin dose and circuit life. ASAIO J 2014;60(1):57–62.
65. Perry R, Stein J, Young G, et al. Antithrombin III administration in neonates with congenital diaphragmatic hernia during the first three days of extracorporeal membrane oxygenation. J Pediatr Surg 2013;48:1837–42.
66. Giglia TM, Massicotte MP, Tweddell JS, et al. Prevention and treatment of thrombosis in pediatric and congenital heart disease: a scientific statement from the American Heart Association. Circulation 2013;128(24):2622–703.
67. Ortmann E, Besser MW, Klein AA. Antifibrinolytic agents in current anesthetic practice. Br J Anaesth 2013;111:549–63.
68. Li JS, Yow E, Berezny KY, et al. Dosing of clopidogrel for platelet inhibition in infants and young children: primary results of the Platelet Inhibition in Children on cLOpidogrel (PICOLO) trial. Circulation 2008;117:553–9.

69. Downard CD, Betit P, Chang RW, et al. Impact of AMICAR on hemorrhagic complications of ECMO: a ten-year review. J Pediatr Surg 2003;38:1212–6.
70. Horwitz JR, Cofer BR, Warner BW, et al. A multicenter trial of ε-aminocaproic acid (Amicar) in the prevention of bleeding in infants on ECMO. J Pediatr Surg 1998;33:1610–3.
71. Long MT, Wagner D, Maslach-Hubbard A, et al. Safety and efficacy of recombinant activated factor VII for refractory hemorrhage in pediatric patients on extracorporeal membrane oxygenation: a single center review. Perfusion 2014;29(2): 163–70.
72. Niebler RA, Punzalan RC, Marchan M, et al. Activated recombinant factor VII for refractory bleeding during extracorporeal membrane oxygenation. Pediatr Crit Care Med 2010;11:98–102.
73. Walker A, Davidosn M, Chalmers E. Letter to the Editor. Pediatr Crit Care Med 2010;11:537–8.
74. Okonta KE, Edwin F, Falase B. Is recombinant activated factor VII effective in the treatment of excessive bleeding after paediatric cardiac surgery. Interact Cardiovasc Thorac Surg 2012;15:690–4.
75. Franchini M, Lippi G. Prothrombin complex concentrates: an update. Blood Transfuse 2010;8:149–54.
76. Dohner ML, Wiedmeyer SE, Staddard RA, et al. Very high users of platelet transfusions in the neonatal intensive care unit. Transfusion 2009;49:869–72.
77. Stiller B, Lemmer J, Merkle F, et al. Consumption of blood products during mechanical circulatory support in children: comparison between ECMO and a pulsatile ventricular assist device. Intensive Care Med 2004;30:1814–20.
78. Smith A, Hardison D, Bridges B, et al. Red blood cell transfusion volume and mortality among patients receiving extracorporeal membrane oxygenation. Perfusion 2013;28:54–60.
79. Thurer RL, Popvsky MA. Blood transfusion and the microcirculation. Transfusion 2011;51:2259–61.
80. Spinella PC, Doctor A, Blumberg N, et al. Does the storage duration of blood products affect outcomes in critically ill patients? Transfusion 2011;51:1644–50.
81. Arslan E, Sierko E, Waters JH, et al. Microcirculatory hemodynamics after acute blood loss followed by fresh and banked blood transfusion. Am J Surg 2005; 190:456–62.

The Influence of Various Patient Characteristics on D-dimer Concentration in Critically Ill Patients and Its Role as a Prognostic Indicator in the Intensive Care Unit Setting

CrossMark

Jenna L. Spring, MD[a], Anne Winkler, MD, MSc[b],
Jerrold H. Levy, MD, FAHA, FCCM[c],*

KEYWORDS

- Bleeding • Safety • D-dimer • Disseminated intravascular coagulation
- Intensive care unit • In-hospital mortality

KEY POINTS

- There is a correlation between increased D-dimer concentration and renal impairment in critically ill patients, with patients in renal failure having the highest D-dimer concentrations.
- Peak D-dimer levels were higher among female patients than in male patients, but there was no association between peak D-dimer levels and other patient characteristics. D-dimer concentration was also not predictive of in-hospital mortality.

INTRODUCTION

D-dimer is a marker of coagulation system activation that was first discovered in the 1970s.[1] Following hemostatic activation, thrombin cleaves fibrinogen to produce fibrin monomers and also activates factor XIII. The fibrin monomers are then covalently cross-linked by activated factor XIII, producing a fibrin mesh. The degradation of the cross-linked fibrin by plasmin leads to the release of various fibrin degradation

Conflict of Interest Statements: Prof. J.H. Levy serves on steering committees for Boehringer Ingelheim, CSL Behring AG, Grifols, Janssen Pharmaceuticals, and The Medicines Company.
[a] Department of Medicine, University of Toronto, Suite RFE 3-805, 200 Elizabeth Street, Toronto, ON M5G 2C4, Canada; [b] Department of Pathology, Emory University, 1364 Clifton Road, NE, Atlanta, GA 30322, USA; [c] Duke University School of Medicine, Divisions of Cardio-thoracic Anesthesiology and Critical Care, Duke University Hospital, 2301 Erwin Road, Durham, NC 27710, USA
* Corresponding author.
E-mail address: jerrold.levy@duke.edu

Clin Lab Med 34 (2014) 675–686
http://dx.doi.org/10.1016/j.cll.2014.06.015
0272-2712/14/$ – see front matter © 2014 Elsevier Inc. All rights reserved.

labmed.theclinics.com

products (FDPs), including D-dimer.[2–5] Numerous conditions, including venous thromboembolism (VTE), trauma, surgery, infection, pregnancy, myocardial infarction, and stroke, are associated with elevations in D-dimer concentration.[4] However, this high molecular weight FDP is only detectable in plasma once it has been released from the fibrin clot. There are several different methods available for detecting D-dimer, the newest of which are automated, quantitative, immunoturbidimetric assays. These assays are sensitive (>90%) but relatively nonspecific (~50%).[6]

Clinically, the D-dimer assay is most commonly used to evaluate patients for potential VTE or to aid in the diagnosis and management of disseminated intravascular coagulation (DIC).[2,4] Given the morbidity and mortality associated with DIC and VTE (especially pulmonary embolism), early diagnosis and treatment are important. The D-dimer assay provides a method to monitor patients with suspected DIC in the critical care setting. This aspect is important because many conditions that lead to admission to the intensive care unit (ICU) also place a patient at increased risk of developing DIC.[7] As a widely available marker of fibrin degradation, D-dimer levels are used as one of the components of both the International Society of Thrombosis and Haemostasis (ISTH) DIC score and the Korean Society on Thrombosis and Hemostasis DIC diagnostic criteria.[8,9] For the more commonly used ISTH score, points are awarded based on the degree of D-dimer elevation, up to a maximum of 3 points for severe elevation. Using these criteria, a score of 5 or higher is consistent with DIC, making D-dimer an important component of the diagnosis.

Given the diagnostic utility of an elevated D-dimer level in certain clinical situations, many studies have examined the influence of various patient characteristics (gender, age, race, and renal function) on D-dimer concentration.[10–18] Using this information, the use of patient-characteristic–adjusted D-dimer cutoffs has been proposed to improve diagnosis.[19,20] However, none of the existing studies were conducted in critically ill patients, and often excluded patients undergoing dialysis or those who had recent exposure to anticoagulation therapy. Heparin exposure, in particular, has been shown to affect the sensitivity of the D-dimer assay,[21] and many critically ill patients receive therapeutic anticoagulation for multiple reasons. In the ICU the initiation or continuation of dialysis is also common, and introduces another variable into the interpretation of hemostatic markers such as D-dimer.

Because of the prevalence of renal dysfunction and dialysis utilization in the ICU, the authors have focused a significant portion of their analysis on the relationship between renal dysfunction and D-dimer concentration. Acute kidney injury has been reported to affect up to 78% of critically ill patients, depending on the patient cohort and definition used,[22] and a significant proportion of these patients ultimately require some form of dialysis.[23] In addition, up to 9% of patients admitted to the ICU are already undergoing chronic dialysis therapy.[24] Furthermore, there are numerous potential causes of D-dimer elevation in critically ill patients, in contrast to results from studies conducted in the ambulatory setting among fairly healthy patients. Thus, it is difficult to make assumptions based on data from existing studies about the factors that may affect D-dimer levels in ICU patients. Additional information is needed regarding the effects of these nonmodifiable variables on D-dimer results in the ICU, as these may influence the interpretation of this important test.

There is also substantial interest in the use of D-dimer as a prognostic marker in a wide range of clinical settings, including various malignancies, pulmonary embolism, and aortic dissection.[25–33] However, few studies have been performed in critically ill patients,[34–36] and the only study in which a fully quantitative D-dimer assay was used found no correlation between D-dimer concentration and in-hospital mortality.[34] Given the limited data available and the constant need for more accurate prognostic indicators, the authors evaluated the impact of D-dimer elevation on in-hospital mortality in their patient population.

MATERIALS AND METHODS
Subjects

Patients admitted to the cardiothoracic ICU at Emory University Hospital (Atlanta, GA) between January 1, 2008 and June 15, 2012 who had at least 1 recorded D-dimer level while in the ICU were identified for inclusion in the study. No patients were excluded, regardless of renal function, exposure to anticoagulation therapy, reason for ICU admission, or known VTE. This study was approved by the hospital's Institutional Review Board, and patient consent was not required as no identifying information was recorded.

In this retrospective chart review, all patient data were obtained from the hospital's electronic medical record. For the comparison of D-dimer concentration and renal function, the most recent D-dimer level was recorded along with the closest preceding creatinine value. With the exception of 3 patients, all creatinine and D-dimer measurements were taken within 24 hours of each other, with the majority occurring within the space of 12 hours. If the D-dimer concentration was outside the reportable range, as was the case for 18 patients, the highest or lowest reportable value was recorded (ie, if the D-dimer was reported as >15,000 ng/mL, it was recorded as 15,000 ng/mL for the purposes of this study). For patients admitted before August 1, 2009, D-dimer testing was performed using the STA Liatest D-dimer assay (Diagnostica Stago, Asnières sur Seine, France). After August 1, 2009, Emory University Hospital switched to the Innovance D-dimer assay (Siemens Medical Solutions, Erlangen, Germany). Both are automated, quantitative, immunoturbidimetric assays, but the Innovance assay is particle-enhanced.

The following information was also recorded for each patient: age, gender, race, in-hospital mortality, peak D-dimer concentration, reason for ICU admission, and whether the patient was undergoing dialysis (hemodialysis or continuous renal replacement therapy [CRRT]) at the time the most recent sample for measurement of D-dimer concentration was collected. The reasons for ICU admission were divided into primarily cardiovascular, primarily pulmonary, and other.

Data Analysis

The estimated glomerular filtration rate (eGFR) was calculated for all patients not undergoing dialysis at the time of D-dimer measurement using the Chronic Kidney Disease Epidemiology Collaboration (CKD-EPI) equation.[37] This formula incorporates age, gender, race, and plasma creatinine level, and has been shown to predict glomerular filtration rate, mortality, and progression to end-stage renal disease more accurately than the better-known Modification of Diet in Renal Disease equation.[37–39] Patients were then categorized into the following 5 eGFR categories in accordance with the Kidney Disease Outcomes Quality Initiative (KDOQI) guidelines: normal eGFR ($\geq$90 mL/min), mildly decreased eGFR (60–89 mL/min), moderately decreased eGFR (30–59 mL/min), severely decreased eGFR (15–30 mL/min), or kidney failure (eGFR <15 mL/min or dialysis).[40]

Continuous variables are expressed as median values with the interquartile range (IQR) listed, while categorical variables are presented as percentages with a 95% confidence interval (CI) for selected values. The Kruskal-Wallis test was used for comparison between categorical and continuous variables, while correlations between

2 continuous variables were carried out using simple linear regression. The Fisher exact test was used for comparison between 2 categorical variables, and the 2-tailed probability reported. Data were assumed to adhere to a non-normal distribution. *P* values of less than .05 were considered statistically significant. All statistical analysis was carried out using JMP software version 10.0 (SAS Institute, Cary, NC, USA).

RESULTS

After identifying patients who had at least 1 D-dimer level recorded during their time in the ICU, a total of 144 patients (19–93 years of age) were included in the analysis. Patient characteristics are outlined in **Table 1**.

Most patients were male (n = 86, 60%), and the median patient age was 61 years (IQR: 48–71 years). There was no statistically significant difference in age between male and female patients (*P* = .21). In terms of race, 83 (58%) of the patients were identified as white, 43 (30%) as black, and 8 (6%) as other. For 10 (7%) of the patients, race was unknown or not disclosed. The reason for ICU admission was primarily cardiovascular for 101 (70%) of the patients and primarily pulmonary for 33 (23%) of the patients. The remaining 10 patients (7%) were admitted for another primary cause. One of the patients in the study was admitted to the ICU on chronic hemodialysis.

The overall in-hospital mortality rate was 29% (95% CI: 22%–37%), which increased to 51% (95% CI: 36%–67%) if only patients undergoing dialysis at the time creatinine and D-dimer levels were measured were considered. The median peak D-dimer level was 3211 ng/mL (IQR: 980–6284 ng/mL), and 87% of patients had at least one D-dimer level recorded that was outside the normal range (0–500 ng/mL).

When the 144 patients were categorized by eGFR according to the CKD-EPI equation and KDOQI guidelines, 18 (13%) had an eGFR of 90 mL/min or higher, 30 (21%) had an eGFR between 60 and 89 mL/min, 38 (26%) had an eGFR between 30 and 59 mL/min, 16 (11%) had an eGFR between 15 and 29 mL/min, and 42 (29%) were undergoing dialysis or had an eGFR of less than 15 mL/min when creatinine and D-dimer levels were measured.

Table 1
Patient characteristics (N = 144)

		% (n)
Age (y)	<40	16 (23)
	40–49	13 (19)
	50–59	18 (26)
	60–69	27 (39)
	≥70	26 (37)
Gender	Female	40 (58)
	Male	60 (86)
Race	White	58 (83)
	Black	30 (43)
	Other	6 (8)
	Unknown	7 (10)
Primary reason for ICU admission	Cardiovascular	70 (101)
	Pulmonary	23 (33)
	Other	7 (10)
Overall in-hospital mortality		29 (42)

Abbreviations: % (n), percentage (number of patients) in each group; ICU, intensive care unit; N, total number of study patients.

D-dimer Concentration and Renal Function

The relationship between the most recent D-dimer concentration and renal function was evaluated using both creatinine levels and eGFR category. Considering all 144 patients, D-dimer concentration increased significantly with increasing creatinine levels ($P = .001$; **Fig. 1**). However, when only patients undergoing dialysis were considered, this relationship was no longer observed ($P = .89$; **Fig. 2**). When evaluating the relationship between D-dimer concentration and eGFR category, the median D-dimer was 1947 ng/mL (IQR: 980–4519 ng/mL) for patients with an eGFR of 90 mL/min or higher, 972 ng/mL (IQR: 302–3808 ng/mL) for patients with an eGFR between 60 and 89 mL/min, 2517 ng/mL (IQR: 585–4759 ng/mL) for patients with an eGFR between 30 and 59 mL/min, 3232 ng/mL (IQR: 1208–6612 ng/mL) for patients with an eGFR between 15 and 29 ng/mL, and 4530 ng/mL (IQR: 2403–15,000 ng/mL) for patients undergoing dialysis when the most recent sample for assessment of D-dimer concentration was drawn or with an eGFR less than 15 ng/mL (**Fig. 3**). These results showed a statistically significant correlation between D-dimer levels and eGFR ($P = .0001$).

Among the 42 patients with renal failure, the median D-dimer concentration was 4326 ng/mL (IQR: 2364–13,009 ng/mL) for patients undergoing dialysis when the most recent sample for measurement of D-dimer concentration was drawn, and 6301 ng/mL (IQR: 3336–16,300 ng/mL) for patients not undergoing dialysis but with an eGFR less than 15 mL/min. However, this difference was not statistically significant ($P = .38$).

When analyzing the relationship between peak D-dimer concentration and patient age, there was an upward trend in peak D-dimer concentration with increasing age, but this was not statistically significant ($P = .21$; **Fig. 4**). There was also no statistically significant relationship between peak D-dimer concentration and race ($P = .32$). The median peak D-dimer concentration was 3091 ng/mL (IQR: 975–6797 ng/mL) for

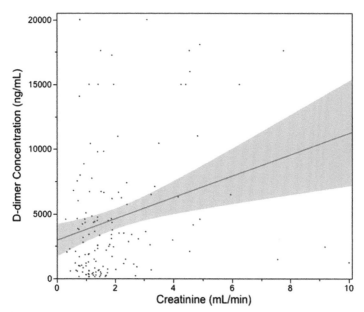

Fig. 1. Relationship between D-dimer concentration and creatinine levels in all patients. There was a significant positive correlation ($P = .001$). Shaded area represents 95% confidence interval of fit.

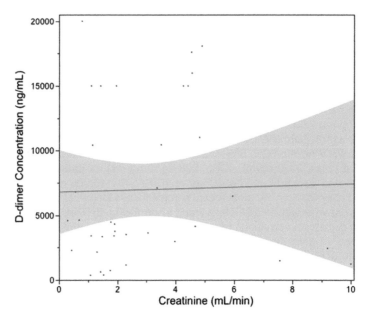

Fig. 2. Relationship between D-dimer concentration and creatinine levels in patients undergoing dialysis at the time creatinine and D-dimer levels were measured. There was no significant correlation ($P = .89$). Shaded area represents 95% confidence interval of fit.

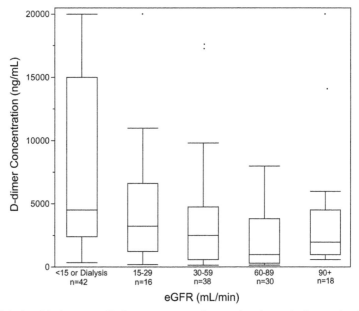

Fig. 3. Relationship between D-dimer concentration and estimated glomerular filtration rate (eGFR). The correlation was significant ($P = .0001$). Median, interquartile range, 95% confidence interval, and outliers are shown for each category.

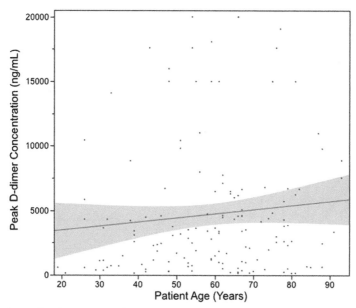

Fig. 4. Relationship between peak D-dimer concentration and patient age. There was no significant correlation ($P = .21$). Shaded area represents 95% confidence interval of fit.

patients identified as black, 3246 ng/mL (IQR: 1028–6232 ng/mL) for those identified as white, 1008 ng/mL (IQR: 523–3565 ng/mL) for those identified as other, and 3770 ng/mL (IQR: 1623–11,984 ng/mL) for patients whose race was unknown.

The only patient demographic analyzed that had a significant relationship with D-dimer concentration was gender. The median peak D-dimer concentration was 4088 ng/mL (IQR: 1083–9097 ng/mL) for female patients and 2702 ng/mL (IQR: 788–4620 ng/mL) for male patients ($P = .04$).

There was no relationship between in-hospital mortality and peak D-dimer concentration ($P = .82$; **Fig. 5**). The median peak D-dimer concentration among patients who survived to hospital discharge was 2814 ng/mL (IQR: 908–6293 ng/mL), whereas the median peak D-dimer concentration among patients who died in hospital was 3456 ng/mL (IQR: 1135–6425 ng/mL). In addition, among the 19 patients who never had an elevated (>500 ng/mL) D-dimer level, there was no improvement in survival ($P = 1.00$). Patients who did not have a recorded D-dimer level greater than 500 ng/mL had a 26% (95% CI: 12%–49%) mortality rate, compared with a 30% (95% CI: 22%–38%) mortality rate among patients who had at least 1 elevated D-dimer measurement.

DISCUSSION

This study is the first to specifically investigate the factors that influence D-dimer concentrations in critically ill patients. The results demonstrate that there is a statistically significant correlation between D-dimer concentration and renal function in the ICU, with patients with renal failure having the highest D-dimer levels. As previously suggested in other studies, it is unlikely that the association between renal dysfunction and increased D-dimer concentration is due to decreased renal clearance alone.[11,13,18,41] With a molecular weight of approximately 180 kDa, D-dimer is too large to be effectively cleared at the glomerulus, or removed by hemodialysis or CRRT. A more likely

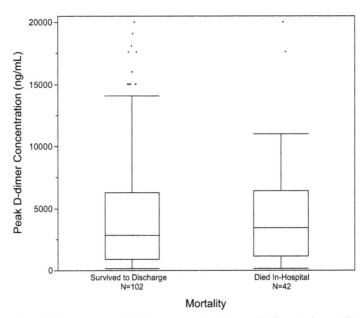

Fig. 5. Relationship between peak D-dimer concentration and in-hospital mortality. The correlation was not significant ($P = .82$). Median, interquartile range, 95% confidence interval, and outliers are shown for each category.

explanation for the association between D-dimer levels and renal failure is increased coagulation system activation and fibrinolysis, which are intrinsic to the renal impairment itself. The results of a study carried out in 1989 by Gordge and colleagues[13] suggest that this effect may be most pronounced in patients with acute renal failure (ARF); much greater D-dimer elevations are seen in patients with ARF than in those with chronic kidney disease. In the present study population, ARF was the predominant reason for dialysis, with only 1 patient known to be undergoing chronic hemodialysis before ICU admission.

One unexpected outcome of this study was that patients with normal renal function (eGFR $\geq$90 mL/min) had a higher median D-dimer concentration than patients with mild renal dysfunction (eGFR between 60 and 89 mL/min). This finding was likely attributable to the small size of the normal renal function group (n = 18) and the presence of statistical outliers, which skewed the data to some extent. Two of the 18 patients in this group had normal renal function but a severely elevated D-dimer. One of these cases involved a patient with thrombosis while the other had no apparent explanation. D-dimer levels otherwise adhered to an inverse relationship with eGFR category.

Results with Patients Undergoing Dialysis

Within the group of patients undergoing dialysis, the lack of correlation between creatinine and D-dimer levels is likely explained by the inability of D-dimer to pass through the dialysis membrane while creatinine can be dialyzed. In fact, several patients in the dialysis group had normal, or near normal, creatinine values in the setting of an extremely elevated D-dimer concentration. Although it was not statistically significant, the trend toward lower D-dimer levels in patients undergoing dialysis in comparison with those with renal failure (eGFR <15 mL/min) was somewhat surprising, given the hypercoagulable state induced by dialysis.[42] One would expect that this would only add to the increased D-dimer level associated with renal failure alone. Possible explanations include a difference in underlying disease between these 2 groups, and the small sample size of patients with renal failure who were not undergoing dialysis.

Further studies are needed to determine the diagnostic utility of D-dimer levels in critically ill patients with renal dysfunction, especially in the case of suspected DIC. Only 13% of patients did not have an elevated D-dimer level, a proportion that is likely reflective of the relative severity of illness in this study population. High D-dimer levels have been reported in medical ICUs in the absence of obvious thromboembolic disease,[43] and the usefulness of checking D-dimer concentration in this setting has been called into question.[44] The high prevalence of D-dimer elevation in this study population supports the limited utility of measuring D-dimer concentration in critically ill patients as a means of ruling out VTE. Careful consideration should be given to carrying out the test for this purpose, as a negative result is unlikely even in the absence of thromboembolic disease. Conversely, in DIC the degree of D-dimer elevation is given significant weight. Therefore, the influence of renal dysfunction in producing moderate to severe D-dimer elevations may be an important diagnostic consideration, especially as diagnostic scoring systems with various D-dimer cutoffs become the norm.

Effect of Gender and Race on D-dimer Concentration

Aside from decreased renal function, female gender was the only other factor analyzed that was significantly associated with increased D-dimer concentration in this patient population. This relationship has also been demonstrated in previous studies of healthier patients,[12,17] and it is unclear as to why this effect was seen in this patient population while the more widely reported correlation between D-dimer concentration and patient age was not.[11,12,15,17,19,20] One possible explanation lies in the severity of illness in the patient population studied, irrespective of age. In the ambulatory setting, in which many previous studies were based, older individuals tend to have more comorbidities and be sicker overall, whereas this is not necessarily the case in the ICU. Meanwhile, the proportion of women and men probably does not change as markedly between the ICU and outpatient settings, preserving the effect of gender on D-dimer concentration.

There is also some evidence to suggest that D-dimer levels may be higher in black patients than in their white counterparts. In a study of more than 1700 elderly individuals by Pieper and colleagues[14] the correlation between race and D-dimer level was marked, and persisted despite controlling for socioeconomic and demographic variations between groups. However, in the present analysis, peak D-dimer levels were almost equal between black and white patients. Although a racial difference in coagulation system activation may exist that the authors were unable to detect, it should be validated in additional studies.

No Connection with In-Hospital Mortality

Finally, in the analysis of D-dimer as a prognostic indicator, there was no association between either peak D-dimer level or the presence of D-dimer elevation and in-hospital mortality. This result supports the findings of Shitrit and colleagues[34] in their 2003 study assessing the prognostic utility of D-dimer levels measured at 24 and 48 hours after ICU admission. In this study, which enrolled a combination of medical and surgical patients, the D-dimer concentrations correlated with illness severity scores and were able to predict the extent of organ failure at 48 hours, but were not independent predictors of in-hospital mortality. As mentioned in the study by Shitrit and colleagues,[34] other studies that have demonstrated a correlation between D-dimer level and mortality were carried out using an older, less reliable version of the assay, and did not include surgical patients.[35,36] Nonetheless, this does not automatically invalidate these older study results. The role for D-dimer concentration as a prognostic marker in the ICU remains unclear, even if it may not predict mortality as a primary endpoint. Further investigation is warranted, given the increasing evidence supporting D-dimer as a prognostic indicator in other clinical settings and the correlation with the illness severity scores observed in the study by Shitrit and colleagues.[34]

The present study has several limitations. It was a retrospective analysis, and the study population was restricted to patients with primarily cardiovascular and pulmonary issues, many of whom had undergone recent surgery and had been exposed to extensive anticoagulation therapy. Thus, these results may not be generalizable to all critically ill patients. In terms of the data collection, 2 different D-dimer assays were used during the study period. Although the assays are similar, they may produce slightly different results. Furthermore, the D-dimer concentrations were occasionally outside the reportable range for the assays used. Therefore, extremely high or low values could not be accurately captured. Using the median rather than the mean for statistical analysis mitigated this issue somewhat, but exact values would have been preferable.

SUMMARY

This study demonstrates that the previously reported correlation between renal dysfunction and elevated D-dimer levels persists in the critically ill patient population, with patients with renal failure having the highest plasma D-dimer levels. Large prospective studies are needed to determine the effect this finding may have on the utility of D-dimer concentration as a diagnostic aid in this patient population, particularly with regard to DIC. Although these results do not support the use of D-dimer as a prognostic marker in critically ill patients, the authors consider that further investigation is warranted, given the discrepancy from earlier studies and the increasing evidence supporting D-dimer concentration as a prognostic marker in other patient populations.

ACKNOWLEDGMENTS

The authors would like to thank Dr Linda Demma for her assistance with the statistical analysis of the data.

REFERENCES

1. Gaffney PJ, Lane DA, Kakkar VV, et al. Characterisation of a soluble D dimer-E complex in crosslinked fibrin digests. Thromb Res 1975;7(1):89–99.
2. Adam SS, Key NS, Greenberg CS. D-dimer antigen: current concepts and future prospects. Blood 2009;113(13):2878–87.
3. Gaffney PJ, Joe F. The lysis of crosslinked human fibrin by plasmin yields initially a single molecular complex, D dimer-E. Thromb Res 1979;15(5–6):673–87.
4. Bates SM. D-dimer assays in diagnosis and management of thrombotic and bleeding disorders. Semin Thromb Hemost 2012;38(7):673–82.
5. Walker JB, Nesheim ME. The molecular weights, mass distribution, chain composition, and structure of soluble fibrin degradation products released from a fibrin clot perfused with plasmin. J Biol Chem 1999;274(8):5201–12.
6. Di Nisio M, Squizzato A, Rutjes AW, et al. Diagnostic accuracy of D-dimer test for exclusion of venous thromboembolism: a systematic review. J Thromb Haemost 2007;5(2):296–304.
7. Levi M. Disseminated intravascular coagulation. Crit Care Med 2007;35(9): 2191–5.

8. Taylor FB Jr, Toh CH, Hoots WK, et al. Towards definition, clinical and laboratory criteria, and a scoring system for disseminated intravascular coagulation. Thromb Haemost 2001;86(5):1327–30.
9. Lee JH, Song JW, Song KS. Diagnosis of overt disseminated intravascular coagulation: a comparative study using criteria from the International Society versus the Korean Society on Thrombosis and Hemostasis. Yonsei Med J 2007;48(4):595–600.
10. Karami-Djurabi R, Klok FA, Kooiman J, et al. D-dimer testing in patients with suspected pulmonary embolism and impaired renal function. Am J Med 2009; 122(11):1050–3.
11. Qasim A, Duggan M, O'Connell N, et al. Clinical conditions and patient factors significantly influence diagnostic utility of D-dimer in venous thromboembolism. Blood Coagul Fibrinolysis 2009;20(4):244–7.
12. Legnani C, Cini M, Cosmi B, et al. Age and gender specific cut-off values to improve the performance of D-dimer assays to predict the risk of venous thromboembolism recurrence. Intern Emerg Med 2013;8:229–36.
13. Gordge MP, Faint RW, Rylance PB, et al. Plasma D dimer: a useful marker of fibrin breakdown in renal failure. Thromb Haemost 1989;61(3):522–5.
14. Pieper CF, Rao KM, Currie MS, et al. Age, functional status, and racial differences in plasma D-dimer levels in community-dwelling elderly persons. J Gerontol A Biol Sci Med Sci 2000;55(11):M649–57.
15. Lee AJ, Fowkes GR, Lowe GD, et al. Determinants of fibrin D-dimer in the Edinburgh Artery Study. Arterioscler Thromb Vasc Biol 1995;15(8):1094–7.
16. Shlipak MG, Fried LF, Crump C, et al. Elevations of inflammatory and procoagulant biomarkers in elderly persons with renal insufficiency. Circulation 2003;107(1):87–92.
17. Kabrhel C, Mark Courtney D, Camargo CA Jr, et al. Factors associated with positive D-dimer results in patients evaluated for pulmonary embolism. Acad Emerg Med 2010;17(6):589–97.
18. Catena C, Zingaro L, Casaccio D, et al. Abnormalities of coagulation in hypertensive patients with reduced creatinine clearance. Am J Med 2000;109(7):556–61.
19. Penaloza A, Roy PM, Kline J, et al. Performance of age-adjusted D-dimer cut-off to rule out pulmonary embolism. J Thromb Haemost 2012;10(7):1291–6.
20. Douma RA, le Gal G, Sohne M, et al. Potential of an age adjusted D-dimer cut-off value to improve the exclusion of pulmonary embolism in older patients: a retrospective analysis of three large cohorts. BMJ 2010;340:c1475.
21. Siragusa S. Plasma D-dimer test accuracy can be affected by heparin administration. Arch Intern Med 2003;163(2):246 [author reply: 247].
22. Hoste EA, Kellum JA. Acute kidney injury: epidemiology and diagnostic criteria. Curr Opin Crit Care 2006;12(6):531–7.
23. Elseviers MM, Lins RL, Van der Niepen P, et al. Renal replacement therapy is an independent risk factor for mortality in critically ill patients with acute kidney injury. Crit Care 2010;14(6):R221.
24. Thompson S, Pannu N. Dialysis patients and critical illness. Am J Kidney Dis 2012;59(1):145–51.
25. Ay C, Dunkler D, Pirker R, et al. High D-dimer levels are associated with poor prognosis in cancer patients. Haematologica 2012;97(8):1158–64.
26. Nagy Z, Horvath O, Kadas J, et al. D-dimer as a potential prognostic marker. Pathol Oncol Res 2012;18(3):669–74.
27. Stender MT, Larsen TB, Sorensen HT, et al. Preoperative plasma D-dimer predicts 1-year survival in colorectal cancer patients with absence of venous thromboembolism (VTE): a prospective clinical cohort study. J Thromb Haemost 2012;10(10): 2027–31.

28. Raj SD, Zhou X, Bueso-Ramos CE, et al. Prognostic significance of elevated D-dimer for survival in patients with sarcoma. Am J Clin Oncol 2012;35(5):462–7.

29. Ohlmann P, Faure A, Morel O, et al. Diagnostic and prognostic value of circulating D-dimers in patients with acute aortic dissection. Crit Care Med 2006;34(5):1358–64.

30. Weber T, Rammer M, Auer J, et al. Plasma concentrations of D-dimer predict mortality in acute type A aortic dissection. Heart 2006;92(6):836–7.

31. Stein PD, Janjua M, Matta F, et al. Prognostic value of D-dimer in stable patients with pulmonary embolism. Clin Appl Thromb Hemost 2011;17(6):E183–5.

32. Aujesky D, Roy PM, Guy M, et al. Prognostic value of D-dimer in patients with pulmonary embolism. Thromb Haemost 2006;96(4):478–82.

33. Ghanima W, Abdelnoor M, Holmen LO, et al. D-dimer level is associated with the extent of pulmonary embolism. Thromb Res 2007;120(2):281–8.

34. Shitrit D, Izbicki G, Shitrit AB, et al. Prognostic value of a new quantitative D-dimer test in critically ill patients 24 and 48 h following admission to the intensive care unit. Blood Coagul Fibrinolysis 2004;15(1):15–9.

35. Shorr AF, Trotta RF, Alkins SA, et al. D-dimer assay predicts mortality in critically ill patients without disseminated intravascular coagulation or venous thromboembolic disease. Intensive Care Med 1999;25(2):207–10.

36. Kollef MH, Eisenberg PR, Shannon W. A rapid assay for the detection of circulating D-dimer is associated with clinical outcomes among critically ill patients. Crit Care Med 1998;26(6):1054–60.

37. Levey AS, Stevens LA, Schmid CH, et al. A new equation to estimate glomerular filtration rate. Ann Intern Med 2009;150(9):604–12.

38. Matsushita K, Mahmoodi BK, Woodward M, et al. Comparison of risk prediction using the CKD-EPI equation and the MDRD study equation for estimated glomerular filtration rate. JAMA 2012;307(18):1941–51.

39. Matsushita K, Tonelli M, Lloyd A, et al. Clinical risk implications of the CKD Epidemiology Collaboration (CKD-EPI) equation compared with the Modification of Diet in Renal Disease (MDRD) Study equation for estimated GFR. Am J Kidney Dis 2012;60(2):241–9.

40. National Kidney Foundation. KDOQI clinical practice guidelines for chronic kidney disease: evaluation, classification, and stratification. Am J Kidney Dis 2002;39(2 Suppl 1):S1–266.

41. Dubin R, Cushman M, Folsom AR, et al. Kidney function and multiple hemostatic markers: cross sectional associations in the multi-ethnic study of atherosclerosis. BMC Nephrol 2011;12:3.

42. Ambuhl PM, Wuthrich RP, Korte W, et al. Plasma hypercoagulability in haemodialysis patients: impact of dialysis and anticoagulation. Nephrol Dial Transplant 1997;12(11):2355–64.

43. Kollef MH, Zahid M, Eisenberg PR. Predictive value of a rapid semiquantitative D-dimer assay in critically ill patients with suspected venous thromboembolic disease. Crit Care Med 2000;28(2):414–20.

44. Goldhaber SZ. The perils of D-dimer in the medical intensive care unit. Crit Care Med 2000;28(2):583–4.

Index

Note: Page numbers of article titles are in **boldface** type.

Clin Lab Med 34 (2014) 687–697
http://dx.doi.org/10.1016/S0272-2712(14)00068-7
0272-2712/14/$ – see front matter © 2014 Elsevier Inc. All rights reserved.

labmed.theclinics.com

Printed and bound by CPI Group (UK) Ltd, Croydon, CR0 4YY

07/10/2024

01040498-0010